Celiac Disease

Guest Editors

BENJAMIN LEBWOHL, MD, MS
PETER H.R. GREEN, MD

GASTROINTESTINAL ENDOSCOPY CLINICS OF NORTH AMERICA

www.giendo.theclinics.com

Consulting Editor
CHARLES J. LIGHTDALE, MD

October 2012 • Volume 22 • Number 4

SAUNDERS an imprint of ELSEVIER, Inc.

W.B. SAUNDERS COMPANY
A Division of Elsevier Inc.

1600 John F. Kennedy Blvd. ● Suite 1800 ● Philadelphia, Pennsylvania 19103-2899

http://www.giendo.theclinics.com

GASTROINTESTINAL ENDOSCOPY CLINICS OF NORTH AMERICA Volume 22, Number 4
October 2012 ISSN 1052-5157, ISBN-13: 978-1-4557-4915-7

Editor: Kerry Holland
Developmental Editor: Donald Mumford

Gastrointestinal Endoscopy Clinics of North America (ISSN 1052-5157) is published quarterly by Elsevier Inc., 360 Park Avenue South, New York, NY 10010-1710. Months of issue are January, April, July, and October. Business and Editorial Offices: 1600 John F. Kennedy Blvd., Suite 1800, Philadelphia, PA, 19103-2899. Periodicals postage paid at New York, NY and additional mailing offices. Subscription prices are $315.00 per year for US individuals, $441.00 per year for US institutions, $168.00 per year for US students and residents, $351.00 per year for Canadian individuals, $538.00 per year for Canadian institutions, $445.00 per year for international individuals, $538.00 per year for international institutions, and $234.00 per year for Canadian and foreign students/residents. To receive student/resident rate, orders must be accompanied by name of affiliated institution, date of term, and the *signature* of program/residency coordinator on institution letterhead. Orders will be billed at individual rate until proof of status is received. Foreign air speed delivery is included in all *Clinics* subscription prices. All prices are subject to change without notice. **POSTMASTER:** Send address change to *Gastrointestinal Endoscopy Clinics of North America*, Elsevier Health Sciences Division, Subscription Customer Service, 3251 Riverport Lane, Maryland Heights, MO 63043. **Customer Service: 1-800-654-2452 (US). From outside the United States, call 1-314-447-8871. Fax: 1-314-447-8029. E-mail: JournalsCustomerService-usa@elsevier.com (for print support) or JournalsOnlineSupport-usa@elsevier.com (for online support)**.

Reprints. For copies of 100 or more, of articles in this publication, please contact the Commercial Reprints Department, Elsevier Inc., 360 Park Avenue South, New York, NY 10010-1710. Tel. (212) 633-3812; Fax: (212) 482-1935; E-mail: reprints@elsevier.com.

Gastrointestinal Endoscopy Clinics of North America is covered in *Excerpta Medica, MEDLINE/PubMed (Index Medicus), and MEDLINE/MEDLARS.*

Printed and bound by CPI Group (UK) Ltd, Croydon, CR0 4YY

Transferred to digital print 2012

Contributors

CONSULTING EDITOR

CHARLES J. LIGHTDALE, MD
Professor, Department of Medicine, Columbia University Medical Center, New York, New York

GUEST EDITORS

BENJAMIN LEBWOHL, MD, MS
Assistant Professor of Clinical Medicine and Epidemiology, Department of Medicine, Mailman School of Public Health, Celiac Disease Center, Columbia University, New York, New York

PETER H.R. GREEN, MD
Professor of Clinical Medicine, Department of Medicine, and Director, Celiac Disease Center, Columbia University, New York, New York

AUTHORS

ARMIN ALAEDINI, PhD
Assistant Professor, Department of Medicine, Celiac Disease Center, and Institute of Human Nutrition, Columbia University Medical Center, New York, New York

ASAAD ASSIRI, MD
Pediatric Gastroenterology, Faculty of Medicine, King Khalid University Hospital, King Saud University, Riyadh, Saudi Arabia

IMRAN AZIZ, MRCP
Clinical Research Fellow in Gastroenterology, Department of Gastroenterology, Royal Hallamshire Hospital, Sheffield, United Kingdom

FEI BAO, MD
Assistant Professor of Clinical Pathology and Cell Biology, Department of Pathology and Cell Biology, Columbia University Medical Center and New York Presbyterian Hospital, New York, New York

KASSEM BARADA, MD
Professor of Medicine, Division of Gastroenterology, Department of Internal Medicine, American University of Beirut Medical Center, Beirut, Lebanon

GOVIND BHAGAT, MBBS
Professor of Clinical Pathology and Cell Biology, Department of Pathology and Cell Biology, Columbia University Medical Center and New York Presbyterian Hospital, New York, New York

CARLO CATASSI, MD
Professor of Medicine, Department of Pediatrics, Università Politecnica delle Marche,
Ancona, Italy; Center for Celiac Research, Mucosal Biology Research Center, University
of Maryland School of Medicine, Baltimore, Maryland

CHRISTOPHE CELLIER, MD, PhD
Professor, Université Paris Descartes; Gastroenterology Department, Hôpital Européen
Georges Pompidou APHP, Paris, France

EDWARD J. CIACCIO, PhD
Celiac Disease Center, Columbia University; Division of Digestive Diseases, College
of Physicians and Surgeons, Columbia University, New York, New York

PAUL J. CICLITIRA, MD
Division of Diabetes and Nutrition, Department of Gastroenterology, Rayne Institute,
St Thomas' Hospitals NHS Trust, London, United Kingdom

HUSSEIN ABU DAYA, MD
Postdoctoral Research Fellow, Division of Gastroenterology, Department of Internal
Medicine, American University of Beirut Medical Center, Beirut, Lebanon; Celiac Disease
Center, Columbia University, New York, New York

ALESSIO FASANO, MD
Mucosal Biology Research Center, Center for Celiac Disease Research, Health Science
Facility II, University of Maryland School of Medicine, Baltimore, Maryland

PETER H.R. GREEN, MD
Professor of Clinical Medicine, Director, Department of Medicine, Celiac Disease Center,
Columbia University, New York, New York

STEFANO GUANDALINI, MD
Section of Gastroenterology, Hepatology and Nutrition, Department of Pediatrics,
University of Chicago, Chicago, Illinois; Pediatric Gastroenterology, Faculty of Medicine,
King Khalid University Hospital, King Saud University, Riyadh, Saudi Arabia

BANA JABRI, MD, PhD
Professor of Medicine, Section of Gastroenterology, Hepatology and Nutrition,
Department of Medicine, University of Chicago, and University of Chicago Celiac Disease
Center, Chicago, Illinois

CIARAN P. KELLY, MD
Professor of Medicine, Division of Gastroenterology, The Celiac Center, Beth Israel
Deaconess Medical Center, Harvard Medical School, Boston, Massachusetts

SONIA S. KUPFER, MD
Assistant Professor of Medicine, Section of Gastroenterology, Hepatology and Nutrition,
Department of Medicine, University of Chicago Medicine, and University of Chicago
Celiac Disease Center, Chicago, Illinois

BENJAMIN LEBWOHL, MD, MS
Assistant Professor of Clinical Medicine and Epidemiology, Department of Medicine,
Celiac Disease Center, Columbia University, New York, New York

DANIEL A. LEFFLER, MD
Division of Gastroenterology, Beth Israel Deaconess Medical Center, Boston,
Massachusetts

SUZANNE K. LEWIS, MD
Assistant Professor of Clinical Medicine, Celiac Disease Center, Columbia University; Division of Digestive Diseases, College of Physicians and Surgeons, Columbia University, New York, New York

JONAS F. LUDVIGSSON, MD, PhD
Department of Pediatrics, Örebro University Hospital, Örebro, Sweden

KNUT E.A. LUNDIN, MD, PhD, FACP
Associate Professor; Consultant Gastroenterologist, Department of Gastroenterology, Oslo University Hospital Rikshospitalet, Center for Immune Regulation, University of Oslo, Oslo, Norway

GEORGIA MALAMUT, MD, PhD
Université Paris Descartes; Gastroenterology Department, Hôpital Européen Georges Pompidou APHP, Paris, France

RUPA MUKHERJEE, MD
Clinical Instructor in Medicine, Division of Gastroenterology, Department of Medicine, The Celiac Center, Beth Israel Deaconess Medical Center, Harvard Medical School, Boston, Massachusetts

JOSEPH A. MURRAY, MD, PhD
Professor, Division of Gastroenterology and Hepatology, Mayo Clinic, Rochester, Minnesota

IKRAM NASR, MD
Department of Gastroenterology, Guy's and St Thomas' Hospitals NHS Trust, London, United Kingdom

CATHERINE NEWLAND, MD
Section of Gastroenterology, Hepatology and Nutrition, Department of Pediatrics, University of Chicago, Chicago, Illinois

NORELLE RIZKALLA REILLY, MD
Assistant Professor, Department of Pediatrics, Celiac Disease Center, Columbia University, New York, New York

KAMRAN ROSTAMI, MD, PhD
Professor of Medicine, College of Medical and Dental Sciences, University of Birmingham, United Kingdom

ALBERTO RUBIO-TAPIA, MD
Division of Gastroenterology and Hepatology, Department of Medicine, Mayo Clinic College of Medicine, Rochester, New York

DAVID S. SANDERS, MD, FRCP, FACG
Professor of Gastroenterology, Department of Gastroenterology, Royal Hallamshire Hospital, Sheffield, United Kingdom

DETLEF SCHUPPAN, MD, PhD
Professor of Medicine, Division of Gastroenterology, The Celiac Center, Beth Israel Deaconess Medical Center, Harvard Medical School, Boston, Massachusetts; Division of Molecular and Translational Medicine, Department of Medicine I, Johannes Gutenberg University, Mainz, Germany

CAROL E. SEMRAD, MD
Professor of Medicine, The University of Chicago Medicine, Chicago, Illinois

SUZANNE SIMPSON, RD
Celiac Disease Center, Columbia University, New York, New York

CHRISTINA A. TENNYSON, MD
Assistant Professor of Clinical Medicine, Celiac Disease Center, Columbia University; Division of Digestive Diseases, College of Physicians and Surgeons, Columbia University, New York, New York

TRICIA THOMPSON, RD, MS
Gluten Free Watchdog, LLC, Manchester, Massachusetts

Contents

> The mode of presentation of patients with celiac disease has changed dramatically over the recent decades, with diarrheal or classic presentations becoming less common. This trend is most markedly seen in children, whose main presentations include recurrent abdominal pain, growth issues, and screening groups at risk. Among adults, presentations include diarrhea, anemia, osteoporosis, and recognition at endoscopy performed for gastroesophageal reflux disease, as well as screening. The groups most commonly screened include family members of patients with celiac disease, Down syndrome, and autoimmune diseases.

> Irritable bowel syndrome (IBS) is a prevalent functional gastrointestinal disorder that has a significant impact on quality of life and health care resources. Celiac disease (CD), a gluten-sensitive enteropathy, can be mistaken for IBS. This article discusses the connection between IBS and CD and the new concept of nonceliac gluten sensitivity (NCGS). NCGS may occur in the presence of a normal or near-normal small bowel biopsy. Some patients with IBS without CD may derive symptomatic benefit from a gluten-free diet. Future research could facilitate a significant impact on the quality of life in this potential subgroup of patients.

> Celiac disease results from the interplay of genetic, environmental, and immunologic factors. An understanding of the pathophysiology of celiac disease, in which the trigger (wheat, rye, and barley) is known, will undoubtedly reveal basic mechanisms that underlie other autoimmune diseases (eg, type 1 diabetes) that share many common pathogenic perturbations. This review describes seminal findings in each of the 3 domains of the pathogenesis of celiac disease, namely genetics, environmental triggers, and immune dysregulation, with a focus on newer areas of investigation such as non-HLA genetic variants, the intestinal microbiome, and the role of the innate immune system.

Gluten sensitivity has been best recognized and understood in the context of two conditions, celiac disease and wheat allergy. However, some individuals complain of symptoms in response to ingestion of "gluten," without histologic or serologic evidence of celiac disease or wheat allergy. The term non-celiac gluten sensitivity (NCGS) has been suggested for this condition, although a role for gluten proteins as the sole trigger of the associated symptoms remains to be established. This article reviews the available information regarding symptomatology, epidemiology and genetics, serology and histology, and in vitro and in vivo experimental data on the pathophysiology of NCGS.

Celiac disease is a common inflammatory disease of the small intestine triggered by gluten in genetically susceptible individuals. Diagnosis is made by serologic testing and upper endoscopy with small bowel biopsy in most individuals. Celiac patients may present with abdominal pain or nonspecific gastrointestinal complaints that result in radiologic imaging before diagnosis of celiac disease. Wireless video capsule endoscopy, device-assisted enteroscopy, and enterography allow careful examination of the entire small bowel and targeted sampling of suspicious lesions. This review focuses on the role of device-assisted enteroscopy and radiologic imaging, in particular enterography, in celiac disease.

Video capsule endoscopy (VCE) provides a safe, non-invasive way to visualize the small intestine and is helpful in celiac disease patients in select situations. VCE can be performed in patients who are unable or unwilling to undergo conventional endoscopy, those with positive celiac serology with normal duodenal biopsies, and also in those who develop alarm symptoms. VCE has limitations including subjective interpretation. Techniques are being developed to standardize assessment of VCE images in patients with known or suspected celiac disease. Pilot studies using computer-based quantification methods have shown promise in examining the 3-dimensional mucosal structure and motility.

A small subset of patients with celiac disease become refractory to a gluten-free diet, with persistent or recurrent symptoms of malabsorption and intestinal villous atrophy. This condition, defined as *refractory celiac disease* (RCD), is diagnosed after other small bowel diseases with villous atrophy are excluded. RCD is subdivided into 2 subgroups: type I RCD and type II RCD (RCDII). This latter condition is considered a low-grade intraepithelial lymphoma and has a poor prognosis. This article reviews the clinical and pathologic features of RCD and recent pathogenic findings in RCDII, offering a model to study how inflammation can drive T-cell lymphomagenesis.

The prevalence of celiac disease (CD) in many developing countries is similar to that of developed areas, in both low- and high-risk groups. The disorder is underestimated because of lack of disease awareness. CD is strongly associated with HLA-DQ2 in developing countries. Clinical presentation may be characterized by chronic diarrhea, anemia, stunting and increased mortality. Few studies have addressed atypical or silent CD. Diagnosis is initially made by serologic tests and is confirmed by small intestinal biopsies. In developing countries the adherence to the treatment is still difficult because of poor availability of dedicated gluten-free food.

The gluten-free diet is currently the only treatment for celiac disease, and patients should be monitored closely by a dietitian who is knowledgeable regarding this diet. Evaluation by a dietitian includes a comprehensive assessment of dietary history, with an emphasis on caloric and micronutrient intake. Patient knowledge of the gluten-free diet is assessed and interpretation of food labels is taught. Identification of micronutrient deficiencies or comorbid gastrointestinal conditions may occur during a comprehensive dietary assessment. In patients with evidence of gluten exposure, a thorough evaluation for cross-contamination is performed.

Currently, the only available therapy for celiac disease is strict lifelong adherence to a gluten-free diet (GFD). Although safe and effective, the GFD is not ideal. It is frequently expensive, of limited nutritional value, and not readily available in many countries. Consequently, a need exists for novel, nondietary therapies for celiac disease. Based on the current understanding of celiac disease pathogenesis, several potential targets of therapeutic intervention exist. These novel strategies provide promise of alternative, adjunctive treatment options but also raise important questions regarding safety, efficacy, and monitoring of long-term treatment effect.

GASTROINTESTINAL ENDOSCOPY CLINICS OF NORTH AMERICA

Foreword

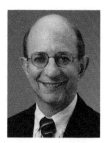

Charles J. Lightdale, MD
Consulting Editor

Celiac disease, long underdiagnosed, is now widely recognized by gastroenterologists and gastrointestinal endoscopists. Current estimates are that up to 1% of the population in the United States may suffer from this autoimmune disease caused by gluten in wheat, rye, barley, and other grains. Along with more accurate diagnosis, celiac disease seems to have actually increased in the United States over the past 50 years, perhaps related to the cross-breeding of hardier wheat plants or to processed foods employing high-gluten flours. Patients with celiac disease who follow a strict gluten-free diet can usually reverse the damage to the small intestinal lining and the related digestive symptoms and nutritional deficiencies. Furthermore, millions of Americans, who don't have the characteristic small intestinal abnormalities required for a diagnosis of celiac disease, seem to have gluten sensitivity and feel better on a gluten-free diet. Gluten-free foods are now ubiquitous, and a multibillion dollar industry supplies highly palatable (often expensive) products online, in supermarkets, in health food stores, and in college cafeterias.

Recent years have seen tremendous advances in understanding the epidemiology, genetics, and pathophysiology of celiac disease, while researchers are still in the early stages of studying the gluten sensitivity phenomenon. With so much public interest, clinicians have become increasingly engaged, and scientific activity has further accelerated. Medical treatments beyond gluten-free diets are being developed. It seemed the right time to devote an entire issue of the *Gastrointestinal Endoscopy Clinics of North America* to "Celiac Disease." Dr Peter H.R. Green and Dr Benjamin Lebwohl, the guest editors for this issue, are at the forefront in celiac disease management, advocacy, and research, based at the Celiac Center at New York–Presbyterian Hospital/Columbia University Medical Center in New York. They have assembled an extraordinary group of international contributors and topics ranging from the latest in diagnosis and management to new insights from the laboratory. Celiac disease and gluten sensitivity have emerged from the shadows to front

http://dx.doi.org/10.1016/j.giec.2012.09.002
1052-5157/12/$ – see front matter
giendo.theclinics.com

and center in gastroenterology. This landmark, comprehensive volume should not be missed.

Charles J. Lightdale, MD
Department of Medicine
Columbia University Medical Center
161 Fort Washington Avenue, Room 812
New York, NY 10032, USA

E-mail address:
CJL18@columbia.edu

Preface
Celiac Disease

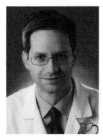 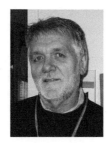

Benjamin Lebwohl, MD, MS   Peter H.R. Green, MD
Guest Editors

Many aspects of the world of celiac disease (CD) are on the rise. The prevalence of CD in the United States has increased 4-fold over the course of the past half-century. Rates of new diagnoses are increasing, including among groups that were previously not thought to be at risk, such as older adults. In parallel with this growth in prevalence and diagnoses, our understanding of CD pathophysiology has increased, and CD is now held up as a unique opportunity in the study of autoimmune diseases, as the triggering antigen (dietary gluten) is known. Also on the rise is awareness of CD, both among patients as well as among physicians and researchers, as evidenced by the growth in research publication output on the subject of CD in the past decade. The popularity and availability of gluten-free food are also on the rise, and gluten sensitivity has hit the mainstream, with the medical community racing to catch up with our patients in terms of understanding the biologic basis for this phenomenon.

The goal of this issue is to summarize and synthesize the latest advances in understanding, diagnosing, and treating CD. The first part of this volume concerns the protean clinical manifestations and pathophysiology of CD, as well as the progress in the diagnosis of CD, which for the majority of patients remains dependent on small intestinal histology. The second section focuses on the monitoring and consequences of CD, as well as an update on our emerging understanding of gluten sensitivity, and the state of CD in the developing world. The third section presents a pair of articles concerning therapy for CD, which at this time is limited to the gluten-free diet, but may soon expand to nondietary therapies based on a variety of promising pharmacologic approaches.

We would like to thank Dr Charles Lightdale, Consulting Editor, for the invitation to develop this volume. We also thank Kerry Holland for her editorial guidance, and the article authors for contributing their expertise to this volume. Last, we thank our

Gastrointest Endoscopy Clin N Am 22 (2012) xv–xvi
http://dx.doi.org/10.1016/j.giec.2012.08.001
1052-5157/12/$ – see front matter © 2012 Published by Elsevier Inc.

patients for inspiring us, for encouraging and assisting us in our research efforts, and for raising awareness of this important disease.

Benjamin Lebwohl, MD, MS
Department of Medicine, Mailman School of Public Health
The Celiac Disease Center at Columbia University
180 Fort Washington Avenue, Suite 936
New York, NY 10032, USA

Peter H.R. Green, MD
Department of Medicine, Director
The Celiac Disease Center at Columbia University
180 Fort Washington Avenue, Suite 936
New York, NY 10032, USA

E-mail addresses:
bl114@columbia.edu (B. Lebwohl)
pg11@columbia.edu (P.H.R. Green)

Presentation of Celiac Disease

Norelle Rizkalla Reilly, MD[a], Alessio Fasano, MD[b],
Peter H.R. Green, MD[c],*

KEYWORDS

• Celiac disease • Diarrhea • Clinical presentation • Autoimmune diseases

KEY POINTS

- Among children, celiac disease has a varied presentation, and is affected especially by the age at presentation.
- In addition to the diverse spectrum of disease presentations and age-related variability of the manifestations of celiac disease in children, the shifting presentation of the disease over time is recognized.
- While the list of conditions associated with celiac disease is quite extensive, there are several groups that are more frequently targeted for celiac disease screening because of their strong association.

CHILDREN

Celiac disease was originally considered a pediatric disorder characterized by malabsorption and steatorrhea.[1–3] Subsequently it was recognized that celiac disease could affect adults at any age,[4,5] and, contrary to opinion at that time, children did not grow out of the disease.[6] Most adults with celiac disease diagnosed before 1980 presented with diarrhea.[7] With the advent of serologic tests in the 1980s, the wide spectrum of clinical manifestations became apparent.

Among children celiac disease has a varied presentation, and is affected especially by the age at presentation. Very young children present more often with "classic" celiac disease, characterized by diarrhea, abdominal distension, and failure to thrive.[8,9] These younger patients are more likely to present with diarrheal or malabsorptive manifestations of the disease,[10] whereas older children and adolescents are more likely to present with atypical gastrointestinal complaints such as pain, vomiting, or constipation. In addition, extraintestinal symptoms such as arthritis, neurologic symptoms,

[a] Department of Pediatrics, Celiac Disease Center, Columbia University, Room 936, 180 Fort Washington Avenue, New York, NY 10032, USA; [b] Mucosal Biology Research Center, Center for Celiac Disease Research, Health Science Facility II, University of Maryland School of Medicine, Room S345, 20 Penn Street, Baltimore, MD 21201, USA; [c] Department of Medicine, Celiac Disease Center, Columbia University, Room 936, 180 Fort Washington Avenue, New York, NY 10032, USA
* Corresponding author.
E-mail address: pg11@columbia.edu

Gastrointest Endoscopy Clin N Am 22 (2012) 613–621
http://dx.doi.org/10.1016/j.giec.2012.07.008
1052-5157/12/$ – see front matter © 2012 Published by Elsevier Inc.

and anemia are not infrequent, as are asymptomatic cases.[11,12] The authors' experience shows that currently the vast majority of children with celiac disease present in 1 of the 3 following ways[13]: (1) growth issues that include failure to thrive in the youngest children or short stature among older children[14]; (2) recurrent abdominal pain the cause of which is unclear, possibly related to episodic or transient intussusceptions that are being increasingly recognized to occur in both adults and children with celiac disease[15–21]; (3) at-risk children screened for the disease because either they were relatives of patients with celiac disease or they had one or more autoimmune disorders or Down syndrome.[13,22] Based on our observation, only 9% of children present with diarrhea.[13] In fact, diarrhea and the malabsorption syndrome are mainly evident in the very young (<2 years old).[23] The authors' experience differs from a series of pediatric patients from Spain in which 62% of the children presented with diarrhea.[8]

In addition to the diverse spectrum of disease presentations and age-related variability of the manifestations of celiac disease in children, the shifting presentation of the disease over time is recognized. An overall decrease in the prevalence of diarrheal presentations over the past 2 decades, accompanied by an increase in atypical manifestations of the disease, has been well described in both adults and children.[7,9,24,25] As an example of how much the presentation of celiac disease has changed, a recent study from the Netherlands revealed that celiac disease was more frequently represented in a cohort of children with chronic constipation fulfilling Rome III criteria for irritable bowel syndrome (IBS); celiac disease was more common than hypothyroidism and hypercalcemia as a cause of the constipation.[26]

Overweight and obese children and adolescents with celiac disease are now frequently identified.[13,27,28] The majority of North American children in the authors' series had a normal body mass index; however, there were children who were overweight, only a minority of children studied were underweight.[13] Similarly, adults may be obese at presentation of celiac disease.[29,30]

More widespread use of serologic markers has facilitated the diagnosis of celiac disease in children.[24] This fact alone does not entirely explain the decrease in diarrheal manifestations, as many long-term studies of adult and pediatric patients predating the use of these markers have documented this shift in clinical presentation.[7,31] Of note, since the advent of sensitive and specific serologic assays over the past 2 decades, the gap between initial presentation of symptoms and diagnosis in symptomatic children has been gradually reduced.[32,33] This reduction in duration of symptoms has also been documented in adults.[7]

Breastfeeding practices appear to influence the mode of presentation in children, because children exclusively breastfed seem to less likely present with failure to thrive and short stature.[34] Breast feeding also contributes to delaying the age of presentation of the disease and possibly preventing the disease.[34–37] In addition, there is an association between cesarean delivery and development of celiac disease.[38,39]

ADULTS

The major mode of presentation of celiac disease in adults is diarrhea, although this presentation occurs in fewer than 50% of patients.[7] Other presentations include anemia, mainly caused by iron deficiency, though anemia due to nutritional factors and chronic disease may also be present at diagnosis of celiac disease.[40,41] Anemia is more frequently seen at presentation in adults than in children.[42]

Osteoporosis is another presentation of celiac disease in adults. Reduced bone density is common in patients with celiac disease,[43,44] and there is increased risk of fracture.[45,46] Research from Argentina demonstrated a high prevalence of bone fractures in the peripheral skeleton, mostly occurring before diagnosis or in noncompliant patients.[45] Of interest, a population-based study from Sweden showed both adults and children with celiac disease were at increased risk of fracture.[47] A study from the United States demonstrated an increased prevalence of celiac disease among osteoporotic patients.[48] However, this finding was not confirmed by other studies from France and among postmenopausal women in Turkey.[49,50]

Another mode of presentation is the incidental recognition of signs of villous atrophy caused by celiac disease during endoscopy performed for other indications.[51] Most upper endoscopy procedures in adults are performed for gastroesophageal reflux disease (GERD). When celiac disease is recognized and treated in patients with GERD, improvement in the reflux is frequently noted.[52] There is a reasonable argument for routine duodenal biopsies during endoscopy for adults, as is the usual practice for pediatric gastroenterologists.[53]

Other presentations in adults include dermatitis herpetiformis, IBS, bloating, and chronic fatigue, as well as a variety of neurologic presentations.[54] Many of the symptoms of celiac disease are common, frequently seen among patients attending primary care physicians.[55] In the authors' multicenter North American primary care screening study involving patients with a variety of symptoms including bloating, fatigue, recurrent abdominal pain, and IBS, screening for celiac disease resulted in a 40-fold increase in the rate of diagnosis of celiac disease.[56]

ASYMPTOMATIC PRESENTATIONS

Serologic screening of groups at risk is undoubtedly responsible for the increased detection of celiac disease in children, some of whom are asymptomatic. Screening was the mode of diagnosis of about 25% of children seen in the authors' center[13]; this includes those identified as a result of serologic screening of family members and those with associated autoimmune conditions.[24] Similarly, for adults there has been an increased number of diagnoses attributable to screening of at-risk groups.[25] At present, about 10% of those adults diagnosed with celiac disease seen in the Celiac Disease Center at Columbia University in New York presented through screening of at-risk groups. Not all of those individuals detected by screening are truly asymptomatic.[57,58]

Several high-risk groups are commonly screened. The most frequently at-risk group screened is the group of family members of individuals with celiac disease.[57] Several studies have shown that about 4% to 10% of first-degree relatives have the disease.[59] The greatest risk is among siblings of affected individuals,[60] but the risk extends to second-degree relatives as well.[57,60] Other frequently screened groups include those with type 1 diabetes (3%–7%)[59] and autoimmune liver disease.[61,62]

The reason why some patients present with diarrhea whereas others are asymptomatic is not clear, for there is no correlation of a diarrheal presentation with severity of villous atrophy,[63] nor length of bowel involved as assessed by video capsule endoscopy.[64] Neurohumoral mechanisms may be important in determining the presence of symptoms, as patients with celiac disease had increased mucosal 5-hydroxytryptamine content and enhanced release from the upper small bowel, which correlated with postprandial dyspepsia.[65]

ASSOCIATED CONDITIONS

Although the list of conditions associated with celiac disease is extensive, several groups are more frequently targeted for celiac disease screening because of their strong association. The association between celiac disease and type 1 diabetes in children is well described.[66] The coexistence of both diseases also occurs in adults.[67,68] The onset of diabetes generally precedes that of celiac disease. An increased prevalence of celiac disease has also been described in adults and children with autoimmune thyroid disease.[69-71]

Children and adolescents with autoimmune liver disease, including biliary disease, have a high prevalence of celiac disease.[72,73] An increased prevalence of celiac disease has additionally been identified in children with Down syndrome (7%),[74] Turner syndrome (6.4%),[75] and Williams syndrome (9.5%).[76]

Several other conditions have been associated with celiac disease, including: autoimmune myocarditis; idiopathic dilated cardiomyopathy; Sjögren syndrome; immunoglobulin A (IgA) deficiency; Addison disease; IgA nephropathy; sarcoidosis; primary hyperparathyroidism; alopecia areata; vitiligo; neurologic abnormalities including epilepsy, ataxia, and neuropathy; atopy; inflammatory bowel disease; psoriasis; and chronic urticaria.

The association with celiac disease and autoimmune disorders is strong. About 30% of adult patients with celiac disease have one or more autoimmune disorder,[77,78] compared with about 3% in the general population.[79] The mechanism of these comorbidities is unclear. It has been suggested that the increase is associated with the duration of exposure to gluten,[78] although this hypothesis has not been corroborated by other studies.[80,81] In a study from France, however, after the diagnosis of celiac disease those who were strictly adherent to the gluten-free diet acquired fewer autoimmune disorders than those who were not compliant with the diet.[82] This finding indicates that the diet may be protective against the development of autoimmune diseases. However, the institution of a gluten-free diet did not prevent progression of established autoimmune thyroid disease after the diagnosis of celiac disease.[83]

Celiac disease is also associated with infertility in both women[84-86] and men.[87] Screening of infertile women detects undiagnosed celiac disease.[88] Fertility improves after diagnosis of celiac disease.[89]

TERMINOLOGY AND DEFINITIONS

There have been several terms used to classify the presentations of celiac disease in both childhood and adulthood. Such terms as typical, atypical, classic, nonclassic, silent, asymptomatic, latent, and potential celiac disease have added confusion to the topic. Two extensive reviews have been published recently in an attempt to bring clarity and agreement to the field.[90,91]

REFERENCES

1. Andersen DH. Celiac syndrome. J Pediatr 1947;30:564–82.
2. Dickie WK. Coeliac disease. Investigation of the harmful effects of certain types of cereal on patients with coeliac disease. Utrecht (The Netherlands): Thesis, University of Utrecht; 1950.
3. Wilson R. The coeliac syndrome with adolescent rickets. Ir J Med Sci 1951; 6(301):39–42.
4. Sleisenger MH, Rynbergen HJ, Pert JH, et al. Treatment of non-tropical sprue: a wheat-, rye-, and oat-free diet. J Am Diet Assoc 1957;33(11):1137–40.
5. Benson GD, Kowlessar OD, Sleisenger MH. Adult celiac disease with emphasis upon response to the gluten-free diet. Medicine (Baltimore) 1964;43:1–40. ·
6. Mortimer PE, Stewart JS, Norman AP, et al. Follow-up study of coeliac disease. Br Med J 1968;3(609):7–9.

7. Rampertab SD, Pooran N, Brar P, et al. Trends in the presentation of celiac disease. Am J Med 2006;119(4):355.e9–355.e14.
8. Vivas S, Ruiz de Morales JM, Fernandez M, et al. Age-related clinical, serological, and histopathological features of celiac disease. Am J Gastroenterol 2008; 103(9):2360–5.
9. Telega G, Bennet TR, Werlin S. Emerging new clinical patterns in the presentation of celiac disease. Arch Pediatr Adolesc Med 2008;162(2):164–8.
10. Llorente-Alonso M, Fernandez-Acenero MJ, Sebastian M. Gluten intolerance: gender and age-related features. Can J Gastroenterol 2006;20(11):719–22.
11. Branski D, Troncone R. Celiac disease: a reappraisal. J Pediatr 1998;133(2): 181–7.
12. Ludvigsson JF, Ansved P, Falth-Magnusson K, et al. Symptoms and signs have changed in Swedish children with coeliac disease. J Pediatr Gastroenterol Nutr 2004;38(2):181–6.
13. Reilly NR, Aguilar K, Hassid BG, et al. Celiac disease in normal-weight and over-weight children: clinical features and growth outcomes following a gluten-free diet. J Pediatr Gastroenterol Nutr 2011;53(5):528–31.
14. Dehghani SM, Asadi-Pooya AA. Celiac disease in children with short stature. Indian J Pediatr 2008;75(2):131–3.
15. Sidhu SK, Koulaouzidis A, Tan CW. Coeliac disease inducing mesenteric lymph-adenopathy and intussusception. Intern Med J 2011;41(5):434.
16. Scholz D, Alzen G, Zimmer KP. Re: small bowel intussusception in celiac disease: revisiting a classic association. J Pediatr Gastroenterol Nutr 2011;52(1):117–8 [author reply: 8].
17. Mirk P, Foschi R, Minordi LM, et al. Sonography of the small bowel after oral administration of fluid: an assessment of the diagnostic value of the technique. Radiol Med 2012;117(4):558–74.
18. Fishman DS, Chumpitazi BP, Ngo PD, et al. Small bowel intussusception in celiac disease: revisiting a classic association. J Pediatr Gastroenterol Nutr 2010; 50(3):237.
19. Altaf MA, Grunow JE. Atypical presentations of celiac disease: recurrent intussus-ception and pneumatosis intestinalis. Clin Pediatr (Phila) 2008;47(3):289–92.
20. Gonda TA, Khan SU, Cheng J, et al. Association of intussusception and celiac disease in adults. Dig Dis Sci 2010;55(10):2899–903.
21. Sanders DS, Azmy IA, Kong SC, et al. Symptomatic small bowel intussusception: a surgical opportunity to diagnose adult celiac disease? Gastrointest Endosc 2004;59(1):161–2.
22. Pueschel SM, Romano C, Failla P, et al. A prevalence study of celiac disease in persons with Down syndrome residing in the United States of America. Acta Paediatr 1999;88(9):953–6.
23. Rizkalla Reilly N, Dixit R, Simpson S, et al. Celiac disease in children: an old disease with new features. Minerva Pediatr 2012;64(1):71–81.
24. McGowan KE, Castiglione DA, Butzner JD. The changing face of childhood celiac disease in north america: impact of serological testing. Pediatrics 2009; 124(6):1572–8.
25. Lo W, Sano K, Lebwohl B, et al. Changing presentation of adult celiac disease. Dig Dis Sci 2003;48(2):395–8.
26. Pelleboer RA, Janssen RL, Deckers-Kocken JM, et al. Celiac disease is overrep-resented in patients with constipation. J Pediatr (Rio J) 2012;88(2):173–6.
27. Venkatasubramani N, Telega G, Werlin SL. Obesity in pediatric celiac disease. J Pediatr Gastroenterol Nutr 2010;51(3):295–7.

28. Arslan N, Esen I, Demircioglu F, et al. The changing face of celiac disease: a girl with obesity and celiac disease. J Paediatr Child Health 2009;45(5):317–8.
29. Kabbani TA, Goldberg A, Kelly CP, et al. Body mass index and the risk of obesity in coeliac disease treated with the gluten-free diet. Aliment Pharmacol Ther 2012; 35(6):723–9.
30. Cheng J, Brar PS, Lee AR, et al. Body mass index in celiac disease: beneficial effect of a gluten-free diet. J Clin Gastroenterol 2010;44(4):267–71.
31. Garampazzi A, Rapa A, Mura S, et al. Clinical pattern of celiac disease is still changing. J Pediatr Gastroenterol Nutr 2007;45(5):611–4.
32. Sun S, Puttha R, Ghezaiel S, et al. The effect of biopsy-positive silent coeliac disease and treatment with a gluten-free diet on growth and glycaemic control in children with type 1 diabetes. Diabet Med 2009;26(12):1250–4.
33. Savilahti E, Pelkonen P, Visakorpi JK. IgA deficiency in children. A clinical study with special reference to intestinal findings. Arch Dis Child 1971;46(249):665–70.
34. D'Amico MA, Holmes J, Stavropoulos SN, et al. Presentation of pediatric celiac disease in the united states: prominent effect of breastfeeding. Clin Pediatr (Phila) 2005;44(3):249–58.
35. Vella C, Grech V. Increasing age at diagnosis of celiac disease in Malta. Indian J Pediatr 2004;71(7):581–2.
36. Ivarsson A, Hernell O, Stenlund H, et al. Breast-feeding protects against celiac disease. Am J Clin Nutr 2002;75(5):914–21.
37. Peters U, Schneeweiss S, Trautwein EA, et al. A case-control study of the effect of infant feeding on celiac disease. Ann Nutr Metab 2001;45(4):135–42.
38. Marild K, Stephansson O, Montgomery S, et al. Pregnancy outcome and risk of celiac disease in offspring: a nationwide case-control study. Gastroenterology 2012;142(1):39–45.e3.
39. Decker E, Hornef M, Stockinger S. Cesarean delivery is associated with celiac disease but not inflammatory bowel disease in children. Gut Microbes 2011; 2(2):91–8.
40. Harper JW, Holleran SF, Ramakrishnan R, et al. Anemia in celiac disease is multi-factorial in etiology. Am J Hematol 2007;82(11):996–1000.
41. Bergamaschi G, Markopoulos K, Albertini R, et al. Anemia of chronic disease and defective erythropoietin production in patients with celiac disease. Haematologica 2008;93(12):1785–91.
42. Rodrigo-Saez L, Fuentes-Alvarez D, Perez-Martinez I, et al. Differences between pediatric and adult celiac disease. Rev Esp Enferm Dig 2011;103(5):238–44.
43. Valdimarsson T, Toss G, Ross I, et al. Bone mineral density in coeliac disease. Scand J Gastroenterol 1994;29(5):457–61.
44. Meyer D, Stavropolous S, Diamond B, et al. Osteoporosis in a North American adult population with celiac disease. Am J Gastroenterol 2001;96(1):112–9.
45. Vasquez H, Mazure R, Gonzalez D, et al. Risk of fractures in celiac disease patients: a cross-sectional, case- control study. Am J Gastroenterol 2000;95(1): 183–9.
46. West J, Logan RF, Card TR, et al. Fracture risk in people with celiac disease: a population-based cohort study. Gastroenterology 2003;125(2):429–36.
47. Ludvigsson JF, Michaelsson K, Ekbom A, et al. Coeliac disease and the risk of fractures—a general population-based cohort study. Aliment Pharmacol Ther 2007;25(3):273–85.
48. Stenson WF, Newberry R, Lorenz R, et al. Increased prevalence of celiac disease and need for routine screening among patients with osteoporosis. Arch Intern Med 2005;165(4):393–9.

49. Legroux-Gerot I, Leloire O, Blanckaert F, et al. Screening for celiac disease in patients with osteoporosis. Joint Bone Spine 2009;76(2):162–5.

50. Kavuncu V, Dundar U, Ciftci IH, et al. Is there any requirement for celiac disease screening routinely in postmenapausal women with osteoporosis? Rheumatol Int 2009;29(7):841–5.

51. Green PH, Shane E, Rotterdam H, et al. Significance of unsuspected celiac disease detected at endoscopy. Gastrointest Endosc 2000;51(1):60–5.

52. Nachman F, Vazquez H, Gonzalez A, et al. Gastroesophageal reflux symptoms in patients with celiac disease and the effects of a gluten-free diet. Clin Gastroenterol Hepatol 2011;9(3):214–9.

53. Green PH, Murray JA. Routine duodenal biopsies to exclude celiac disease? Gastrointest Endosc 2003;58(1):92–5.

54. Chin RL, Latov N, Green PH, et al. Neurologic complications of celiac disease. J Clin Neuromuscul Dis 2004;5(3):129–37.

55. Hin H, Bird G, Fisher P, et al. Coeliac disease in primary care: case finding study. BMJ 1999;318(7177):164–7.

56. Catassi C, Kryszak D, Louis-Jacques O, et al. Detection of celiac disease in primary care: a multicenter case-finding study in North America. Am J Gastroenterol 2007;102(7):1454–60.

57. Fasano A, Berti I, Gerarduzzi T, et al. Prevalence of celiac disease in at-risk and not-at-risk groups in the United States: a large multicenter study. Arch Intern Med 2003;163(3):286–92.

58. Aggarwal S, Lebwohl B, Green PH. Screening for celiac disease in average-risk and high-risk populations. Therap Adv Gastroenterol 2012;5(1):37–47.

59. Murray JA. Celiac disease in patients with an affected member, type 1 diabetes, iron-deficiency, or osteoporosis? Gastroenterology 2005;128(4 Pt 2):S52–6.

60. Book L, Zone JJ, Neuhausen SL. Prevalence of celiac disease among relatives of sib pairs with celiac disease in U.S. families. Am J Gastroenterol 2003;98(2):377–81.

61. Dickey W, McMillan SA. Co-screening for primary biliary cirrhosis and coeliac disease. Association between primary biliary cirrhosis and coeliac disease. Gut 1998;43(2):300.

62. Volta U, Rodrigo L, Granito A, et al. Celiac disease in autoimmune cholestatic liver disorders. Am J Gastroenterol 2002;97(10):2609–13.

63. Brar P, Kwon GY, Egbuna I, et al. Lack of correlation of degree of villous atrophy with severity of clinical presentation of coeliac disease. Dig Liver Dis 2007;39(1):26–9.

64. Murray JA, Rubio-Tapia A, Van Dyke CT, et al. Mucosal atrophy in celiac disease: extent of involvement, correlation with clinical presentation, and response to treatment. Clin Gastroenterol Hepatol 2008;6(2):186–93 [quiz: 25].

65. Coleman NS, Foley S, Dunlop SP, et al. Abnormalities of serotonin metabolism and their relation to symptoms in untreated celiac disease. Clin Gastroenterol Hepatol 2006;4(7):874–81.

66. Carlsson AK, Axelsson IE, Borulf SK, et al. Prevalence of IgA-antiendomysium and IgA-antigliadin autoantibodies at diagnosis of insulin-dependent diabetes mellitus in Swedish children and adolescents. Pediatrics 1999;103(6 Pt 1):1248–52.

67. Walsh CH, Cooper BT, Wright AD, et al. Diabetes mellitus and coeliac disease: a clinical study. Q J Med 1978;47(185):89–100.

68. Bouguerra R, Ben Salem L, Chaabouni H, et al. Celiac disease in adult patients with type 1 diabetes mellitus in Tunisia. Diabetes Metab 2005;31(1):83–6.

69. Sategna-Guidetti C, Volta U, Ciacci C, et al. Prevalence of thyroid disorders in untreated adult celiac disease patients and effect of gluten withdrawal: an Italian multicenter study. Am J Gastroenterol 2001;96(3):751–7.

70. Sategna-Guidetti C, Bruno M, Mazza E, et al. Autoimmune thyroid diseases and coeliac disease. Eur J Gastroenterol Hepatol 1998;10(11):927–31.

71. Sattar N, Lazare F, Kacer M, et al. Celiac disease in children, adolescents, and young adults with autoimmune thyroid disease. J Pediatr 2011;158(2):272–275.e1.

72. Caprai S, Vajro P, Ventura A, et al. Autoimmune liver disease associated with celiac disease in childhood: a multicenter study. Clin Gastroenterol Hepatol 2008;6(7):803–6.

73. Diamanti A, Basso MS, Pietrobattista A, et al. Prevalence of celiac disease in children with autoimmune hepatitis. Dig Liver Dis 2008;40(12):965.

74. George EK, Hertzberger-ten Cate R, van Suijlekom-Smit LW, et al. Juvenile chronic arthritis and coeliac disease in The Netherlands. Clin Exp Rheumatol 1996;14(5):571–5.

75. Bonamico M, Pasquino AM, Mariani P, et al. Prevalence and clinical picture of celiac disease in turner syndrome. J Clin Endocrinol Metab 2002;87(12):5495–8.

76. Bonamico M, Mariani P, Danesi HM, et al. Prevalence and clinical picture of celiac disease in Italian Down syndrome patients: a multicenter study. J Pediatr Gastroenterol Nutr 2001;33(2):139–43.

77. Bai D, Brar P, Holleran S, et al. Effect of gender on the manifestations of celiac disease: evidence for greater malabsorption in men. Scand J Gastroenterol 2005;40(2):183–7.

78. Ventura A, Magazzu G, Greco L. Duration of exposure to gluten and risk for autoimmune disorders in patients with celiac disease. SIGEP Study Group for Autoimmune Disorders in Celiac Disease. Gastroenterology 1999;117(2):297–303.

79. Jacobson DL, Gange SJ, Rose NR, et al. Epidemiology and estimated population burden of selected autoimmune diseases in the United States. Clin Immunol Immunopathol 1997;84(3):223–43.

80. Sategna-Guidetti C, Solerio E, Scaglione N, et al. Duration of gluten exposure in adult coeliac disease does not correlate with the risk for autoimmune disorders. Gut 2001;49(4):502–5.

81. Viljamaa M, Kaukinen K, Huhtala H, et al. Coeliac disease, autoimmune diseases and gluten exposure. Scand J Gastroenterol 2005;40(4):437–43.

82. Cosnes J, Cellier C, Viola S, et al. Incidence of autoimmune diseases in celiac disease: protective effect of the gluten-free diet. Clin Gastroenterol Hepatol 2008;6(7):753–8.

83. Metso S, Hyytia-Ilmonen H, Kaukinen K, et al. Gluten-free diet and autoimmune thyroiditis in patients with celiac disease. A prospective controlled study. Scand J Gastroenterol 2012;47(1):43–8.

84. Molteni N, Bardella MT, Bianchi PA. Obstetric and gynecological problems in women with untreated celiac sprue. J Clin Gastroenterol 1990;12(1):37–9.

85. Sher KS, Mayberry JF. Female fertility, obstetric and gynaecological history in coeliac disease. A case control study. Digestion 1994;55(4):243–6.

86. Stazi AV, Mantovani A. A risk factor for female fertility and pregnancy: celiac disease. Gynecol Endocrinol 2000;14(6):454–63.

87. Baker PG, Read AE. Reversible infertility in male coeliac patients. Br Med J 1975;02(5966):316–7.

88. Choi JM, Lebwohl B, Wang J, et al. Increased prevalence of celiac disease in patients with unexplained infertility in the United States. J Reprod Med 2011;56(5–6):199–203.

89. Zugna D, Richiardi L, Akre O, et al. A nationwide population-based study to determine whether coeliac disease is associated with infertility. Gut 2010; 59(11):1471–5.

90. Ludvigsson JF, Leffler DA, Bai JC, et al. The Oslo definitions for coeliac disease and related terms. Gut 2012. [Epub ahead of print] PMID: 22345659.

91. Sapone A, Bai JC, Ciacci C, et al. Spectrum of gluten-related disorders: consensus on new nomenclature and classification. BMC Med 2012;10(1):13.

The Irritable Bowel Syndrome-Celiac Disease Connection

Imran Aziz, MRCP*, David S. Sanders, MD, FRCP, FACG

KEYWORDS

- Celiac disease • Gluten sensitivity • Irritable bowel syndrome
- Gluten-sensitive irritable bowel syndrome

KEY POINTS

- The burden of illness of irritable bowel syndrome (IBS) is significant.
- Identification of patients with IBS is no longer considered to be a diagnosis based on the exclusion of organic disease but a positive diagnosis using symptom-based criteria.
- Recent evidence suggests the classification of 3 gluten-induced and heterogeneous conditions: celiac disease (CD), wheat allergy, and nonceliac gluten sensitivity (NCGS), a form of gluten intolerance that meets neither the diagnostic criteria for CD nor those for wheat allergy.
- Although NCGS has started to gain recognition and credibility within the medical profession, it is still the most common and under-recognized form of gluten disorder.

IRRITABLE BOWEL SYNDROME

Irritable bowel syndrome (IBS) is a functional gastrointestinal disorder, as defined by no identifiable structural or biochemical abnormality. Epidemiologic surveys suggest that IBS is a common condition, with the prevalence reported to range between 5% to 30%.[1,2] IBS is frequently encountered in clinical practice, accounting for almost a third of all gastroenterology cases seen in primary care, with a subsequent third of these being referred on to secondary care for further evaluation.[2] The condition predominantly affects young to middle-aged adults,[3,4] with the natural history of the disorder often following a chronic remitting-relapsing course.[5]

Disclosures: None.
Funding: None.
Conflict of interests: Professor Sanders has received an educational grant from Dr Schär (a gluten-free food manufacturer) to undertake an investigator-led research study on gluten-sensitive irritable bowel syndrome. This research hypothesis was generated by Professor Sanders and the data collected will only be analyzed and published by the Sheffield (United Kingdom) research team.
Department of Gastroenterology, Royal Hallamshire Hospital, Sheffield, UK
* Corresponding author. Department of Gastroenterology, Royal Hallamshire Hospital, Room P39, Sheffield S10 2JF, UK.
E-mail address: imran.aziz@sth.nhs.uk

The burden of illness of IBS is significant. Patients have decreased health-related quality of life (HRQOL) scores compared with healthy individuals and even those with chronic disorders such as diabetes and end-stage renal failure.[6] In addition, patients with IBS generate a substantial economic burden, both because of direct health care costs and impaired work productivity.[7] A systematic review addressing the economic cost of IBS in the United States and United Kingdom in the year 2002 found total direct and indirect costs per patient per year reaching $8750 and $3344, respectively.[8]

The pathophysiologic mechanism of IBS is not completely understood, but is thought to be a dysregulation in the brain-gut axis manifested by alterations in the cerebral and autonomic response, immune function, visceral sensitivity and motility.[9] Triggers of such alterations include genetic factors,[10] chronic stress,[11] enteric infections,[12,13] and diet.[14] Infectious gastroenteritis can lead to long-lasting alterations in gut immunity and function, and the clinical entity is commonly recognized as post-infectious IBS.[12,13] Similar bottom-up mechanisms have been proposed for dietary triggers. Roughly two-thirds of patients with IBS perceive their symptoms to be related to meals, in particular foods rich in carbohydrates, as well as fatty foods, coffee, alcohol, and hot spices.[15] However, identifying the dietary component triggering these IBS symptoms is difficult, with one method being that of dietary exclusion followed by selective rechallenges.[14] The positive response rate for such a technique varies from 15% to 72%. It has been suggested that there may be a significant placebo effect, and such dietary approaches may be time consuming and cumbersome; for this reason, dietary approaches have not always been widely adopted into routine clinical practice.[16] However, increased immunoglobulin (Ig)-G antibodies against dietary antigens such as wheat, beef, pork, and lamb were found to be more common in subjects with IBS than in controls,[17] with subsequent selective dietary exclusion showing significant clinical benefit.[18,19] This contemporary work has generated new interest in this dietetic approach to IBS.

Identification of patients with IBS is no longer considered to be a diagnosis based on the exclusion of organic disease but a positive diagnosis using symptom-based criteria. In 1978, Manning and colleagues[20] first described specific symptoms, which were considered to increase diagnostic confidence. These key symptoms have been incorporated by a multinational working party into the Rome criteria. The Rome I criteria were revised as the Rome II Diagnostic Criteria for Functional Gastrointestinal Disorders and these have been used widely in clinical gastroenterology.[21,22] More recently, the Rome III criteria have been devised and application in clinical studies has begun (**Box 1**).[23,24] The validity of symptom-based criteria has been substantiated

---

Box 1
Rome III criteria

Rome III diagnostic criteria[a] for IBS.

Recurrent abdominal pain or discomfort at least 3 days a month in the past 3 months, associated with 2 or more of the following:

- Improvement with defecation
- Onset associated with a change in frequency of stool
- Onset associated with a change in form (appearance) of stool

[a] Criteria fulfilled for the past 3 months with symptom onset at least 6 months before diagnosis.
  From Longstreth GF, Thompson WG, Chey WD, et al. Functional bowel disorders. Gastroenterology 2006;130(5):1480–91; with permission.

by patient studies,[20] long-term follow-up evaluation of patients with IBS,[25] and factor analysis on healthy volunteers.[26]

However, patients referred from primary care may not represent most IBS sufferers within the community and may be those with refractory symptoms, poorer HRQOL, more psychological distress, or reduced coping mechanisms.[2,27–29] Knowing which patients will benefit from further investigations is challenging because the diagnostic yield in patients with IBS may be low. Nevertheless, previous studies have described disorders in patients who fulfill IBS diagnostic criteria. Examples of conditions that may mimic IBS include bile acid malabsorption,[30] exocrine pancreatic insufficiency,[31] and celiac disease (CD).[32]

CD

CD, a chronic inflammatory disorder of the small bowel, can be defined as a state of heightened immunologic responsiveness to ingested gluten (from wheat, barley, or rye) in genetically susceptible individuals.[33] In the past, CD was thought to be a rare condition with an estimated prevalence of 1 in 8000.[34] With the advent of endoscopic small bowel biopsies and new serologic assays, the prevalence of this condition is now widely appreciated to be around 1%.[35] Furthermore, it is now recognized that patients do not always have to present with classic gastrointestinal symptoms of malabsorption but may have nonclassic symptoms,[36] including atypical gastrointestinal symptoms (such as bloating, abdominal discomfort, gas, or altered defecation),[37] or may present insidiously with iron deficiency anemia,[38] osteoporosis,[39] ataxia, or peripheral neuropathy.[40] Hence, because of symptom overlap, it can be clinically difficult to distinguish CD from IBS.[41] The cornerstone of treatment of CD is lifelong adherence to a strict gluten-free diet (GFD). For most patients, a GFD leads to clinical and histologic remission, normalization of standardized mortality,[42,43] a reduction in long-term health complications (ie, osteoporosis),[44–46] and, in some studies, an improvement in psychological well-being and quality of life.[47,48]

The diagnosis of CD requires a small bowel biopsy showing villous atrophy.[33,49] There are several serologic tests that have been reported to be accurate in identifying patients who should then be referred for a duodenal biopsy. Serologic testing for CD has evolved over the years, starting with antigliadin antibodies (AGA) followed by endomysial (EMA) and tissue transglutaminase (tTG) antibodies. Because of their poor diagnostic accuracy, as shown by their lower sensitivity and specificity, AGA have largely been superseded by EMA and tTG for routine serologic testing in CD. However, AGA still plays a role in diagnosing non–celiac-related neurologic conditions (for example, gluten ataxia) in the absence of enteropathy.[50]

HLA DQ2 or DQ8 are closely linked with CD, occurring in up to 98% of cases, but are also present in 25% of the normal population.[51,52] Hence, an absence of these haplotypes could have a negatively predictive role when trying to exclude CD, particularly in patients who are already on a GFD before presentation and testing. However, testing for these susceptibility genes is not recommended in routine clinical practice because it is an expensive test, not readily available, and thus should be reserved for equivocal cases.[53]

CD AND IBS CROSSOVER

The association between CD and IBS was first reported in 2001, when sequential patients presenting with IBS in secondary care (n = 300) were investigated for CD.[32] Participants were initially investigated for CD with immunoglobulins, IgA/IgG AGA and IgA EMA. Any participant who had a positive IgA AGA, IgA EMA, or IgG AGA in the presence of IgA deficiency was offered a small bowel biopsy to confirm the diagnosis of CD. Our group found CD to be present in 4.7% (14/300) of patients referred to secondary care fulfilling the Rome II criteria for IBS, a 7-fold increase compared with non–IBS-matched controls (0.67%, 95% confidence interval [CI] 1.6-28.0, $P = 0.004$). We then compared our findings with a population of healthy volunteers recruited from primary care (n = 1200). From 1200 volunteers in primary care, there were 12 new cases of CD. The prevalence of CD in this general population sample was 1% (95% CI 0.4-1.3%). The prevalence of CD among patients with IBS in primary care was 3.3%.[54] These studies highlight the importance of a case-finding approach when considering patients with symptoms of IBS, in whom the diagnosis of CD may be missed. Since that time, others have published supportive evidence/validation studies from other international cohorts (**Table 1**).[32, 54–69]

A recent systematic review and large meta-analysis found that the prevalence of biopsy-proven CD in cases meeting the diagnostic criteria for IBS was more than 4-fold that in controls without IBS.[70] The recognized association between IBS and CD has led to a change in practice and guidelines. The National Institute for Health and Clinical Excellence in the United Kingdom and the British Society of Gastroenterology guidelines recommend the routine exclusion of CD in all patients referred with IBS.[53,71] The American College of Gastroenterology (ACG) advise testing for CD in those with diarrhea-predominant IBS (D-IBS) or mixed bowel pattern IBS (M-IBS).[72] However, this has recently been challenged by Cash and colleagues,[69] who found the prevalence of CD in 492 US patients with nonconstipated IBS to be 0.41%, similar to that of healthy controls (0.44%).[69] Given that testing for CD in IBS is cost-effective in areas where the prevalence of CD is 1% or greater,[42,43] this may have implications on future ACG recommendations. However, this study is the first of its kind in the United States and further validation studies are required. What adds to the debate is that a primary care study in the United States noted the prevalence of CD in patients with IBS to be 2.7%.[60] It may be that there is an ascertainment bias: in the United Kingdom, it is estimated that IBS accounts for at least 25% of a gastroenterologist's workload in the out-patient department.[73] The referral pattern in the United States seems to be significantly different to that seen in the United Kingdom, because Cash and colleagues[69] recruited 492 patients from 4 centers over 5 years. Does this suggest that IBS is not a condition commonly referred to secondary care in the United States? Perhaps primary care physicians have already investigated patients for CD before referral?[60] In addition, Cash and colleagues[69] and others did not include patients investigated with constipation predominant IBS (C-IBS) for CD (see **Table 1**), but the largest multicenter CD epidemiologic screening study in the United States (involving 13,145 patients from 32 states) found CD to be present in 2.63% of patients complaining of constipation (40/1530). Furthermore, this group also noted constipation to be prevalent in 20.2% of newly diagnosed CD cases.[74] Therefore, should patients with C-IBS be included or excluded from identifying CD cases? There is variation in the international literature. Jadallah and Khader recently noted that, in their group, the prevalence of CD in D-IBS was 6.8% (95% CI 3.36–10.23) but only 1.68% (95% CI 0.35–3.01) in C-IBS.[65] Similar data were also noted by Shahbazkhani and colleagues,[62] who found that C-IBS accounted for a third of the subsequently diagnosed CD cases. The diversity in the diagnostic criteria, referral patterns, number of patients, IBS subtypes, serologic tests, and histologic confirmation that are used to investigate patients with IBS for CD may account for the varying results seen in **Table 1**. A standardized method would help to elucidate this.

The association of CD and IBS symptoms is biologically plausible, with many mechanisms being reported; for example, autonomic dysfunction, intussusception, exocrine pancreatic disease, small intestinal ulceration, and associated microscopic colitis.[75]

Table 1
Studies of celiac disease in cohorts of patients with IBS

Report	Year	Country	Setting	N	Criteria	IBS Subtype Investigated (%)	Initial Tests	Biopsy	Prevalence (%)
Hin et al[55]	1999	United Kingdom	Primary care	132	NR	NR	EMA	Yes	0
Agréus et al[56]	2000	Sweden	Primary care	50	NR	NR	AGA, EMA	Yes	0
Holt et al[57]	2001	United Kingdom	Primary care	138	Rome I	NR	AGA, EMA	No	0.7
Sanders et al[54]	2003	United Kingdom	Primary care	123	Rome II	NR	AGA, EMA	Yes	3.3
Locke[58]	2004	United States	Primary care	50	Manning	D-IBS (38)	tTG, EMA	No	–
Kennedy et al[59]	2006	United Kingdom	Primary care	141	Rome I	NR	AGA, EMA	No	0.7
Catassi et al[60]	2007	United States	Primary care	264	NR	NR	EMA, tTG	Yes	2.7
Sanders et al[32]	2001	United Kingdom	Secondary care	300	Rome II	D-IBS (28), C-IBS (21), M-IBS (51)	AGA, EMA	Yes	4.7
Demarchi et al[61]	2002	Italy	Secondary care	257	Rome II	NR	AGA, EMA	Yes	8.2
Shahbazkhani et al[62]	2003	Iran	Secondary care	105	Rome II	D-IBS (23), C-IBS (34), M-IBS (43)	AGA, EMA	Yes	11.4
v d Wouden et al[63]	2007	Holland	Secondary care	148	Rome II	NR	EMA	No	0
Ozdil et al[64]	2008	Turkey	Secondary care	60	Rome II	D-IBS (22), C-IBS (55), M-IBS (23)	AGA, EMA, tTG	Yes	0
Jadallah et al[65]	2009	Jordan	Secondary care	742	Rome II	D-IBS (28), C-IBS (48), M-IBS (24)	tTG	Yes	3.2
Z-Wcisio et al[66]	2009	Poland	Secondary care	200	Rome II	D-IBS (100)	tTG	Yes	7
Korkut et al[67]	2010	Turkey	Secondary care	100	Rome III	D-IBS (21), C-IBS (63), M-IBS (16)	POCT, AGA, tTG	Yes	2
El-Salhy et al[68]	2011	Norway	Secondary care	968	Rome III	NR	D2 biopsy	Yes	0.4
Cash et al[69]	2011	United States	Secondary care	492	Rome II	D-IBS and M-IBS	AGA, EMA, tTG	Yes	0.41

Abbreviations: AGA, antigliadin antibodies; C-IBS, constipation; D-IBS, diarrhea; EMA, endomysial antibodies; M-IBS, mixed pattern predominant IBS; NR, not reported; POCT, point of care test; tTG tissue transglutaminase antibodies.

Our group found an increased prevalence of CD in patients referred with surgical abdominal pain, notably in those with unexplained or nonspecific abdominal pain.[75]

The association between IBS and CD seems to operate in both directions, because patients with CD (on a GFD) are more likely than controls to describe IBS symptoms. A study by O'Leary and colleagues found 20% of patients with CD to also fulfill the Rome criteria for IBS, compared with 5% of healthy controls.[76] This study also showed that patients with CD with IBS have a markedly lower HRQOL than their counterparts without IBS. This novel observation is also supported by research from our own group who recently reported in a cross-sectional study (n = 1031) that patients with CD and persisting IBS symptoms have worse Short Form 36 (SF-36) scores than those who only have CD.[77]

These patients also report a higher frequency of medical consultations compared with CD patients without IBS.[78] Predictors of IBS-type symptoms among adults with CD include mental disorder, female sex, and occasional nonadherence to a GFD.[78] These data offer further support to the biopsychosocial model of IBS, with CD possibly playing its part by having a sensitizing effect on the bowel through mucosal inflammation.

NCGS: A NEW CONDITION IN THE SPECTRUM OF GLUTEN-RELATED DISORDERS

Until recently, the terms gluten sensitivity and CD were synonymous in the literature.[79] Gluten was associated only with CD and wheat allergy; therefore, patients with gluten-induced gastrointestinal symptoms who produced normal values of tTG and IgE and showed normal histology were advised to continue integrating gluten foods into their diet, because gluten was not regarded as the cause for their condition.[80]

However, most of those seeking medical attention for gluten-induced gastrointestinal symptoms do not have CD or wheat allergy. In a study with 94 adults affected by abdominal symptoms after cereal ingestion, Kaukinen and colleagues reported a prevalence of 9% with CD, 8% with latent CD, and 20% with cereal allergy. Sixty-three percent of study subjects could not be classified as allergic or as having CD, but were affected by gluten foods and clinically benefitted from a GFD.[81]

Meanwhile, more recent evidence suggests the classification of 3 gluten-induced and heterogeneous conditions: CD, wheat allergy, and nonceliac gluten sensitivity (NCGS), a form of gluten intolerance that meets neither the diagnostic criteria for CD nor those for wheat allergy.[82] NCGS is an umbrella term and can incorporate a wide range of symptoms including abdominal discomfort, bloating, pain, or diarrhea; it may also present with a variety of extraintestinal symptoms that may include headaches and migraines, lethargy and tiredness, attention deficit syndrome and hyperactivity, autism and schizophrenia, muscular disturbances, and bone and joint pain (see **Table 2**).[82–86] For the purpose of this article, NCGS is referred to only in the context of gastrointestinal symptoms.

Table 2	
Symptoms and associations in gluten sensitivity	
Symptoms	Bloating
	Abdominal discomfort or pain
	Diarrhea or constipation
Extraintestinal symptoms	Headaches and migraines, lethargy, and tiredness
Associations	Attention deficit syndrome
	Autism
	Muscular disturbances as well as bone and joint pain

In an article by Verdu and colleagues, NCGS is defined by "one or more of a variety of immunologic, morphologic, or symptomatic manifestations that may also be shared by CD and IBS" and thus, in some quarters, is referred to as the no-man's land between these two conditions.[87]

Patients with NCGS are unable to tolerate gluten and develop an adverse reaction when eating gluten that usually, and differently from CD, does not lead to severe small intestinal damage. Although the gastrointestinal symptoms in NCGS may resemble those associated with CD, the overall clinical picture is not accompanied by the concurrence of tTG autoantibodies, villous atrophy, or autoimmune disease. The diversity of gluten-induced conditions indicates that the immune system manages gliadin in different ways.[88]

CD, characterized by the presence of specific autoantibodies to tTG, is considered an autoimmune and Th1-mediated disorder with strong genetic association; although virtually all patients with CD carry the genetic markers HLA DQ2 or DQ8, only 50% of patients with NCGS, few more than in the general population, carry either the HLA DQ2 or DQ8 haplotypes.[88,89] In contrast with patients with CD, patients with NCGS do not present with significant histologic mucosal alterations in the small intestine. These individuals also show a lower increment in intraepithelial CD3 lymphocytes and are always anti-tTG negative as well as EMA negative. A recent retrospective review found the serologic pattern of patients with NCGS to be characterized by IgG AGA positivity in more than half of cases associated to IgA AGA in a few patients, but without EMA, tTG, and deamidated gliadin peptide antibodies (DGP-AGA), which are the specific markers of CD and were highly prevalent in the CD comparison group.[90]

Furthermore, patients with NCGS show normal intestinal permeability and activation of the innate immunity instead of adaptive immune mechanisms compared with patients with CD.[91] The immune mechanism underpinning this is complex and as yet not fully understood. Gliadin has been shown to activate the release of interleukin (IL)-15 in both healthy individuals and those with CD.[92] IL-15 is considered to be the first triggering signal of CD.[93] However, in healthy individuals, the IL-15 does not reach the response threshold to elicit an inflammatory cascade, presumably because of decreased duodenal IL-15 receptor (IL-15R) expression. In patients with CD, an inflammatory response is triggered after the release of IL-15, because there is an increased IL-15R expression coupled with a decreased immune response threshold against this cytokine[94]; this subsequently leads to both an innate and a secondary adaptive immune response, ultimately manifesting as small intestinal damage. Patients with NCGS have been proposed to fulfill the criteria to stimulate an innate immune response but seemingly fall short of triggering the adaptive immune response, presumably because they lack the associated machinery to do so, such as HLA typing and epithelial permeability. As a result the inflammatory small bowel response is halted and mucosal manifestations absent.[95] Recent work by Sapone and colleagues comparing mucosal expression in patients with CD and NCGS supports this hypothesis, as shown by significantly higher levels of adaptive immune markers (interferon-γ, IL-6, IL-21, and IL-17) in CD compared with NCGS. In contrast, the NCGS group had significantly higher expression of innate markers, such as the Toll-like receptor (TLR) 2, and, to a lesser extent, TLR 1.[88,91]

Although NCGS has started to gain recognition and credibility within the medical profession, it is still the most common and under-recognized form of gluten disorder. Based on the results of their cohort study investigating the mortality of patients with NCGS and CD in Northern Ireland, Anderson and colleagues estimated that, for every person with CD, there could be at least 6 or 7 people with NCGS.[96] NCGS may therefore affect 6% to 10% of the general population, whereas CD is thought to affect only

1%. In total, all three gluten sensitivity disorders affect about 10% of the general population.

Although immunoassays like the EMA and anti-tTG assays are being successfully used for the diagnosis of CD, the diagnosis of NCGS is difficult because of the lack of diagnostic criteria.[81,97] In the current absence of specific markers for NCGS, the gold standard of NCGS testing is still the gluten elimination diet, which involves strict avoidance of gluten-containing foods for 2 to 3 months. Remission of symptoms on elimination and return of symptoms on the reintroduction of gluten are indicators for NCGS.

IS THERE A RELATIONSHIP BETWEEN IBS AND GLUTEN SENSITIVITY?

Our group previously reported that AGA were present in ~12% of the general population and ~17% in IBS (both in the presence of a normal small bowel biopsy).[32,54] Cash and colleagues found that, in their cohort of patients with IBS, despite only 0.41% being found to have CD, slightly more than 7% had CD-associated antibodies, predominantly IgG AGA (4.88%) and IgA AGA antibodies (1.63%).[69] Kaukinen and colleagues noted that most patients with cereal-induced gastrointestinal symptoms complained of bloating (83%), diarrhea (63%), and abdominal discomfort (34%), symptoms seemingly consistent with the Rome criteria; of those in whom CD was excluded, AGA were present in 40%.[81] This finding further supports the hypothesis of gluten-sensitivity IBS (GS-IBS) (**Fig. 1**).[87,98] What this may suggest is that, in susceptible individuals, the consumption of gluten results in an immune response that is manifested by the production of AGA.

Wahnschaffe and colleagues also described an association between CD-like abnormalities and a subgroup of patients with IBS. This investigating group used the presence of intestinal antibodies (to gluten) on small bowel aspirate to define an IBS subgroup (n = 26).[99] These patients then agreed to commence a GFD for 6 months. During this time, they reported an improvement in their stool frequency and there was also a reduction in intestinal antibody levels. However, the investigators concluded that this test is invasive, not a standard procedure, and is probably not feasible in routine clinical practice.

The investigators have provided further, more recent work suggesting that serum celiac-associated antibodies and HLA DQ2 or DQ8 pattern may predict a response to a GFD in D-IBS.[100] At first, out of a total 145 patients with D-IBS, 36% were found

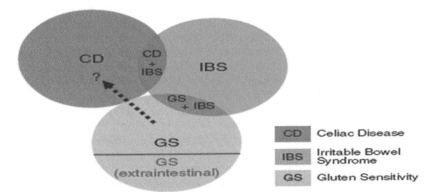

Fig. 1. A model for the relationship between celiac disease, IBS, and gluten sensitivity. (*From* Ball AJ, Hadjivassiliou M, Sanders DS. Is gluten sensitivity a "No Man's Land" or a "Fertile Crescent" for research? Am J Gastroenterol 2010;105(1):222–3 [author reply: 223–4]; with permission.)

to be IgG AGA/TTG positive and 39% DQ2 positive. This percentage was significantly less than in the untreated celiac group, but significantly more than among patients with inflammatory bowel disease and healthy controls. Furthermore, 41 (n = 41) patients with D-IBS then agreed to participate in a 6-month GFD. Positive IgG AGA/TTG and HLA DQ2 were all independent factors for a symptomatic response to a GFD. The combination of both a positive serum IgG AGA/TTG and HLA for a clinical response to a GFD had a sensitivity, specificity, positive predictive value, and negative predictive value of 75%, 76%, 56%, and 88%, respectively. However, this study was not blinded and had 11/41 (25%) patients with D-IBS with increased intraepithelial lymphocytes (IEL), although this was shown not to correlate with a clinical response and neither was there a significant change in the IEL count after a GFD in responders and nonresponders. There are many potential causes of increased duodenal IEL, including CD, and therefore a gluten challenge may have been useful in inducing further histologic deterioration and identifying whether these patients belonged to the celiac spectrum.[101]

In addition, a study by an Australian group adds to the debate.[102] The investigators undertook a double-blind, randomized, placebo-controlled rechallenge trial in patients with IBS fulfilling the Rome III criteria (n = 34). The patients were recruited through a newspaper advertisement and were already taking a self-imposed GFD because of symptomatic gastrointestinal benefit. CD was excluded by a negative HLA DQ2 or DQ8 pattern, or a normal duodenal biopsy (on gluten challenge) in the presence of a positive HLA. Patients were randomized according to a computer-generated list of random numbers held by an independent observer to either the gluten or the placebo treatment group. Over the 6-week study period, the severity scores of pain, satisfaction with stool consistency, and tiredness were significantly higher for those consuming the gluten diet compared with the placebo group. Despite this, there was no evidence of intestinal inflammation or damage while being challenged with gluten (using fecal lactoferrin and intestinal permeability). Thus, these patients could not be viewed as having latent CD. This study is the first to describe an NCGS that may cause IBS. Based on the current data, gluten may cause symptoms in patients with IBS. However, 2 different research groups have published opposing studies. How can this be explained? Perhaps there are many mechanisms by which gluten can cause symptoms in patients with IBS-type symptoms? GS-IBS now seems to be part of the spectrum of gluten-related disorders.

SUMMARY

Although gluten induced, NCGS differs from other gluten-related disorders. Whilst, in wheat allergy and NCGS, the immune response to the dietary component gliadin results in immunity toward it, CD involves self-directed adaptive response mechanisms leading to an autoimmune process and possibly to the onset of other autoimmune conditions.[88,103]

CD is considered to be a condition that requires lifelong avoidance of gliadin; NCGS can vary in duration and gluten threshold sensitivity.[104] However, little is known about the pathogenic mechanism behind NCGS. At present, it is unclear whether patients with NCGS may tolerate a minimum of gluten. Furthermore, it is questionable whether NCGS is a reversible condition and whether patients can tolerate gluten products after an extended period of gluten avoidance.

In light of its high prevalence and the difficulties involved with its diagnosis, there is a need for highly sensitive and specific serologic markers alongside other markers such as anti-tTG, already in use for CD. AGA may have an essential role to play, but on this occasion to identify the subgroup of patients with IBS who have GS-IBS. Whether routinely testing patients with IBS for their HLA typing is clinically beneficial and ultimately cost-effective also needs to be determined. The current plight of patients with IBS is one of great economic burden associated with a poor HRQOL. Determining the prevalence of GS-IBS in clinical practice may allow correct identification of a subgroup of patients with IBS who may benefit from a GFD. The recognition of GS-IBS could benefit patients in terms of symptoms and quality of life.

Therefore, NCGS should no longer be seen as the no-man's land but as a fertile crescent for further research, to elucidate GS-IBS and improve its diagnosis to support patients affected by GS-IBS in the most clinically efficient way possible.

REFERENCES

1. Hillilä MT, Färkkilä MA. Prevalence of irritable bowel syndrome according to different diagnostic criteria in a non-selected adult population. Aliment Pharmacol Ther 2004;20(3):339–45.
2. Thompson WG, Heaton KW, Smyth GT, et al. Irritable bowel syndrome in general practice: prevalence, characteristics, and referral. Gut 2000;46(1):78–82.
3. Chang L, Toner BB, Fukudo S, et al. Gender, age, society, culture, and the patient's perspective in the functional gastrointestinal disorders. Gastroenterology 2006;130(5):1435–46.
4. Drossman DA, Camilleri M, Mayer EA, et al. AGA technical review on irritable bowel syndrome. Gastroenterology 2002;123(6):2108–31.
5. Agréus L, Svärdsudd K, Talley NJ, et al. Natural history of gastroesophageal reflux disease and functional abdominal disorders: a population-based study. Am J Gastroenterol 2001;96(10):2905–14.
6. Gralnek IM, Hays RD, Kilbourne A, et al. The impact of irritable bowel syndrome on health-related quality of life. Gastroenterology 2000;119(3):654–60.
7. Sandler RS, Everhart JE, Donowitz M, et al. The burden of selected digestive diseases in the United States. Gastroenterology 2002;122(5):1500–11.
8. Maxion-Bergemann S, Thielecke F, Abel F, et al. Costs of irritable bowel syndrome in the UK and US. Pharmacoeconomics 2006;24(1):21–37.
9. Crowell MD, Harris L, Jones MP, et al. New insights into the pathophysiology of irritable bowel syndrome: implications for future treatments. Curr Gastroenterol Rep 2005;7(4):272–9.
10. Morris-Yates A, Talley NJ, Boyce PM, et al. Evidence of a genetic contribution to functional bowel disorder. Am J Gastroenterol 1998;93(8):1311–7.
11. Ford MJ, Miller PM, Eastwood J, et al. Life events, psychiatric illness and the irritable bowel syndrome. Gut 1987;28(2):160–5.
12. Rodríguez LA, Ruigómez A. Increased risk of irritable bowel syndrome after bacterial gastroenteritis: cohort study. BMJ 1999;318(7183):565–6.
13. Ruigómez A, García Rodríguez LA, Panés J. Risk of irritable bowel syndrome after an episode of bacterial gastroenteritis in general practice: influence of comorbidities. Clin Gastroenterol Hepatol 2007;5(4):465–9.
14. Jones VA, McLaughlan P, Shorthouse M, et al. Food intolerance: a major factor in the pathogenesis of irritable bowel syndrome. Lancet 1982;2(8308):1115–7.
15. Simrén M, Månsson A, Langkilde AM, et al. Food-related gastrointestinal symptoms in the irritable bowel syndrome. Digestion 2001;63(2):108–15.
16. Niec AM, Frankum B, Talley NJ. Are adverse food reactions linked to irritable bowel syndrome? Am J Gastroenterol 1998;93(11):2184–90.

17. Zar S, Benson MJ, Kumar D. Food-specific serum IgG4 and IgE titers to common food antigens in irritable bowel syndrome. Am J Gastroenterol 2005;100(7): 1550–7.
18. Zar S, Mincher L, Benson MJ, et al. Food-specific IgG4 antibody-guided exclusion diet improves symptoms and rectal compliance in irritable bowel syndrome. Scand J Gastroenterol 2005;40(7):800–7.
19. Atkinson W, Sheldon TA, Shaath N, et al. Food elimination based on IgG antibodies in irritable bowel syndrome: a randomised controlled trial. Gut 2004; 53(10):1459–64.
20. Manning AP, Thompson WG, Heaton KW, et al. Towards positive diagnosis of the irritable bowel. Br Med J 1978;2(6138):653–4.
21. Thompson WG, Longstreth GF, Drossman DA, et al. Functional bowel disorders and functional abdominal pain. Gut 1999;45(Suppl 2):II43–7.
22. Drossman DA, Thompson WG, Talley NJ, et al. Identification of subgroups of functional bowel disorders. Gastroenterol Int 1990;3:159–72.
23. Drossman DA. The functional gastrointestinal disorders and the Rome III process. Gastroenterology 2006;130(5):1377–90.
24. Longstreth GF, Thompson WG, Chey WD, et al. Functional bowel disorders. Gastroenterology 2006;130(5):1480–91.
25. Harvey RF, Mauad EC, Brown AM. Prognosis in the irritable bowel syndrome: a 5-year prospective study. Lancet 1987;1(8539):963–5.
26. Whitehead WE, Crowell MD, Bosmajian L, et al. Existence of irritable bowel syndrome supported by factor analysis of symptoms in two community samples. Gastroenterology 1990;98(2):336–40.
27. Heaton KW, O'Donnell LJ, Braddon FE, et al. Symptoms of irritable bowel syndrome in a British urban community: consulters and nonconsulters. Gastroenterology 1992;102(6):1962–7.
28. Frank L, Kleinman L, Rentz A, et al. Health-related quality of life associated with irritable bowel syndrome: comparison with other chronic diseases. Clin Ther 2002;24(4):675–89 [discussion: 674].
29. Koloski NA, Talley NJ, Boyce PM. Predictors of health care seeking for irritable bowel syndrome and nonulcer dyspepsia: a critical review of the literature on symptom and psychosocial factors. Am J Gastroenterol 2001;96(5):1340–9.
30. Smith MJ, Cherian P, Raju GS, et al. Bile acid malabsorption in persistent diarrhoea. J R Coll Physicians Lond 2000;34(5):448–51.
31. Leeds JS, Hopper AD, Sidhu R, et al. Some patients with irritable bowel syndrome may have exocrine pancreatic insufficiency. Clin Gastroenterol Hepatol 2010;8(5):433–8.
32. Sanders DS, Carter MJ, Hurlstone DP, et al. Association of adult coeliac disease with irritable bowel syndrome: a case-control study in patients fulfilling Rome II criteria referred to secondary care. Lancet 2001;358(9292):1504–8.
33. AGA Institute. AGA Institute Medical Position Statement on the Diagnosis and Management of Celiac Disease. Gastroenterology 2006;131(6):1977–80.
34. Davidson LS, Fountain JR. Incidence of the sprue syndrome; with some observations on the natural history. Br Med J 1950;1(4663):1157–61.
35. West J, Logan RF, Hill PG, et al. Seroprevalence, correlates, and characteristics of undetected coeliac disease in England. Gut 2003;52(7):960–5.
36. Ludvigsson JF, Leffler DA, Bai JC, et al. The Oslo definitions for coeliac disease and related terms. Gut 2012, in press.
37. Zipser RD, Patel S, Yahya KZ, et al. Presentations of adult celiac disease in a nationwide patient support group. Dig Dis Sci 2003;48(4):761–4.

38. Corazza GR, Valentini RA, Andreani ML, et al. Subclinical coeliac disease is a frequent cause of iron-deficiency anaemia. Scand J Gastroenterol 1995; 30(2):153–6.
39. Kemppainen T, Kröger H, Janatuinen E, et al. Osteoporosis in adult patients with celiac disease. Bone 1999;24(3):249–55.
40. Hadjivassiliou M, Gibson A, Davies-Jones GA, et al. Does cryptic gluten sensitivity play a part in neurological illness? Lancet 1996;347(8998):369–71.
41. Frissora CL, Koch KL. Symptom overlap and comorbidity of irritable bowel syndrome with other conditions. Curr Gastroenterol Rep 2005;7(4):264–71.
42. West J, Logan RF, Smith CJ, et al. Malignancy and mortality in people with coeliac disease: population based cohort study. BMJ 2004;329(7468):716–9.
43. Corrao G, Corazza GR, Bagnardi V, et al. Mortality in patients with coeliac disease and their relatives: a cohort study. Lancet 2001;358(9279):356–61.
44. Tau C, Mautalen C, De Rosa S, et al. Bone mineral density in children with celiac disease. Effect of a gluten-free diet. Eur J Clin Nutr 2006;60(3):358–63.
45. Dewar DH, Ciclitira PJ. Clinical features and diagnosis of celiac disease. Gastroenterology 2005;128(4 Suppl 1):S19–24.
46. Green PH, Fleischauer AT, Bhagat G, et al. Risk of malignancy in patients with celiac disease. Am J Med 2003;115(3):191–5.
47. Zarkadas M, Cranney A, Case S, et al. The impact of a gluten-free diet on adults with coeliac disease: results of a national survey. J Hum Nutr Diet 2006;19(1):41–9.
48. Mustalahti K, Lohiniemi S, Collin P, et al. Gluten-free diet and quality of life in patients with screen-detected celiac disease. Eff Clin Pract 2002;5(3):105–13.
49. Revised criteria for diagnosis of coeliac disease. Report of Working Group of European Society of Paediatric Gastroenterology and Nutrition. Arch Dis Child 1990;65(8):909–11.
50. Hadjivassiliou M, Grünewald RA, Davies-Jones GA. Gluten sensitivity as a neurological illness. J Neurol Neurosurg Psychiatry 2002;72(5):560–3.
51. Sollid LM, Markussen G, Ek J, et al. Evidence for a primary association of celiac disease to a particular HLA-DQ alpha/beta heterodimer. J Exp Med 1989; 169(1):345–50.
52. Murdock AM, Johnston SD. Diagnostic criteria for coeliac disease: time for change? Eur J Gastroenterol Hepatol 2005;17(1):41–3.
53. Coeliac disease: recognition and assessment of coeliac disease. London: National Institute for Health and Clinical Excellence; 2009. Available at: http://www.nice.org.uk/CG86.
54. Sanders DS, Patel D, Stephenson TJ, et al. A primary care cross-sectional study of undiagnosed adult coeliac disease. Eur J Gastroenterol Hepatol 2003;15(4):407–13.
55. Hin H, Bird G, Fisher P, et al. Coeliac disease in primary care: case finding study. BMJ 1999;318(7177):164–7.
56. Agréus L, Svärdsudd K, Tibblin G, et al. Endomysium antibodies are superior to gliadin antibodies in screening for coeliac disease in patients presenting supposed functional gastrointestinal symptoms. Scand J Prim Health Care 2000;18(2):105–10.
57. Holt R, Darnley S, Kennedy T, et al. Screening for coeliac disease in patients with a clinical diagnosis of irritable syndrome. Gastroenterology 2001;120(Suppl 1): A757 [abstract 4064].
58. Locke GR, Murray JA, Zinsmeister AR, et al. Celiac disease serology in irritable bowel syndrome and dyspepsia: a population-based case-control study. Mayo Clin Proc 2004;79(4):476–82.

59. Kennedy TM, Chalder T, McCrone P, et al. Cognitive behavioural therapy in addition to antispasmodic therapy for irritable bowel syndrome in primary care: randomised controlled trial. Health Technol Assess 2006;10(19):iii–iv, ix–x, 1–67.

60. Catassi C, Kryszak D, Louis-Jacques O, et al. Detection of celiac disease in primary care: a multicenter case-finding study in North America. Am J Gastroenterol 2007;102(7):1454–60.

61. Demarchi B, Astegiano M, Sapone N, et al. Prevalence of coeliac disease in IBS patients in Turin [abstract]. Gastroenterology 2002;122(Suppl 4):A193.

62. Shahbazkhani B, Forootan M, Merat S, et al. Coeliac disease presenting with symptoms of irritable bowel syndrome. Aliment Pharmacol Ther 2003;18(2):231–5.

63. van der Wouden EJ, Nelis GF, Vecht J. Screening for coeliac disease in patients fulfilling the Rome II criteria for irritable bowel syndrome in a secondary care hospital in The Netherlands: a prospective observational study. Gut 2007; 56(3):444–5.

64. Ozdil K, Sokmen M, Ersoy O, et al. Association of gluten enteropathy and irritable bowel syndrome in adult Turkish population. Dig Dis Sci 2008;53(7): 1852–5.

65. Jadallah KA, Khader YS. Celiac disease in patients with presumed irritable bowel syndrome: a case-finding study. World J Gastroenterol 2009;15(42):5321–5.

66. Zwolińska-Wcisło M, Galicka-Latała D, Rozpondek P, et al. Frequency of celiac disease and irritable bowel syndrome coexistence and its influence on the disease course. Przegl Lek 2009;66(3):126–9 [in Polish].

67. Korkut E, Bektas M, Oztas E, et al. The prevalence of celiac disease in patients fulfilling Rome III criteria for irritable bowel syndrome. Eur J Intern Med 2010; 21(5):389–92.

68. El-Salhy M, Lomholt-Beck B, Gundersen D. The prevalence of celiac disease in patients with irritable bowel syndrome. Mol Med Report 2011;4(3):403–5.

69. Cash BD, Rubenstein JH, Young PE, et al. The prevalence of celiac disease among patients with nonconstipated irritable bowel syndrome is similar to controls. Gastroenterology 2011;141(4):1187–93.

70. Ford AC, Chey WD, Talley NJ, et al. Yield of diagnostic tests for celiac disease in individuals with symptoms suggestive of irritable bowel syndrome: systematic review and meta-analysis. Arch Intern Med 2009;169(7):651–8.

71. Spiller R, Aziz Q, Creed F, et al. Guidelines on the irritable bowel syndrome: mechanisms and practical management. Gut 2007;56(12):1770–98.

72. American College of Gastroenterology Functional Gastrointestinal Disorders Task Force. Evidence-based position statement on the management of irritable bowel syndrome in North America. Am J Gastroenterol 2002;97(Suppl 11):S1–5.

73. Harvey RF, Salih SY, Read AE. Organic and functional disorders in 2000 gastroenterology outpatients. Lancet 1983;1(8325):632–4.

74. Fasano A, Berti I, Gerarduzzi T, et al. Prevalence of celiac disease in at-risk and not-at-risk groups in the United States: a large multicenter study. Arch Intern Med 2003;163(3):286–92.

75. Sanders DS, Hopper AD, Azmy IA, et al. Association of adult celiac disease with surgical abdominal pain: a case-control study in patients referred to secondary care. Ann Surg 2005;242(2):201–7.

76. O'Leary C, Wieneke P, Buckley S, et al. Celiac disease and irritable bowel-type symptoms. Am J Gastroenterol 2002;97(6):1463–7.

77. Barratt SM, Leeds JS, Robinson K, et al. Reflux and irritable bowel syndrome are negative predictors of quality of life in coeliac disease and inflammatory bowel disease. Eur J Gastroenterol Hepatol 2011;23(2):159–65.

78. Häuser W, Musial F, Caspary WF, et al. Predictors of irritable bowel-type symptoms and healthcare-seeking behavior among adults with celiac disease. Psychosom Med 2007;69(4):370–6.
79. Hadjivassiliou M, Williamson CA, Woodroofe N. The immunology of gluten sensitivity: beyond the gut. Trends Immunol 2004;25(11):578–82.
80. Rostami K, Villanacci V. Microscopic enteritis: novel prospect in coeliac disease clinical and immuno-histogenesis. Evolution in diagnostic and treatment strategies. Dig Liver Dis 2009;41(4):245–52.
81. Kaukinen K, Turjanmaa K, Mäki M, et al. Intolerance to cereals is not specific for coeliac disease. Scand J Gastroenterol 2000;35(9):942–6.
82. Sapone A, Bai JC, Ciacci C, et al. Spectrum of gluten-related disorders: consensus on new nomenclature and classification. BMC Med 2012;10(1):13.
83. Ford RP. The gluten syndrome: a neurological disease. Med Hypotheses 2009; 73(3):438–40.
84. Elder JH, Shankar M, Shuster J, et al. The gluten-free, casein-free diet in autism: results of a preliminary double blind clinical trial. J Autism Dev Disord 2006; 36(3):413–20.
85. Dickerson F, Stallings C, Origoni A, et al. Markers of gluten sensitivity and celiac disease in recent-onset psychosis and multi-episode schizophrenia. Biol Psychiatry 2010;68(1):100–4.
86. Hadjivassiliou M, Chattopadhyay AK, Grünewald RA, et al. Myopathy associated with gluten sensitivity. Muscle Nerve 2007;35(4):443–50.
87. Verdu EF, Armstrong D, Murray JA. Between celiac disease and irritable bowel syndrome: the "no man's land" of gluten sensitivity. Am J Gastroenterol 2009; 104(6):1587–94.
88. Sapone A, Lammers KM, Mazzarella G, et al. Differential mucosal IL-17 expression in two gliadin-induced disorders: gluten sensitivity and the autoimmune enteropathy celiac disease. Int Arch Allergy Immunol 2010;152(1):75–80.
89. Bizzaro N, Tozzoli R, Villalta D, et al. Cutting-edge issues in celiac disease and in gluten intolerance. Clin Rev Allergy Immunol 2012;42(3):279–87.
90. Volta U, Tovoli F, Cicola R, et al. Serological tests in gluten sensitivity (nonceliac gluten intolerance). J Clin Gastroenterol 2012;46(8):680–5.
91. Sapone A, Lammers KM, Casolaro V, et al. Divergence of gut permeability and mucosal immune gene expression in two gluten-associated conditions: celiac disease and gluten sensitivity. BMC Med 2011;9:23.
92. Bernardo D, Garrote JA, Fernández-Salazar L, et al. Is gliadin really safe for non-coeliac individuals? Production of interleukin 15 in biopsy culture from non-coeliac individuals challenged with gliadin peptides. Gut 2007;56(6): 889–90.
93. Di Sabatino A, Ciccocioppo R, Cupelli F, et al. Epithelium derived interleukin 15 regulates intraepithelial lymphocyte Th1 cytokine production, cytotoxicity, and survival in coeliac disease. Gut 2006;55(4):469–77.
94. Bernardo D, Garrote JA, Allegretti Y, et al. Higher constitutive IL15R alpha expression and lower IL-15 response threshold in coeliac disease patients. Clin Exp Immunol 2008;154(1):64–73.
95. Bernardo D, Garrote JA, Arranz E. Are non-celiac disease gluten-intolerant patients innate immunity responders to gluten? Am J Gastroenterol 2011; 106(12):2201 [author reply: 2201–2].
96. Anderson LA, McMillan SA, Watson RG, et al. Malignancy and mortality in a population-based cohort of patients with coeliac disease or "gluten sensitivity". World J Gastroenterol 2007;13(1):146–51.

97. Carroccio A, Vitale G, Di Prima L, et al. Comparison of anti-transglutaminase ELISAs and an anti-endomysial antibody assay in the diagnosis of celiac disease: a prospective study. Clin Chem 2002;48(9):1546–50.

98. Ball AJ, Hadjivassiliou M, Sanders DS. Is gluten sensitivity a "No Man's Land" or a "Fertile Crescent" for research? Am J Gastroenterol 2010;105(1):222–3 [author reply: 223–4].

99. Wahnschaffe U, Ullrich R, Riecken EO, et al. Celiac disease-like abnormalities in a subgroup of patients with irritable bowel syndrome. Gastroenterology 2001; 121(6):1329–38.

100. Wahnschaffe U, Schulzke JD, Zeitz M, et al. Predictors of clinical response to gluten-free diet in patients diagnosed with diarrhea-predominant irritable bowel syndrome. Clin Gastroenterol Hepatol 2007;5(7):844–50 [quiz: 769].

101. Aziz I, Evans KE, Hopper AD, et al. A prospective study into the aetiology of lymphocytic duodenosis. Aliment Pharmacol Ther 2010;32(11–12):1392–7.

102. Biesiekierski JR, Newnham ED, Irving PM, et al. Gluten causes gastrointestinal symptoms in subjects without celiac disease: a double-blind randomized placebo-controlled trial. Am J Gastroenterol 2011;106(3):508–14 [quiz: 515].

103. Catassi C, Fasano A. Celiac disease. Curr Opin Gastroenterol 2008;24(6): 687–91.

104. Catassi C, Fabiani E, Iacono G, et al. A prospective, double-blind, placebo-controlled trial to establish a safe gluten threshold for patients with celiac disease. Am J Clin Nutr 2007;85(1):160–6.

Pathophysiology of Celiac Disease

Sonia S. Kupfer, MD[a,b,*], Bana Jabri, MD, PhD[a,b]

KEYWORDS

- Celiac disease • HLA-DQ2 and HLA-DQ8 • Single-nucleotide polymorphisms
- Intestinal microbiome • Gluten • Deamidation • Adaptive and innate immunity

KEY POINTS

- Celiac disease results from the interplay of genetic, environmental, and immunologic factors.
- HLA-DQ2 and HLA-DQ8 are the strongest and best-characterized genetic susceptibility factors in celiac disease, although recent genome-wide association studies have identified additional susceptibility variants, many involved in the immune system and overlapping with other immune-mediated disease.
- Environmental factors implicated in disease pathogenesis include gluten, commensal and pathogenic microorganisms, timing of gluten introduction, mode of delivery, and duration of breastfeeding; however, the mechanisms underlying these associations are incompletely understood.
- Both the adaptive and innate immune systems are dysregulated in the pathophysiology of celiac disease.
- Improved understanding of the pathophysiology of celiac disease will help uncover new potential therapeutic targets and provide insight into disease mechanisms relevant to other immune-mediated disease such as type 1 diabetes.

INTRODUCTION

Celiac disease is an intestinal inflammatory disease that is triggered by dietary gluten, a protein found in wheat, barley, and rye, in genetically susceptible individuals.[1] Descriptions of a celiac disease–like phenotype can be traced back to the Greek physician Aretaeus in the first and second century AD (reviewed in Ref.[2]). Gluten was identified as the culprit of celiac disease by Dutch physicians who observed that, during the 1944-1945 famine when wheat and rye were scarce, celiac children symptomatically improved.[3] Subsequent studies characterized many features of celiac disease, and while disease pathogenesis and pathophysiology remain incompletely

[a] University of Chicago Celiac Disease Center, Chicago, IL, USA; [b] Section of Gastroenterology, Hepatology and Nutrition, Department of Medicine, University of Chicago Medicine, 900 East 57th Street, MB#9, Chicago, IL 60637, USA
* Corresponding author.
E-mail address: skupfer@medicine.bsd.uchicago.edu

Gastrointest Endoscopy Clin N Am 22 (2012) 639–660
http://dx.doi.org/10.1016/j.giec.2012.07.003
1052-5157/12/$ – see front matter © 2012 Elsevier Inc. All rights reserved.

understood, the disease is thought to arise from the interplay of genetic, environmental, and immunologic factors (**Fig. 1**). An understanding of the pathophysiology of celiac disease, in which the trigger (wheat, rye, and barley) is known, will undoubtedly reveal basic mechanisms that underlie other autoimmune diseases (eg, type 1 diabetes) that share many common pathogenic perturbations. This review describes seminal findings in each of the 3 domains of the pathogenesis of celiac disease, namely genetics, environmental triggers, and immune dysregulation, with a focus on newer areas of investigation such as non–human leukocyte antigen (HLA) genetic variants, the intestinal microbiome, and the role of the innate immune system.

GENETICS

Celiac disease has a strong hereditary component. Epidemiologic studies show that up to 20% of first-degree relatives are affected by the disease,[4] with concordance rates of 75% to 80% in monozygotic twins and 10% in dizygotic twins.[5] The strongest and best-characterized genetic susceptibility factors in celiac disease are the HLA class II genes known as HLA-DQ2 and HLA-DQ8, molecules responsible for presentation of antigens to immune cells. However, although HLA-DQ2 or -DQ8 are necessary for disease to develop, they are not sufficient thus implicating other genetic or environmental factors in disease development. Approximately 25% to 30% of individuals of European descent carry HLA-DQ2 susceptibility, but only about 4% of these individuals will develop celiac disease in their lifetime,[6] underscoring the role of additional factors. Recent large-scale genetics studies known as genome-wide association studies (GWAS) have identified several common non-HLA genetic factors (many in genes involved in immunity) associated with celiac disease which, on their own, contribute a small amount to overall risk but have great potential in discovering important and novel pathways involved in disease pathogenesis.

HLA-DQ2 and HLA-DQ8 Genetics and Disease Risk

HLA is the name of the major histocompatibility complex (MHC) in humans.[7] These genes reside on chromosome 6 and are divided into 3 classes (I–III) (**Fig. 2**). HLA-DQ

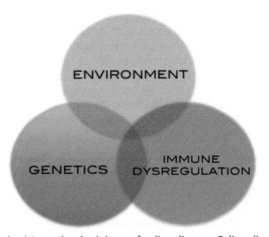

Fig. 1. Factors involved in pathophysiology of celiac disease. Celiac disease is thought to arise from the interplay of genetic, environmental, and immunologic factors. This review highlights seminal findings in each of these domains.

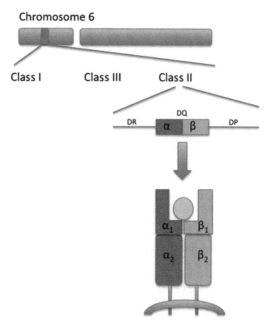

Fig. 2. Class II HLA-DQ. The genes encoding for HLA molecules are found in the major histocompatibility (MHC) complex on chromosome 6. HLA molecules involved in celiac disease are encoded in a region known as class II; by genes known as -DQ (other class II genes include -DR and -DP). Class II HLA-DQ genes encode for α and β chains that are associated as heterodimers on the surface of antigen-presenting cells and that form a cleft that binds antigens. HLA-DQA1 genes code for 2 α chains (α_1 and α_2) and HLA-DQB1 genes code for 2 β chains (β_1 and β_2).

is a class II molecule on chromosome 6p21.3 responsible for presentation of peptides from outside cells (compared with class I molecules that present peptides from within cells and class III molecules that encode complement proteins). HLA-DQ is composed of an $\alpha\beta$ heterodimer encoded by HLA-DQA1 and HLA-DQB1 genes, respectively. The $\alpha\beta$ heterodimer is a cell-surface receptor located on antigen-presenting cells (APCs).

The genetics of celiac disease is complex because the number, type, and configuration of the DQA1 and DQB1 alleles determine disease risk. Current World Health Organization nomenclature is HLA followed by a hyphen followed by the gene (eg, DQA1, DQB1, and so forth), an asterisk (separator), allele group (field 1), colon (field separator), and protein (field 2),[8] for example, HLA-DQB1*02:01 refers to the HLA gene DQB1, allele group 02 and protein 01. The isoform encoded by a specific combination of DQA1 and DQB1 genes can be expressed as HLAx.y, where x refers to DQB1 and y to DQA1. For example, DQ2.5 is the protein encoded by DQB1*02 and DQA1*05 inherited in either *cis* (on the same chromosome) or *trans* (on different chromosomes). When these alleles are located on the same chromosome (ie, in *cis*), they are often inherited in a haplotype with another class II molecule, DRB1*03 (DR3).

Fig. 3A and B highlights HLA configurations associated with celiac disease. The highest risk group are those that carry DQB1*02 on both chromosomes (ie, homozygotes), known as the gene dose effect.[4,5] DQB1*02 homozygosity (carrying 2 DQB1*02 alleles) has an estimated prevalence of 2% in the population but represents 25% of all celiac patients, because of an estimated 5-fold increased risk of celiac

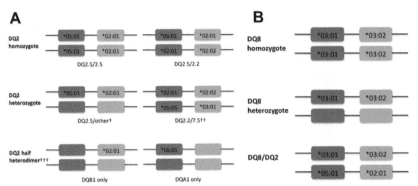

Fig. 3. HLA configurations in celiac disease. (*A*) HLA-DQ2 homozygotes, heterozygotes and half-heterodimers, and (*B*) HLA-DQ8 homozygotes, heterozygotes and DQ8/DQ2. Red boxes denote the DQA1 gene encoding the alpha-chain and orange boxes denote the DQB1 gene encoding the beta-chain (see **Fig. 2**). Shown in the boxes are the specific alleles for each gene. Current WHO nomenclatures uses an asterix followed by the allele group (eg, 05), a colon then the protein group (eg, 01). An empty box refers to other HLA alleles not associated with celiac disease. Shown below the genes are the isoforms. † cis acting (ie, on the same chromosome); †† trans acting (ie, on opposite chromosomes); ††† risk of celiac disease for DQ2 half heterodimers is lower than the general population especially individuals carrying only DQA1*05.[15]

disease in comparison with heterozygotes (carrying 1 DQB1*02 allele).[6,9] Studies have shown that the CD4+ helper T-cell response from DQB1*02 homozygous individuals is stronger than the response from heterozygous individuals.[4,10] Moreover, DQB1*02 homozygosity may be associated with younger age of onset[11,12] and a more complicated clinical course, including refractory sprue.[13] DQ2.5 (DQB1*02/DQA1*05) heterozygotes are the most common HLA configurations, and represent up to 50% of the HLA types found in celiac disease patients.[9] While DQ2.2 (DQB1*02/DQA1*02) is highly homologous to DQ2.5, it alone carries little risk of celiac disease because of the decreased stability of bound peptides.[14]

A small minority of celiac patients carries only 1 of the alleles of the risk HLA-DQ2 heterodimer: HLA-DQA1*05 (05:01 or 05:05) or HLA-DQB1*02 (02:01 or 02:02); this is called the half-heterodimer. The European Genetic Cluster on Celiac Disease typed more than 1000 celiac patients and found that 6% carried neither HLA-DQ2 nor HLA-DQ8. Of these patients, 93% (57/61) carried the DQ2.5 half-heterodimer with almost three-quarters carrying only the DQB1*02 allele.[15] The prevalence of individuals carrying only 1 copy of DQB1*02 was increased in celiac patients compared with controls, while the prevalence of those carrying only 1 DQA1*05 was higher in controls than in patients, indicating a negative association for the DQA1*05 half-heterodimer.[9]

DQ8 is a heterodimer composed of α chains encoded by DQA1*03:01 and β chains encoded by DQB1*03:02. When they are inherited on the same chromosome, they are found on a haplotype with DRB1*04 notated as DR4-DQ8. The prevalence of HLA-DQ8 in the general population varies geographically, with higher rates in individuals from the Middle East and South America.[16] In celiac disease overall, HLA-DQ8 is found in 5% to 10% of patients.[9,15] As with DQ2, the risk of disease with HLA-DQ8 follows a gradient. The highest risk appears to be in individuals who inherit DQ8 and DQ2, although the overall prevalence of carrying both DQ8 and DQ2 is low, at 2.5%.[9] In individuals with HLA-DQ8 and DQ2.2 or DQ2.5 the risk is estimated at 1:24, whereas in those with

HLA-DQ8 but not DQ2.2 or DQ2.5 the risk is estimated at 1:89.[9] DQ8 homozygosity confers increased risk in comparison with DQ8 heterozygotes.[17]

Development of celiac disease in individuals who are HLA-DQ2 and HLA-DQ8 negative is extremely rare. In a large European collaborative study, only 4 of 1008 patients (0.4%) fulfilled criteria for celiac disease but did not carry DQ2 (including half-heterodimer) or DQ8.[15] No other class I or II associations were identified in this small group. In support of these findings, 2 additional studies in the United States and Italy found the prevalence of DQ2/8 negativity in celiac disease to range from 0.16% to 0.9%.[9,17] Therefore in a very small group of patients, if clinical suspicion is high with supporting serologic and histologic findings, celiac disease can be diagnosed in the absence HLA-DQ2 or HLA-DQ8. However, the overall risk of celiac disease in individuals who do not carry DQ2 or DQ8 is very low. These findings support the use of HLA testing for its high negative predictive value (**Fig. 4**).

HLA Peptide Binding

HLA-DQ2 and HLA-DQ8 play a key role in celiac disease owing to their physiochemical properties and binding of specific peptides deamidated by tissue transglutaminase 2 (tTG2). Both HLA-DQ2 and HLA-DQ8 contain positively charged pockets with a preference for binding negatively charged particles. Specifically, in DQ2, the

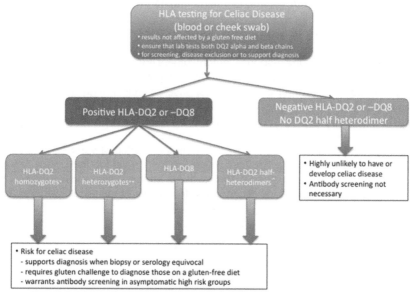

*HLA-DQ2 homozygotes carry either DQ2.5/2.5 or DQ2.5/2.2
**HLA-DQ2 heterozygotes carry either DQ2.5/other allele or DQ2.2/7.5
^HLA-DQ2 half-heterodimers carry either an alpha chain (DQA1*05) or a beta chain (DQB1*02) but no other susceptibility alleles; Risk to develop celiac disease *much lower* than with other susceptibility alleles

Fig. 4. Clinical application of HLA testing. HLA testing should be considered for screening or disease exclusion, or to support a diagnosis. Testing is unaffected by a gluten-free diet. Providers should ensure that both DQ2 α and β chains are tested. If a patient carries HLA-DQ2 or -DQ8, they carry a risk factor (or varying magnitude) for celiac disease, and additional workup should be considered. Individuals carrying HLA-DQ2 half-heterodimers are also at risk for celiac disease (albeit substantially lower than other HLA-DQ2 and HLA-DQ8 positive patients). If HLA-DQ2 and -DQ8 are not present, then celiac disease risk is highly unlikely and antibody screening is not necessary.

lysine position at β71 has a preference for binding negatively charged residues at positions P4, P6, and P7 (**Fig. 5**).[18] The DQ8 β57 polymorphism creates a basic environment with a preference for binding the negatively charged residue at P9 (see **Fig. 5**).[19]

In celiac disease, these HLA molecules on APCs present gluten peptides to CD4[+] T cells, thereby activating them.[20,21] The size of the peptide fragment defines stimulatory activity, with larger fragments showing increased CD4[+] T-cell stimulation compared with smaller fragments.[22–26] While deamidation favors binding to HLA-DQ2 or HLA-DQ8,[14] studies have suggested that it is not an absolute requirement for stimulation of CD4[+] T cells, especially in the case of HLA-DQ8.[19,27] The mechanism for recognition of native peptides is that the polymorphism at position β57 allows DQ8 to switch from an interaction with a negatively charged residue in the T cell receptor (TCR) to one in the peptide.[19]

Non-HLA Genetic Susceptibility Factors and Role in Disease Pathogenesis

HLA is the best-characterized genetic susceptibility factor in celiac disease, but does not account for all disease heritability, suggesting that additional genetic factors play a role. GWAS have identified several candidate genetic susceptibility factors in celiac disease. The results of GWAS shed light on new genes and genetic pathways involved in disease pathogenesis. The immediate challenge is to identify variants within these regions that are functionally important, to elucidate their role in celiac disease pathogenesis. To date, non-HLA genetic loci harboring 115 genes have been associated with celiac disease using GWAS.[28–31] Of these genes, 28 are immune related, which can be broadly grouped into categories based on function and pathways (reviewed in Refs.[32,33]). Enrichment analysis indicates that these genes are broadly involved in adaptive and innate immune response, among others (**Fig. 6**). Taken as a whole, these results underscore the importance of immune dysregulation in celiac disease by confirming the role of the adaptive immune response as well as highlighting pathways involved in innate immune response. Post-GWAS studies will need to focus on elucidating the functional basis of these genetic variants, in particular the role of regulatory variation.

An intriguing finding to emerge from GWAS is the overlap of variants identified in several diseases and traits, including several immune-related diseases. Common loci have been identified with type 1 diabetes, rheumatoid arthritis, and Crohn disease, suggesting common genetic backgrounds for these immune-related diseases.

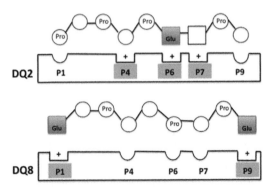

Fig. 5. MHC class II–gluten peptide complexes. MHC class II molecules HLA-DQ2 and -DQ8 preferentially bind a glutamate residue of the gluten peptide at position 6 and position 1/9, respectively. This binding is enhanced by a negatively charged glutamate and positively charged pocket of the HLA molecule.

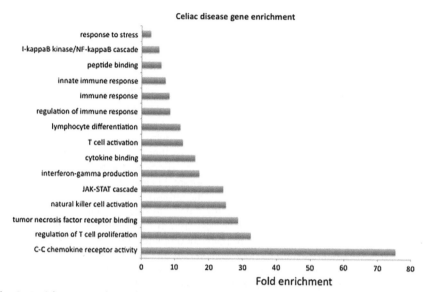

Fig. 6. Enrichment analysis of non-HLA genes associated with celiac disease. GeneTrail was used to test for enrichment of functional annotations among non-HLA genes associated with celiac disease from genome-wide association studies published through 2012. The graph shows the fold enrichment (x-axis) and significantly enriched biological functions (y-axis). Background expectations were based on all human genes. P values were calculated using a hypergeometric distribution using the approach by Backes C et al[143] to control the false discovery rate. P values for enrichment shown here ranged from 4.8×10^{-2} to 3.2×10^{-11}.

However, non-HLA loci in celiac disease are estimated to account for a small portion of overall genetic risk. The reason for "missing heritability" is still under investigation, and could be explained by the contribution of highly penetrant genetic variants with lower allele frequencies than those studied in GWAS. These rare variants may have greater impact on disease susceptibility than common variants discovered to date and, as large-scale sequencing studies are completed, the role played by rare genetic variants in the pathogenesis of celiac disease will become clear. Moreover, the role of gene-gene and gene-environment interactions needs to be explored further in celiac disease.

ENVIRONMENT

Environmental factors clearly play an important role in celiac disease pathogenesis. The primary trigger in the disease is gluten, and over the past decade many studies have contributed to our understanding of gluten biochemistry and antigenic epitopes, transport through the small intestinal epithelium, modification by tTG, and binding to APCs in the lamina propria with subsequent activation of adaptive immunity. Moreover, it has become clear that gluten is associated with innate immune responses in the gut epithelium and that cytotoxic intraepithelial lymphocytes appear to play a central role. In addition, emerging data implicate microbiota (both commensal and pathogenic) in disease pathogenesis, while epidemiologic studies have suggested that early (and possibly late) gluten introduction to children, cesarean-section delivery, and lack of breastfeeding are important risk factors in the development of celiac disease.

Gluten and Epithelial Transport of Peptide Fragments

Wheat, rye, and barley belong to the same tribe called Triticeae, which diverged from oats belonging to the Aveneae tribe (**Fig. 7**). Although "gluten" is used as the general term to describe the trigger of celiac disease, gluten technically refers to the disease-activating peptides found only in wheat. Gluten comprises 2 different protein types, gliadins and glutenins, capable of triggering disease.[34–36] The peptides in barley and rye, hordeins and secalins respectively, are also capable of activating disease.[37] By contrast, oats, comprising more distantly related peptides called avenins, rarely trigger celiac disease.[38] Gliadins, glutenins, hordein, and secalins contain high contents of prolines and glutamines, which makes them resistant to degradation by gastric acid, pancreatic, and brush-border enzymes because these are lacking in prolyl endopeptidase activity.[39,40] There is ongoing interest in leveraging certain bacterial or fungal endopeptidase activities as a therapeutic strategy.[39–42]

Transport of peptide fragments across the small intestinal epithelium and intestinal permeability have been areas of intense research in celiac disease, although their primary role in disease pathogenesis remains incompletely understood. Peptide fragments that have been resistant to degradation can be transported across the epithelium primarily by transcellular pathways (reviewed in Ref.[43]). Tight junctions play a role in peptide transport, and GWAS in celiac disease have found susceptibility single-nucleotide polymorphisms in tight junction–associated genes.[29,44,45]

However, it is unclear whether altered intestinal permeability is a primary cause or a consequence of intestinal inflammation. Moreover, the role of tight-junction blockade as a therapeutic strategy has been studied using prehaptoglobin-2, an analogue of the zonula occludens toxin.[46–48] However, this study did not directly measure intestinal permeability, therefore the mechanism of action remains unclear. An alternative mechanism of transcellular transport of gliadin involves abnormal retrotransport of immunoglobulin A (IgA)-gliadin by the CD71 receptor.[49] CD71, a transferrin receptor, was shown to be upregulated and apically expressed in active celiac disease, leading to escape of gliadin degradation and translocation to the lamina propria, known as the "Trojan horse" phenomenon.[49] Further study is required to determine the role of peptide fragment transport and intestinal permeability in pathogenesis.

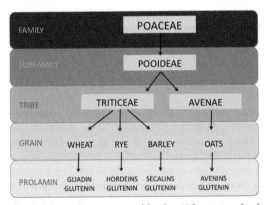

Fig. 7. Divergence of oats from wheat, rye, and barley. Wheat, rye, barley, and oats belong to the same grain family (Poaceae) and subfamily (Pooideae). However, they belong to distinct tribes: wheat, rye, and barley (Triticeae), and oats (Avenae). The prolamins from the Triticeae tribe are immunogenic and contribute to celiac disease, whereas avenins from pure, uncontaminated oats are safe for the vast majority of celiac patients.

Microbiota

An emerging field of investigation is the role of the human microbiome in human health and disease.[50] The human intestine harbors a vast number and variety of commensal microorganisms that are complex and dynamic (reviewed in Ref.[51]). In the past 5 years there have been important technological developments in high-throughput sequencing that have enabled investigators to characterize the human microbiome using culture-free methods known as metagenomics.[52] Although an individual's microbiome is unique, there is evidence of sharing among family members.[53] The microbiome is influenced by diet,[54] and the interplay between diet and the microbiome affects metabolic function.[55] There are important interactions between the gut microbiome, diet, and the immune system that appear to contribute to phenotypes such as obesity,[53] inflammatory bowel disease,[56] and celiac disease.

Studies of the gut microbiome in celiac disease are still in their early stages and have yielded conflicting results, likely due to different experimental approaches on fecal or biopsy samples in various patient populations from different countries. All of these factors can bias microbiome results. In 2004, a study identified rod-shaped bacteria in intestinal biopsies of celiac patients, suggesting a role for the microbiome in celiac disease.[57] Further studies analyzed samples for metabolic readouts of the gut microbiome (eg, short-chain fatty acid and volatile compounds) in celiac patients[58,59] as well as first-degree relatives of celiac patients,[60] and found significant differences when compared with controls. Additional studies using various methodologies found differences in fecal and/or mucosal-associated composition primarily of *Bacteroides, Clostridium, Bifidobacterium, Lactobacillus, Escherichia coli*, and *Staphylococcus*[59,61–65] between celiac patients (both untreated and treated) and controls. Differences in microbial composition were also found between adults and children with celiac disease.[66] However, other studies have failed to find differences in the microbiome among cases and controls.[67] A recent article hypothesized that the intestinal microbiome as a whole determines the switch from tolerance to immune response in genetically susceptible infants, and found a lack of Bacteroidetes and an increased abundance of Firmicutes in a longitudinal study of at-risk infants followed from birth to 24 months.[68] Further studies using combined genomic approaches are needed to clarify the role of the microbiome in celiac disease.

Consistent with the role of diet in modulating the gut microbiome, the gluten-free diet alone in healthy individuals led to decreases in *Bifidobacterium* and *Lactobacillus*.[69] Moreover, animal and human studies suggest possible interactions between commensal bacteria and immune responses in celiac disease.[70,71] Animal studies have suggested that the microbiome in celiac disease might alter intestinal permeability, thereby contributing to disease pathogenesis.[72] To date, probiotic studies in celiac disease investigated the proteolytic activity of VSL#3 or sourdough lactobacilli,[42,73] but none has studied the role in modulating commensal flora, although there are data for the therapeutic effect of probiotics in irritable bowel syndrome.[74] Animal and human studies in this area are ongoing.

Despite technological advances in studying the human intestinal microbiome, many questions remain to be answered about the role of commensal bacteria in immune-mediated gastrointestinal diseases such as celiac disease or inflammatory bowel diseases (reviewed in Ref.[75]). First, and perhaps most important, among these is whether the intestinal microbiota is a cause or a consequence of intestinal inflammation. There is evidence to support both sides, and additional studies are needed to elucidate cause and effect. Moreover, there is interest in how microbial alterations could be used for therapeutic interventions, although clinical trials are lacking in celiac disease. There are questions about how diet affects and alters intestinal microbiota as well as on the effect of different microbes on immune function. Finally the role of commensal fungi and viruses has not been studied in celiac disease.

Other Environmental Risk Factors

Besides the commensal microbiome, several other factors including childhood infections (notably rotavirus), mode of delivery, gluten introduction to infants, and breastfeeding have been studied in celiac disease. The data on these factors stems primarily from epidemiologic and ecological studies, and their role in disease pathogenesis remains to be fully elucidated.

The role of pathogenic organisms in celiac disease had been suggested in the 1980s when Kagnoff and colleagues[76] described a 12-amino-acid sequence homology between A-gliadin and the E1b protein from human adenovirus type 12, and that celiac patients had a significantly higher rate of previous adenovirus type 12 infection compared with controls.[77] It was hypothesized that there may be immunologic crossreactivity between antigenic elements shared by viruses and α-gliadin.[78] However, follow-up studies are inconsistent in their findings regarding adenovirus type 12 and celiac disease.[79–81] The finding of a seasonal pattern of higher rates of summer births in children with celiac disease also suggests a role for infectious agents.[82] More recent studies implicate rotavirus in the pathogenesis of celiac disease. Stene and colleagues[83] prospectively followed children with HLA risk and determined that frequent rotavirus infections (as measured by rotavirus antibody titers) showed a moderate, but statistically significant increased risk of celiac disease. Zanoni and colleagues[84] used a peptide-library approach with sera of active celiac patients, and found an autoantigen peptide to recognize rotavirus serotype 1 major neutralizing protein VP7 as well as HSP60, desmoglein 1, and toll-like receptor 4 (TLR4). Antipeptide antibodies altered intestinal permeability and activated monocytes via TLR4 signaling, suggesting a role of innate immunity and viral infection in disease pathogenesis.

Mode of delivery has also been studied as a possible risk factor for celiac disease, perhaps because of altered exposure to commensal bacteria in the perinatal period. Though not confirmed in all studies,[85] cesarean section, particularly performed electively, is associated with a modest increased risk of later celiac disease.[86,87] Intriguingly a recent study found that children born vaginally have microbiota in various tissues that resemble their mother's vaginal flora including *Lactobacillus*, *Prevotella*, and *Sneathia* spp., whereas children born by cesarean section harbored flora resembling skin bacterial communities such as *Staphylococcus*, *Corynebacterium*, and *Propionibacterium* spp.[88] Additional work is needed to correlate neonatal bacterial colonization with future risk of celiac disease.

The effect of timing of gluten introduction on the risk of celiac disease came to the forefront with the Swedish celiac "epidemic" in the 1980s and 1990s. Prospective, population-based data noted that in 1985, there was a 4-fold increase in the incidence of celiac disease in children younger than 2 years that precipitously dropped to pre-1985 rates a decade later.[89,90] Ten years later, the prevalence of celiac disease in Swedish children born during the epidemic remained 3 times higher than the population prevalence.[91] This rapid rise and decline in disease incidence correlated with changes in infant feeding practices including younger age of gluten introduction, increased amount of gluten in diet, and reduced breastfeeding.[89,92] A prospective 10-year observational study in children at risk for celiac disease noted a 5-fold increased risk of celiac disease autoimmunity when gluten was introduced in the first 3 months of life compared with introduction at 4 to 6 months, further evidence that early gluten introduction is a risk factor.[93] Despite these ecological and epidemiologic studies, the reasons why early gluten introduction causes a higher risk of celiac disease remain unexplained.

Breastfeeding has also been shown in some studies to be protective against celiac disease. A meta-analysis pooled 5 case-control studies and found a 52% reduction in celiac disease correlating with duration of breastfeeding.[94] Hypotheses for the protective effect of breastfeeding on celiac disease include avoidance of early gluten introduction, protection against infections, decreased immune response due to IgA antibodies in breast milk, and T-cell–specific suppressive effects. Mothers with at-risk infants are therefore counseled to continue breastfeeding as long as possible and introduce gluten between 4 and 6 months of age.[95]

IMMUNE DYSREGULATION
Introduction

Celiac disease requires genetic susceptibility (primarily HLA-DQ2 or HLA-DQ8) as well as environmental exposures (gluten ingestion foremost), but these alone are insufficient to trigger the disease and do not explain ongoing inflammation of the small intestine. Immune dysregulation, therefore, is a core feature of the pathogenesis of celiac disease and has been the subject of intense research over the last few decades. The role of tTG in the deamidation of specific toxic epitopes and the initiation of gluten-specific T-cell adaptive immune responses has been elucidated. Moreover, the role of innate immune responses in disease pathogenesis has recently received attention, especially in small intestinal epithelial damage via $CD8^+CD4^-$ intraepithelial lymphocytes.

Toxic Epitopes and Tissue Transglutaminase

Once undigested peptide fragments from wheat, rye, and barley are transported to the lamina propria they are subject to deamidation by tTG2, which converts glutamine to glutamate, thereby introducing negative charges that have stronger binding affinity for HLA-DQ2 and HLA-DQ8 on APCs. tTG2 belongs to a family of calcium-dependent transamidating enzymes that catalyze covalent and irreversible cross-linking of proteins expressed in all cell types. In an inactive, closed form, tTG2 is located intracellularly and is enzymatically inactive.[96] For reasons that are incompletely understood, tTG2 is transported extracellularly where, in the presence of calcium, tTG2 is in an open reduced form and is enzymatically active.[97] Under normal physiologic conditions, tTG2 is rapidly inactivated via oxidation. While in a reducing environment such as ongoing inflammation tTG2 remains active extracellularly, which might facilitate ongoing tTG2 activity (**Fig. 8**).[98]

Certain glutamine residues, so-called toxic epitopes, have higher specificity for tTG2 deamidation in the small intestine. Peptides derived from wheat, rye, and barley are heterogeneous populations. Gliadin peptides are subdivided into α-, γ-, and ω-gliadins, whereas glutenins are characterized as high molecular weight or low molecular weight. Among gliadin, glutenin, hordein, and secalin peptides (as well as a few avenin peptides derived from oats), toxic epitopes composed of a 9-amino-acid core sequence elicit gluten-specific T-cell responses in celiac disease dependent on HLA type. A nomenclature system has been proposed recently for celiac disease–relevant gluten epitopes, based on specific criteria.[99]

A hallmark of celiac disease is the presence of anti-tTG2 antibodies that can be detected in the serum by enzyme-linked immunosorbent assay. Anti-tTG2 antibodies (especially IgA) are highly sensitive and specific for the disease.[100] However, the mechanism of autoantibody formation remains incompletely understood (reviewed in Ref.[101]). Furthermore, there is controversy about the role of anti-tTG2 antibodies

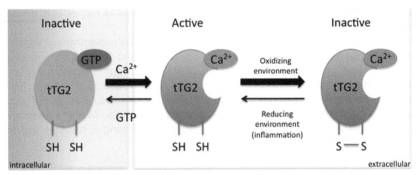

Fig. 8. Active and inactive states of tissue transglutaminase (tTG2). tTG2 is active in an open conformation in a reduced state. In the presence of guanosine triphosphate (GTP) and in the absence of Ca^{2+} (ie, intracellular environment), tTG2 is in a reduced, closed state and the enzyme is inactive. On release to the extracellular environment with low GTP and high Ca^{2+}, tTG2 takes on an open conformation and is active. Usually oxidizing conditions in the extracellular environment render tTG2 inactivated in its open conformation by the formation of a disulfide bond between 2 vicinal cysteine residues in the enzyme. On creation of reducing conditions (ie, inflammation), the disulfide bond is reduced and the enzyme can again take an active open conformation.

in disease pathogenesis (reviewed in Refs.[102,103]). A recent study[104] provided evidence favoring a T-cell–dependent model of antibody formation in celiac disease, suggesting that tTG-specific B cells act as APCs for the gluten-specific T-cell immune response. Additional studies suggest that autoantibodies could modulate small intestinal biology by enhancing the passage of gliadin peptides,[49] inhibiting angiogenesis,[105,106] or altering tTG2 activity[104–110]; although there are conflicting data as to whether tTG2 activity is inhibited or enhanced. Support for a role of autoantibodies in disease pathogenesis is provided by extraintestinal manifestations of celiac disease, notably dermatitis herpetiformis. In this dermatologic condition associated with celiac disease, anti-tTG3 antibodies are expressed in the dermal papillae and are thought to mediate lesion formation.[111]

Adaptive Immune Response

The role of the adaptive immune system in the gut is to distinguish between harmful and beneficial antigens derived from microorganisms (commensal and pathogenic) as well as ingested food peptides. As a result, the intestinal mucosa holds a large proportion of all immune cells in the body that reside in gut-associated lymphoid tissue (GALT) where naïve T and B cells are found (reviewed in Ref.[112]). Immune cells residing in the lamina propria and epithelial layer, by contrast, have effector and memory function. APCs patrol areas of naïve B or T cells and give costimulatory signals that induce T-cell or B-cell differentiation that, in turn, leads to elimination of harmful antigens or tolerance of harmless antigens. Maintenance of an adaptive tolerogenic T-cell response to a soluble protein antigen is termed oral tolerance. Under normal physiologic conditions, oral tolerance is maintained in an environment of retinoic acid along with the cytokine transforming growth factor β, which together induce development of regulatory T cells to suppress proinflammatory effector T cells.[113,114] However, in celiac disease it appears that retinoic acid, in the context of high interleukin (IL)-15, promotes destructive immune responses to gluten rather than oral tolerance.[115] These findings also underscore the close association between adaptive and innate immunity in the pathogenesis of celiac disease (see subsequent section on innate immunity). An integrative model of immune dysregulation in celiac disease is shown in **Fig. 9**.

The role of adaptive immunity in the pathogenesis of celiac disease was first described in the 1970s when Ferguson and MacDonald[116,117] reported an association of celiac disease with a lymphocyte-mediated immunity to gluten in the small intestine, and that T-cell–mediated immunity led to characteristic pathologic changes such as villous atrophy in an allograft rejection model. Further studies found that T cells recognize gluten peptides presented by HLA-DQ2 or HLA-DQ8 molecules on APCs in the lamina propria.[118,119] Gluten-specific T cells from small intestines of celiac patients reveal high levels of interferon-γ (IFN-γ),[120] and messenger RNA for IFN-γ was high in biopsies from celiac patients treated with short-term gluten in vitro.[121] In celiac disease, IFN-γ is produced by T-helper 1 (Th1) cells induced by IL-15, IFN-α and, possibly, IL-18.[115,122,123] IFN-α, in particular, is highly expressed in small bowel from celiac patients, and it likely plays an important role in differentiation of

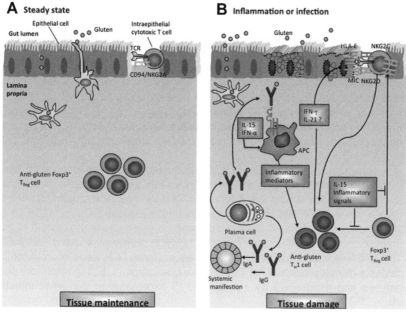

Fig. 9. Immune dysregulation in celiac disease. (A) In health, gluten is tolerated in the presence of antigluten Foxp^{3+} regulatory T cells. Moreover, intraepithelial lymphocytes (IELs) express inhibitory natural killer (NK) receptors that prevent uncontrolled T-cell activation. (B) With inflammation (eg, celiac disease shown here) or infection, HLA-DQ2 or -DQ8 bind gluten on antigen-presenting cells and present to T cells leading to an antigluten T-cell response, which releases interferon (IFN)-γ and possibly interleukin (IL)-21, leading to epithelial damage. The upregulation of IL-15 and IFN-α in the lamina propria induce dendritic cells to acquire a proinflammatory phenotype. The innate immune system is also dysregulated in celiac disease in that IELs undergo reprogramming to acquire an NK phenotype characterized by upregulation of NKG2D and CD94/NKG2C receptors that recognize MHC class I–related chains A and B (MICA, MICB), and HLA-E on epithelial cells mediating tissue damage. IL-15 upregulates NK receptors and promotes T-cell receptor–independent killing as well as blocking Foxp^{3+} regulatory T-cell action on IELs. Finally, the humoral immune system produces gluten-specific antibodies that mediate systemic manifestations. notably dermatitis herpetiformis. IgA, immunoglobulin A; IgG, immunoglobulin G; TCR, T-cell receptor.

proinflammatory dendritic cells. In support of this hypothesis, clinical observations have been made of development of celiac disease after IFN-α treatment for hepatitis C,[124] and higher risk of celiac disease in patients with Down syndrome in whom IFN-α receptor expression and type I IFN response are increased as chromosome 21 harbors the IFN-α receptor.[125,126]

Innate Immune Response

Although gluten-specific CD4[+] T cells play a central role in celiac disease, they are not sufficient to produce characteristic epithelial damage and villous atrophy. This damage is mediated by innate immune signals, with intraepithelial lymphocytes (IELs) playing a primary role (reviewed in Ref.[127]). IELs are a prominent histologic feature in the spectrum of celiac disease, and aberrant IEL populations underlie refractory sprue (polyclonal in type I and monoclonal in type II) as well as enteropathy-associated lymphoma.[128] Intestinal IELs are a heterogeneous population composed primarily of TCRαβ[+] CD8[+] cells, but also TCRγδ[+] and few natural killer (NK)-like cells.[129]

Epithelial stress can be triggered by inflammation, infection, and gluten peptides leading to expression of stress signals on enterocytes, primarily MHC class I–related chains A and B (MICA and MICB) molecules and HLA-E (see **Fig. 9**).[130] In healthy intestine, IELs typically express inhibitory CD94/NKG2A receptors. In celiac disease, on the other hand, IELs express NK receptors NKG2D[131] and CD94/NKG2C[132] that recognize MICA and MICB[133] and HLA-E on epithelial cells,[134] which mediate epithelial destruction. IL-15 plays a key role here by upregulating NK receptors on cytotoxic IELs and enabling TCR independent killing.[131,135,136] Cytokine secretion (eg, IFN-γ) and proliferation is mediated by CD94-NKG2C.[132] Activation of cytotoxic IELs might also be induced by gluten-specific CD4[+] T cells through IL-21[123,137] and IFN-γ.[121,138]

In refractory sprue, IELs acquire a highly activated NK-like phenotype.[128] In this condition, the inflammatory state in the small intestine persists despite avoidance of wheat, rye, and barley. There are 2 types (RCD I and II) characterized by their IEL phenotypes (reviewed in Ref.[139]). In RCD type I, IELs express CD3 and CD8 as well as TCRβ, similar to that found in celiac disease. In these cases, prognosis is good with immunosuppressive therapy.[128,140] RCD type II, on the other hand, lacks CD8, CD4, and TCRαβ, has intracellular CD3ε, has a clonal TCR gene rearrangement, and carries a dismal prognosis.[140] The NK-like phenotype of IELs in refractory sprue is promoted and maintained by elevated IL-15 expression in the small intestinal epithelium.[141,142]

UNANSWERED QUESTIONS AND FUTURE DIRECTIONS

We have come a long way in our understanding of celiac disease pathogenesis since Dicke's first clinical observations in the 1950s. However, several questions remain unanswered in all 3 domains of genetics, environment, and immunology. In the genetics of celiac disease, there has been an explosion in the number of identified susceptibility variants because of the technological improvements in genotyping. The next phase of study will need to elucidate the functional consequences of these variants and their contribution to disease pathogenesis. The full impact of rare variants in celiac disease has not yet been studied, and could explain some of the missing heritability. In addition, the role of epigenetics (eg, methylation) in celiac disease has not been investigated, and could play an important role in disease susceptibility. Finally, the application of genetics discoveries in clinical practice remains undetermined. At present, HLA genetic testing is used primarily for its negative predictive value, and it is not clear whether additional low or moderately penetrant susceptibility variants will alter clinical diagnosis and management.

Regarding environmental factors, it remains unclear how microorganisms (both commensal and pathogenic) contribute to disease. To date, investigators have been unable to tease apart cause versus consequence in microbiome studies in celiac disease. Moreover, it remains to be studied how modulation of the microbiome, through use of probiotics, for example, could alter disease onset or course. Of importance, the role of viruses and fungi has been understudied in celiac disease to date. While epidemiologic studies suggest certain protective factors such as breastfeeding and timing of gluten introduction, mechanistic underpinnings of these observations remain incompletely understood.

Our immunologic understanding of celiac disease now encompasses both adaptive and innate immunity. However, questions remain about transport of gluten peptides across the epithelium into the lamina propria. Moreover, the pathogenic role of anti-TG antibodies continues to be debated. In addition, the role of TCR$\gamma\delta^+$ IELs in disease pathogenesis remains unexplored. Improved understanding of the pathogenesis of celiac disease is crucial to the development of novel and effective treatment strategies.

REFERENCES

1. Troncone R, Jabri B. Coeliac disease and gluten sensitivity. J Intern Med 2011; 269:582–90.
2. Losowsky MS. A history of coeliac disease. Dig Dis 2008;26:112–20.
3. Dicke WK, Weijers HA, van de Kamer JH. Coeliac disease. II. The presence in wheat of a factor having a deleterious effect in cases of coeliac disease. Acta Paediatr 1953;42:34–42.
4. Ploski R, Ek J, Thorsby E, et al. On the HLA-DQ(alpha 1*0501, beta 1*0201)-associated susceptibility in celiac disease: a possible gene dosage effect of DQB1*0201. Tissue Antigens 1993;41:173–7.
5. van Belzen MJ, Koeleman BP, Crusius JB, et al. Defining the contribution of the HLA region to cis DQ2-positive coeliac disease patients. Genes Immun 2004;5: 215–20.
6. Mearin ML, Biemond I, Pena AS, et al. HLA-DR phenotypes in Spanish coeliac children: their contribution to the understanding of the genetics of the disease. Gut 1983;24:532–7.
7. Janeway CA, Travers P. 3rd edition. Immunobiology: the immune system in health and disease, vol. 1. London and New York: Current Biology Ltd./Garland Publishing Inc; 1997. p. 24–1, 25.
8. Marsh SG, for the WHO Nomenclature Committee for Factors of the HLA System. Nomenclature for factors of the HLA system, update January 2012. Tissue Antigens 2012;79:393–7.
9. Megiorni F, Mora B, Bonamico M, et al. HLA-DQ and risk gradient for celiac disease. Hum Immunol 2009;70:55–9.
10. Vader W, Stepniak D, Kooy Y, et al. The HLA-DQ2 gene dose effect in celiac disease is directly related to the magnitude and breadth of gluten-specific T cell responses. Proc Natl Acad Sci U S A 2003;100:12390–5.
11. Zubillaga P, Vidales MC, Zubillaga I, et al. HLA-DQA1 and HLA-DQB1 genetic markers and clinical presentation in celiac disease. J Pediatr Gastroenterol Nutr 2002;34:548–54.

12. Congia M, Cucca F, Frau F, et al. A gene dosage effect of the DQA1*0501/DQB1*0201 allelic combination influences the clinical heterogeneity of celiac disease. Hum Immunol 1994;40:138–42.

13. Al-Toma A, Goerres MS, Meijer JW, et al. Human leukocyte antigen-DQ2 homozygosity and the development of refractory celiac disease and enteropathy-associated T-cell lymphoma. Clin Gastroenterol Hepatol 2006;4:315–9.

14. Fallang LE, Bergseng E, Hotta K, et al. Differences in the risk of celiac disease associated with HLA-DQ2.5 or HLA-DQ2.2 are related to sustained gluten antigen presentation. Nat Immunol 2009;10:1096–101.

15. Karell K, Louka AS, Moodie SJ, et al. HLA types in celiac disease patients not carrying the DQA1*05-DQB1*02 (DQ2) heterodimer: results from the European Genetics Cluster on Celiac Disease. Hum Immunol 2003;64:469–77.

16. The Allele Frequency Net Database. 2012. Available at: www.allelefrequencies.net. Accessed March 19, 2012.

17. Pietzak MM, Schofield TC, McGinniss MJ, et al. Stratifying risk for celiac disease in a large at-risk United States population by using HLA alleles. Clin Gastroenterol Hepatol 2009;7:966–71.

18. Kim CY, Quarsten H, Bergseng E, et al. Structural basis for HLA-DQ2-mediated presentation of gluten epitopes in celiac disease. Proc Natl Acad Sci U S A 2004;101:4175–9.

19. Hovhannisyan Z, Weiss A, Martin A, et al. The role of HLA-DQ8 beta57 polymorphism in the anti-gluten T-cell response in coeliac disease. Nature 2008;456:534–8.

20. Molberg O, Kett K, Scott H, et al. Gliadin specific, HLA DQ2-restricted T cells are commonly found in small intestinal biopsies from coeliac disease patients, but not from controls. Scand J Immunol 1997;46:103–9.

21. Molberg O, Mcadam SN, Korner R, et al. Tissue transglutaminase selectively modifies gliadin peptides that are recognized by gut-derived T cells in celiac disease. Nat Med 1998;4:713–7.

22. Arentz-Hansen H, Korner R, Molberg O, et al. The intestinal T cell response to alpha-gliadin in adult celiac disease is focused on a single deamidated glutamine targeted by tissue transglutaminase. J Exp Med 2000;191:603–12.

23. Arentz-Hansen H, McAdam SN, Molberg O, et al. Celiac lesion T cells recognize epitopes that cluster in regions of gliadins rich in proline residues. Gastroenterology 2002;123:803–9.

24. Qiao SW, Bergseng E, Molberg O, et al. Antigen presentation to celiac lesion-derived T cells of a 33-mer gliadin peptide naturally formed by gastrointestinal digestion. J Immunol 2004;173:1757–62.

25. van de Wal Y, Kooy YM, van Veelen PA, et al. Small intestinal T cells of celiac disease patients recognize a natural pepsin fragment of gliadin. Proc Natl Acad Sci U S A 1998;95:10050–4.

26. Shan L, Qiao SW, Arentz-Hansen H, et al. Identification and analysis of multivalent proteolytically resistant peptides from gluten: implications for celiac sprue. J Proteome Res 2005;4:1732–41.

27. Henderson KN, Tye-Din JA, Reid HH, et al. A structural and immunological basis for the role of human leukocyte antigen DQ8 in celiac disease. Immunity 2007;27:23–34.

28. van Heel DA, Franke L, Hunt KA, et al. A genome-wide association study for celiac disease identifies risk variants in the region harboring IL2 and IL21. Nat Genet 2007;39:827–9.

29. Hunt KA, Zhernakova A, Turner G, et al. Newly identified genetic risk variants for celiac disease related to the immune response. Nat Genet 2008;40:395–402.

30. Dubois PC, Trynka G, Franke L, et al. Multiple common variants for celiac disease influencing immune gene expression. Nat Genet 2010;42:295–302.
31. Trynka G, Hunt KA, Bockett NA, et al. Dense genotyping identifies and localizes multiple common and rare variant association signals in celiac disease. Nat Genet 2011;43:1193–201.
32. Trynka G, Wijmenga C, van Heel DA. A genetic perspective on coeliac disease. Trends Mol Med 2010;16:537–50.
33. Abadie V, Sollid LM, Barreiro LB, et al. Integration of genetic and immunological insights into a model of celiac disease pathogenesis. Annu Rev Immunol 2011; 29:493–525.
34. van de Wal Y, Kooy YM, van Veelen P, et al. Glutenin is involved in the gluten-driven mucosal T cell response. Eur J Immunol 1999;29:3133–9.
35. Molberg O, Solheim Flaete N, Jensen T, et al. Intestinal T-cell responses to high-molecular-weight glutenins in celiac disease. Gastroenterology 2003;125:337–44.
36. Dewar DH, Amato M, Ellis HJ, et al. The toxicity of high molecular weight glutenin subunits of wheat to patients with coeliac disease. Eur J Gastroenterol Hepatol 2006;18:483–91.
37. Vader LW, Stepniak DT, Bunnik EM, et al. Characterization of cereal toxicity for celiac disease patients based on protein homology in grains. Gastroenterology 2003;125:1105–13.
38. Arentz-Hansen H, Fleckenstein B, Molberg O, et al. The molecular basis for oat intolerance in patients with celiac disease. PLoS Med 2004;1:e1.
39. Shan L, Molberg O, Parrot I, et al. Structural basis for gluten intolerance in celiac sprue. Science 2002;297:2275–9.
40. Hausch F, Shan L, Santiago NA, et al. Intestinal digestive resistance of immunodominant gliadin peptides. Am J Physiol Gastrointest Liver Physiol 2002;283: G996–1003.
41. Stepniak D, Spaenij-Dekking L, Mitea C, et al. Highly efficient gluten degradation with a newly identified prolyl endoprotease: implications for celiac disease. Am J Physiol Gastrointest Liver Physiol 2006;291:G621–9.
42. De Angelis M, Rizzello CG, Fasano A, et al. VSL#3 probiotic preparation has the capacity to hydrolyze gliadin polypeptides responsible for celiac sprue. Biochim Biophys Acta 2006;1762:80–93.
43. Heyman M, Abed J, Lebreton C, et al. Intestinal permeability in coeliac disease: insight into mechanisms and relevance to pathogenesis. Gut 2011;61:1355–64.
44. Wapenaar MC, Monsuur AJ, van Bodegraven AA, et al. Associations with tight junction genes PARD3 and MAGI2 in Dutch patients point to a common barrier defect for coeliac disease and ulcerative colitis. Gut 2008;57:463–7.
45. Monsuur AJ, de Bakker PI, Alizadeh BZ, et al. Myosin IXB variant increases the risk of celiac disease and points toward a primary intestinal barrier defect. Nat Genet 2005;37:1341–4.
46. Fasano A, Baudry B, Pumplin DW, et al. *Vibrio cholerae* produces a second enterotoxin, which affects intestinal tight junctions. Proc Natl Acad Sci U S A 1991;88:5242–6.
47. Paterson BM, Lammers KM, Arrieta MC, et al. The safety, tolerance, pharmacokinetic and pharmacodynamic effects of single doses of AT-1001 in coeliac disease subjects: a proof of concept study. Aliment Pharmacol Ther 2007;26: 757–66.
48. Tripathi A, Lammers KM, Goldblum S, et al. Identification of human zonulin, a physiological modulator of tight junctions, as prehaptoglobin-2. Proc Natl Acad Sci U S A 2009;106:16799–804.

49. Matysiak-Budnik T, Moura IC, Arcos-Fajardo M, et al. Secretory IgA mediates retrotranscytosis of intact gliadin peptides via the transferrin receptor in celiac disease. J Exp Med 2008;205:143–54.
50. Turnbaugh PJ, Ley RE, Hamady M, et al. The human microbiome project. Nature 2007;449:804–10.
51. Kau AL, Ahern PP, Griffin NW, et al. Human nutrition, the gut microbiome and the immune system. Nature 2011;474:327–36.
52. Petrosino JF, Highlander S, Luna RA, et al. Metagenomic pyrosequencing and microbial identification. Clin Chem 2009;55:856–66.
53. Turnbaugh PJ, Hamady M, Yatsunenko T, et al. A core gut microbiome in obese and lean twins. Nature 2009;457:480–4.
54. Muegge BD, Kuczynski J, Knights D, et al. Diet drives convergence in gut microbiome functions across mammalian phylogeny and within humans. Science 2011;332:970–4.
55. Wikoff WR, Anfora AT, Liu J, et al. Metabolomics analysis reveals large effects of gut microflora on mammalian blood metabolites. Proc Natl Acad Sci U S A 2009; 106:3698–703.
56. Murphy SF, Kwon JH, Boone DL. Novel players in inflammatory bowel disease pathogenesis. Curr Gastroenterol Rep 2012;14:146–52.
57. Forsberg G, Fahlgren A, Horstedt P, et al. Presence of bacteria and innate immunity of intestinal epithelium in childhood celiac disease. Am J Gastroenterol 2004;99:894–904.
58. Tjellstrom B, Stenhammar L, Hogberg L, et al. Gut microflora associated characteristics in children with celiac disease. Am J Gastroenterol 2005;100: 2784–8.
59. Di Cagno R, De Angelis M, De Pasquale I, et al. Duodenal and faecal microbiota of celiac children: molecular, phenotype and metabolome characterization. BMC Microbiol 2011;11:219.
60. Tjellstrom B, Stenhammar L, Hogberg L, et al. Gut microflora associated characteristics in first-degree relatives of children with celiac disease. Scand J Gastroenterol 2007;42:1204–8.
61. Calvert VS, Collantes R, Elariny H, et al. A systems biology approach to the pathogenesis of obesity-related nonalcoholic fatty liver disease using reverse phase protein microarrays for multiplexed cell signaling analysis. Hepatology 2007;46:166–72.
62. Collado MC, Donat E, Ribes-Koninckx C, et al. Specific duodenal and faecal bacterial groups associated with paediatric coeliac disease. J Clin Pathol 2009;62:264–9.
63. Sanz Y, Sanchez E, Marzotto M, et al. Differences in faecal bacterial communities in coeliac and healthy children as detected by PCR and denaturing gradient gel electrophoresis. FEMS Immunol Med Microbiol 2007;51:562–8.
64. Schippa S, Iebba V, Barbato M, et al. A distinctive 'microbial signature' in celiac pediatric patients. BMC Microbiol 2010;10:175.
65. Sanchez E, Donat E, Ribes-Koninckx C, et al. Intestinal *Bacteroides* species associated with coeliac disease. J Clin Pathol 2010;63:1105–11.
66. Nistal E, Caminero A, Herran AR, et al. Differences of small intestinal bacteria populations in adults and children with/without celiac disease: effect of age, gluten diet, and disease. Inflamm Bowel Dis 2012;18(4):649–56.
67. Kalliomaki M, Satokari R, Lahteenoja H, et al. Expression of microbiota, Toll-like receptors and their regulators in the small intestinal mucosa in celiac disease. J Pediatr Gastroenterol Nutr 2012;54(6):727–32.

68. Sellitto M, Bai G, Serena G, et al. Proof of concept of microbiome-metabolome analysis and delayed gluten exposure on celiac disease autoimmunity in genetically at-risk infants. PLoS One 2012;7:e33387.
69. De Palma G, Nadal I, Collado MC, et al. Effects of a gluten-free diet on gut microbiota and immune function in healthy adult human subjects. Br J Nutr 2009;102:1154–60.
70. De Palma G, Cinova J, Stepankova R, et al. Pivotal advance: bifidobacteria and gram-negative bacteria differentially influence immune responses in the proinflammatory milieu of celiac disease. J Leukoc Biol 2010;87:765–78.
71. D'Arienzo R, Maurano F, Lavermicocca P, et al. Modulation of the immune response by probiotic strains in a mouse model of gluten sensitivity. Cytokine 2009;48:254–9.
72. Cinova J, De Palma G, Stepankova R, et al. Role of intestinal bacteria in gliadin-induced changes in intestinal mucosa: study in germ-free rats. PLoS One 2011; 6:e16169.
73. De Angelis M, Rizzello CG, Scala E, et al. Probiotic preparation has the capacity to hydrolyze proteins responsible for wheat allergy. J Food Prot 2007;70:135–44.
74. Ringel Y, Ringel-Kulka T. The rationale and clinical effectiveness of probiotics in irritable bowel syndrome. J Clin Gastroenterol 2011;45(Suppl):S145–8.
75. Sartor RB. Key questions to guide a better understanding of host-commensal microbiota interactions in intestinal inflammation. Mucosal Immunol 2011;4:127–32.
76. Kagnoff MF, Austin RK, Hubert JJ, et al. Possible role for a human adenovirus in the pathogenesis of celiac disease. J Exp Med 1984;160:1544–57.
77. Kagnoff MF, Paterson YJ, Kumar PJ, et al. Evidence for the role of a human intestinal adenovirus in the pathogenesis of coeliac disease. Gut 1987;28:995–1001.
78. Kagnoff MF. Celiac disease: adenovirus and alpha gliadin. Curr Top Microbiol Immunol 1989;145:67–78.
79. Mahon J, Blair GE, Wood GM, et al. Is persistent adenovirus 12 infection involved in coeliac disease? A search for viral DNA using the polymerase chain reaction. Gut 1991;32:1114–6.
80. Lahdeaho ML, Lehtinen M, Rissa HR, et al. Antipeptide antibodies to adenovirus E1b protein indicate enhanced risk of celiac disease and dermatitis herpetiformis. Int Arch Allergy Immunol 1993;101:272–6.
81. Vesy CJ, Greenson JK, Papp AC, et al. Evaluation of celiac disease biopsies for adenovirus 12 DNA using a multiplex polymerase chain reaction. Mod Pathol 1993;6:61–4.
82. Ivarsson A, Hernell O, Nystrom L, et al. Children born in the summer have increased risk for coeliac disease. J Epidemiol Community Health 2003;57:36–9.
83. Stene LC, Honeyman MC, Hoffenberg EJ, et al. Rotavirus infection frequency and risk of celiac disease autoimmunity in early childhood: a longitudinal study. Am J Gastroenterol 2006;101:2333–40.
84. Zanoni G, Navone R, Lunardi C, et al. In celiac disease, a subset of autoantibodies against transglutaminase binds toll-like receptor 4 and induces activation of monocytes. PLoS Med 2006;3:e358.
85. Roberts SE, Williams JG, Meddings D, et al. Perinatal risk factors and coeliac disease in children and young adults: a record linkage study. Aliment Pharmacol Ther 2009;29:222–31.
86. Decker E, Engelmann G, Findeisen A, et al. Cesarean delivery is associated with celiac disease but not inflammatory bowel disease in children. Pediatrics 2010; 125:e1433–40.

87. Marild K, Stephansson O, Montgomery S, et al. Pregnancy outcome and risk of celiac disease in offspring: a nationwide case-control study. Gastroenterology 2012;142:39–45.e3.

88. Dominguez-Bello MG, Costello EK, Contreras M, et al. Delivery mode shapes the acquisition and structure of the initial microbiota across multiple body habitats in newborns. Proc Natl Acad Sci U S A 2010;107:11971–5.

89. Ivarsson A, Persson LA, Nystrom L, et al. Epidemic of coeliac disease in Swedish children. Acta Paediatr 2000;89:165–71.

90. Ivarsson A, Persson LA, Nystrom L, et al. The Swedish coeliac disease epidemic with a prevailing twofold higher risk in girls compared to boys may reflect gender specific risk factors. Eur J Epidemiol 2003;18:677–84.

91. Myleus A, Ivarsson A, Webb C, et al. Celiac disease revealed in 3% of Swedish 12-year-olds born during an epidemic. J Pediatr Gastroenterol Nutr 2009;49:170–6.

92. Ivarsson A. The Swedish epidemic of coeliac disease explored using an epidemiological approach—some lessons to be learnt. Best Pract Res Clin Gastroenterol 2005;19:425–40.

93. Norris JM, Barriga K, Hoffenberg EJ, et al. Risk of celiac disease autoimmunity and timing of gluten introduction in the diet of infants at increased risk of disease. JAMA 2005;293:2343–51.

94. Akobeng AK, Ramanan AV, Buchan I, et al. Effect of breast feeding on risk of coeliac disease: a systematic review and meta-analysis of observational studies. Arch Dis Child 2006;91:39–43.

95. Guandalini S. The influence of gluten: weaning recommendations for healthy children and children at risk for celiac disease. Nestle Nutr Workshop Ser Pediatr Program 2007;60:139–51 [discussion: 151–5].

96. Liu S, Cerione RA, Clardy J. Structural basis for the guanine nucleotide-binding activity of tissue transglutaminase and its regulation of transamidation activity. Proc Natl Acad Sci U S A 2002;99:2743–7.

97. Pinkas DM, Strop P, Brunger AT, et al. Transglutaminase 2 undergoes a large conformational change upon activation. PLoS Biol 2007;5:e327.

98. Sollid LM, Jabri B. Celiac disease and transglutaminase 2: a model for post-translational modification of antigens and HLA association in the pathogenesis of autoimmune disorders. Curr Opin Immunol 2011;23:732–8.

99. Sollid LM, Qiao SW, Anderson RP, et al. Nomenclature and listing of celiac disease relevant gluten T-cell epitopes restricted by HLA-DQ molecules. Immunogenetics 2012;64(6):455–60.

100. Rostom A, Dube C, Cranney A, et al. The diagnostic accuracy of serologic tests for celiac disease: a systematic review. Gastroenterology 2005;128:S38–46.

101. Sollid LM, Jabri B. Is celiac disease an autoimmune disorder? Curr Opin Immunol 2005;17:595–600.

102. Lindfors K, Maki M, Kaukinen K. Transglutaminase 2-targeted autoantibodies in celiac disease: pathogenetic players in addition to diagnostic tools? Autoimmun Rev 2010;9:744–9.

103. Di Sabatino A, Vanoli A, Giuffrida P, et al. The function of tissue transglutaminase in celiac disease. Autoimmun Rev 2012;11:746–53.

104. Di Niro R, Mesin L, Zheng NY, et al. High abundance of plasma cells secreting transglutaminase 2-specific IgA autoantibodies with limited somatic hypermutation in celiac disease intestinal lesions. Nat Med 2012;18:441–5.

105. Caja S, Myrsky E, Korponay-Szabo IR, et al. Inhibition of transglutaminase 2 enzymatic activity ameliorates the anti-angiogenic effects of celiac disease autoantibodies. Scand J Gastroenterol 2010;45:421–7.

106. Myrsky E, Kaukinen K, Syrjanen M, et al. Coeliac disease-specific autoanti-bodies targeted against transglutaminase 2 disturb angiogenesis. Clin Exp Immunol 2008;152:111–9.
107. Barone MV, Caputo I, Ribecco MT, et al. Humoral immune response to tissue transglutaminase is related to epithelial cell proliferation in celiac disease. Gastroenterology 2007;132:1245–53.
108. Esposito C, Paparo F, Caputo I, et al. Expression and enzymatic activity of small intestinal tissue transglutaminase in celiac disease. Am J Gastroenterol 2003; 98:1813–20.
109. Dieterich W, Trapp D, Esslinger B, et al. Autoantibodies of patients with coeliac disease are insufficient to block tissue transglutaminase activity. Gut 2003;52: 1562–6.
110. Kiraly R, Vecsei Z, Demenyi T, et al. Coeliac autoantibodies can enhance trans-amidating and inhibit GTPase activity of tissue transglutaminase: dependence on reaction environment and enzyme fitness. J Autoimmun 2006;26:278–87.
111. Sardy M, Karpati S, Merkl B, et al. Epidermal transglutaminase (TGase 3) is the autoantigen of dermatitis herpetiformis. J Exp Med 2002;195:747–57.
112. du Pre MF, Samsom JN. Adaptive T-cell responses regulating oral tolerance to protein antigen. Allergy 2011;66:478–90.
113. Coombes JL, Siddiqui KR, Arancibia-Carcamo CV, et al. A functionally special-ized population of mucosal CD103+ DCs induces Foxp3+ regulatory T cells via a TGF-beta and retinoic acid-dependent mechanism. J Exp Med 2007;204: 1757–64.
114. Sun CM, Hall JA, Blank RB, et al. Small intestine lamina propria dendritic cells promote de novo generation of Foxp3 T reg cells via retinoic acid. J Exp Med 2007;204:1775–85.
115. DePaolo RW, Abadie V, Tang F, et al. Co-adjuvant effects of retinoic acid and IL-15 induce inflammatory immunity to dietary antigens. Nature 2011;471:220–4.
116. MacDonald TT, Ferguson A. Hypersensitivity reactions in the small intestine. 2. Effects of allograft rejection on mucosal architecture and lymphoid cell infiltrate. Gut 1976;17:81–91.
117. Ferguson A, MacDonald TT, McClure JP, et al. Cell-mediated immunity to gliadin within the small-intestinal mucosa in coeliac disease. Lancet 1975;1:895–7.
118. Lundin KE, Scott H, Hansen T, et al. Gliadin-specific, HLA-DQ(alpha 1*0501, beta 1*0201) restricted T cells isolated from the small intestinal mucosa of celiac disease patients. J Exp Med 1993;178:187–96.
119. Lundin KE, Gjertsen HA, Scott H, et al. Function of DQ2 and DQ8 as HLA susceptibility molecules in celiac disease. Hum Immunol 1994;41:24–7.
120. Nilsen EM, Lundin KE, Krajci P, et al. Gluten specific, HLA-DQ restricted T cells from coeliac mucosa produce cytokines with Th1 or Th0 profile dominated by interferon gamma. Gut 1995;37:766–76.
121. Nilsen EM, Jahnsen FL, Lundin KE, et al. Gluten induces an intestinal cytokine response strongly dominated by interferon gamma in patients with celiac disease. Gastroenterology 1998;115:551–63.
122. Salvati VM, MacDonald TT, Bajaj-Elliott M, et al. Interleukin 18 and associated markers of T helper cell type 1 activity in coeliac disease. Gut 2002;50:186–90.
123. Monteleone G, Pender SL, Alstead E, et al. Role of interferon alpha in promoting T helper cell type 1 responses in the small intestine in coeliac disease. Gut 2001;48:425–9.
124. Cammarota G, Cuoco L, Cianci R, et al. Onset of coeliac disease during treat-ment with interferon for chronic hepatitis C. Lancet 2000;356:1494–5.

125. George EK, Mearin ML, Bouquet J, et al. High frequency of celiac disease in Down syndrome. J Pediatr 1996;128:555–7.

126. Gerdes AM, Horder M, Bonnevie-Nielsen V. Increased IFN-alpha-induced sensitivity but reduced reactivity of 2′,5′-oligoadenylate synthetase (2,5AS) in trisomy 21 blood lymphocytes. Clin Exp Immunol 1993;93:93–6.

127. Jabri B, Sollid LM. Mechanisms of disease: immunopathogenesis of celiac disease. Nat Clin Pract Gastroenterol Hepatol 2006;3:516–25.

128. Cellier C, Delabesse E, Helmer C, et al. Refractory sprue, coeliac disease, and enteropathy-associated T-cell lymphoma. French Coeliac Disease Study Group. Lancet 2000;356:203–8.

129. Jabri B, Ebert E. Human CD8+ intraepithelial lymphocytes: a unique model to study the regulation of effector cytotoxic T lymphocytes in tissue. Immunol Rev 2007;215:202–14.

130. Hue S, Mention JJ, Monteiro RC, et al. A direct role for NKG2D/MICA interaction in villous atrophy during celiac disease. Immunity 2004;21:367–77.

131. Meresse B, Chen Z, Ciszewski C, et al. Coordinated induction by IL15 of a TCR-independent NKG2D signaling pathway converts CTL into lymphokine-activated killer cells in celiac disease. Immunity 2004;21:357–66.

132. Meresse B, Curran SA, Ciszewski C, et al. Reprogramming of CTLs into natural killer-like cells in celiac disease. J Exp Med 2006;203:1343–55.

133. Bauer S, Groh V, Wu J, et al. Activation of NK cells and T cells by NKG2D, a receptor for stress-inducible MICA. Science 1999;285:727–9.

134. Braud VM, Allan DS, O'Callaghan CA, et al. HLA-E binds to natural killer cell receptors CD94/NKG2A, B and C. Nature 1998;391:795–9.

135. Roberts AI, Lee L, Schwarz E, et al. NKG2D receptors induced by IL-15 costimulate CD28-negative effector CTL in the tissue microenvironment. J Immunol 2001;167:5527–30.

136. Tang F, Chen Z, Ciszewski C, et al. Cytosolic PLA2 is required for CTL-mediated immunopathology of celiac disease via NKG2D and IL-15. J Exp Med 2009;206: 707–19.

137. Kasaian MT, Whitters MJ, Carter LL, et al. IL-21 limits NK cell responses and promotes antigen-specific T cell activation: a mediator of the transition from innate to adaptive immunity. Immunity 2002;16:559–69.

138. Perera L, Shao L, Patel A, et al. Expression of nonclassical class I molecules by intestinal epithelial cells. Inflamm Bowel Dis 2007;13:298–307.

139. Rubio-Tapia A, Murray JA. Classification and management of refractory coeliac disease. Gut 2010;59:547–57.

140. Rubio-Tapia A, Kelly DG, Lahr BD, et al. Clinical staging and survival in refractory celiac disease: a single center experience. Gastroenterology 2009;136: 99–107 [quiz: 352–3].

141. Malamut G, El Machhour R, Montcuquet N, et al. IL-15 triggers an antiapoptotic pathway in human intraepithelial lymphocytes that is a potential new target in celiac disease-associated inflammation and lymphomagenesis. J Clin Invest 2010;120:2131–43.

142. Mention JJ, Ben Ahmed M, Begue B, et al. Interleukin 15: a key to disrupted intraepithelial lymphocyte homeostasis and lymphomagenesis in celiac disease. Gastroenterology 2003;125:730–45.

143. Backes C, Keller A, Kuentzer J, et al. GeneTrail-advanced gene set enrichment analysis. Nucleic Acid Research, Web Server Issue 2007.

Diagnosis of Celiac Disease

Benjamin Lebwohl, MD, MS[a],*, Alberto Rubio-Tapia, MD[b],
Asaad Assiri, MD[c], Catherine Newland, MD[d],
Stefano Guandalini, MD[c,d]

KEYWORDS

- Celiac disease • Population screening • Esophagogastroduodenoscopy
- Undiagnosed celiac disease

KEY POINTS

- Diagnoses of celiac disease (CD) are increasing in the United States and worldwide.
- Despite evidence of increasing rates of diagnosis, the majority of patients in the United States remain undiagnosed.
- One approach to address the relatively low rates of CD diagnosis in the United States is to institute a program of population screening, whereby all individuals regardless of symptoms undergo serologic testing for CD, and those who screen positive subsequently undergo esophagogastroduodenoscopy with small intestinal biopsy.
- Despite calls for general population screening, problems with this approach have led to targeted case finding becoming the preferred method of increasing diagnosis rates.
- The conflicting data with regard to mortality risk in undiagnosed CD are likely due to differences in age, definitions of seropositivity, and follow-up time, but given this residual uncertainty in magnitude of risk, if any, these data do not justify population screening.

INTRODUCTION

This article reviews issues related to identifying the appropriate patient to test for celiac disease (CD), the performance characteristics of serologic testing, the role of gene testing for human leukocyte antigen (HLA) DQ2 and DQ8 haplotypes, and issues

Funding: B.L.: The National Center for Research Resources, a component of the National Institutes of Health (KL2 RR024157). A.R.T.: American College of Gastroenterology Junior Faculty Development Award.
[a] Department of Medicine, Mailman School of Public Health, Celiac Disease Center, Columbia University, 180 Fort Washington Avenue, Suite 936, New York, NY 10032, USA; [b] Division of Gastroenterology and Hepatology, Department of Medicine, Mayo Clinic College of Medicine, Rochester, MN, USA; [c] Pediatric Gastroenterology, Faculty of Medicine, King Khalid University Hospital, King Saud University Riyadh, Riyadh, Saudi Arabia; [d] Section of Gastroenterology, Hepatology and Nutrition, Department of Pediatrics, University of Chicago, Chicago, IL, USA
* Corresponding author.
E-mail address: bl114@columbia.edu

related to the performance of small intestinal biopsy. The article concludes with a review of special diagnostic considerations in pediatric patients.

IDENTIFYING THE APPROPRIATE PATIENT TO TEST FOR CELIAC DISEASE

Diagnoses of CD are increasing in the United States and worldwide. In a population-based study of individuals in Olmsted County, Minnesota, the annual incidence of CD increased dramatically from 0.9 per 100,000 individuals in the years before the availability of serologic tests (1950–1989) to 9.1 per 100,000 in the years 2000 to 2001.[1] Analysis of claims data from a national insurance company found that diagnoses of CD continued to increase through the year 2003, the last year of the analysis.[2]

Despite evidence of increasing rates of diagnosis, the majority of patients in the United States remain undiagnosed. Population-based data are sparse, but inferences on the ratio of undiagnosed to diagnosed individuals can be made based on what is known regarding the seroprevalence of CD in the general population (0.8%–1%).[3–5] In 2001, the point prevalence of diagnosed CD in Olmsted County was 0.04%.[1] If the seroprevalence of CD is 0.8%, then approximately 95% of patients with CD were undiagnosed at that time. While diagnosis rates are increasing, the fact that the seroprevalence of CD is also increasing[4,6] may result in a persistently high undiagnosed-to-diagnosed ratio. The high fraction of undiagnosed patients in the United States stands in contrast to parts of Europe, including Italy and Finland, where the threshold to test for CD is lower and thus the fraction of diagnosed patients is substantially higher.[7,8]

One approach to address the relatively low rates of CD diagnosis in the United States is to institute a program of population screening, whereby all individuals regardless of symptoms undergo serologic testing for CD, and those who screen positive subsequently undergo esophagogastroduodenoscopy (EGD) with small intestinal biopsy. Advocates for this approach note that CD meets World Health Organization criteria for diseases that warrant mass screening: early clinical detection is difficult; the condition is common; screening tests are highly sensitive and specific; effective treatment is available; and untreated disease can lead to complications.[9] Given the reduction in mortality risk that occurs in the years after diagnosis and institution of the gluten-free diet (GFD),[10] and the reduced health care expenditures after diagnosis of CD,[2] screening for CD may be cost effective, and was found to be so in 3 quantitative analyses.[11–13]

Despite calls for general population screening, problems with this approach have led to targeted case finding becoming the preferred method of increasing diagnosis rates. Apart from unresolved questions regarding the logistics of screening (such as deciding on the appropriate age and interval of screening), limitations of the currently available serologic tests pose a significant problem. Given that the prevalence of CD in the general population is 1%, any test with an imperfect specificity will result in a large number of false positives. Assuming that the specificity of tissue transglutaminase (TTG) immunoglobulin A (IgA) is 98%,[14] its positive predictive value when used in the general population is only 34%; as a result, two-thirds of screened individuals who have a positive result will undergo EGD with biopsy and not be diagnosed with CD. This false-positive rate may be reduced by performing a biopsy only on patients with dual positive serologies of TTG endomysial antibody (EMA), but difficulties with the latter serology (see later section Serologic and Genetic Testing) makes this approach less than ideal.

In addition to the technical limitations of serologic screening and its attendant false-positive rate, one objection to routine screening for CD is based on the persistent uncertainty regarding the long-term prognosis of asymptomatic, undiagnosed CD. A major argument for screening is that CD is associated with an increased mortality risk, which declines in the years following diagnosis,[10] a decrease that is attributed to the protective effects of the GFD. The evidence for a mortality risk in undiagnosed CD is less consistent. In an analysis of thawed serum, Rubio-Tapia and colleagues[4] identified individuals with positive CD serologies (both TTG and EMA) in 14 out of 9133 (0.2%) participants in the Warren Air Force cohort. With a follow-up period of 45 years, the patients with seropositivity (who all remained undiagnosed) had a nearly 4-fold risk of death compared with seronegative individuals (hazard ratio [HR] 3.9; 95% confidence interval [CI] 2.0–7.5). In a second cohort study, healthy volunteers with a positive TTG had an increased mortality compared with seronegative subjects (HR 2.53; 95% CI 1.50–4.25).[15] However, in 4 other studies in England,[16] Finland,[17] Ireland,[18] and individuals older than 50 years in Olmsted county,[19] no increase in mortality was noted in undiagnosed seropositive individuals in comparison with their seronegative counterparts. A recent meta-analysis found a modestly increased mortality risk in patients with CD based on serology alone (odds ratio [OR] 1.16; 95% CI 1.02–1.31),[20] but this pooled analysis included seropositive patients who underwent small intestinal biopsy that was normal,[10] raising the possibility of confounding by indication.

The conflicting data with regard to mortality risk in undiagnosed CD are likely due to differences in age, definitions of seropositivity, and follow-up time, but given this residual uncertainty in magnitude of risk, if any, these data do not justify population screening. Although enteropathy-associated T-cell lymphoma appears to be rising in incidence in the United States, possibly as a result of the increased number of patients with undiagnosed CD,[21] given the rarity of this condition it would not justify population screening for CD based on this consideration alone. At the other end of the spectrum of clinical severity, apparently asymptomatic patients may report improved quality of life after screen-detected diagnosis of CD,[22] but data on this topic are insufficient to establish that widespread screening of the population is cost effective.

The favored alternative to population screening at this time is a case-finding approach, whereby health care providers order serologic testing for CD in patients who exhibit one or more of the symptoms, signs, or other diseases closely associated with CD. In this approach, the problem of high false-positive rates of serologic tests is reduced, because the underlying prevalence of CD in a symptomatic or high-risk group is likely to be higher than that of the general population. The feasibility and effectiveness of the case-finding approach was demonstrated in a multicenter study in which adult patients attending a primary care office were given a questionnaire soliciting symptoms (such as diarrhea, abdominal pain, chronic fatigue, and infertility), abnormal laboratory values (including anemia and abnormal liver tests), or associated diseases (such as irritable bowel syndrome, any autoimmune disease, Down syndrome, and Turner syndrome).[23] Individuals responding affirmatively to 1 or more of these items were offered serologic testing for CD and, if positive, EGD with small intestinal biopsy. During the 3-year period, 976 of 2568 eligible patients (38%) responded affirmatively and agreed to serologic testing. Of these 2568 patients, 22 (2.3%) were ultimately diagnosed with CD based on serology and biopsy. Of note, the overall diagnosis rate markedly increased. Compared with the 12-month period preceding the case-finding initiative, the diagnosis rate increased from 0.27 cases per 1000 visits to 8.6 cases per 1000 visits. Such an approach, while increasing diagnosis rates, may still leave the majority of patients undiagnosed.

Although the case-finding approach is the favored strategy, it remains a matter of controversy as to which symptoms and associated diseases should prompt evaluation for CD. Given the protean clinical manifestations of CD and the expanding list of associated conditions,[24] the strategy of testing for CD for one associated symptom or condition may approach that of screening the general population, because nearly 100% of respondents may respond affirmatively to at least one item. For example, in the case-finding study by Catassi and colleagues,[23] 64% of all participants were eligible for CD testing, and this questionnaire did not include additional items that may be justifiably included in a CD symptom checklist, such as peripheral neuropathy,[25] migraines,[26] gastroesophageal reflux,[27] low bone density,[28] and low levels of high-density lipoprotein.[29]

A recent study set at a health fair in Caspar, Wyoming sheds light on the fine line between case finding and screening of the general population.[5] In this study, 3850 individuals attending the health fair submitted a blood sample that was tested for TTG, and serum with positive results then underwent confirmatory EMA testing. These individuals also completed a questionnaire querying respondents for gastrointestinal symptoms including bloating, abdominal pain, heartburn, nausea, diarrhea, and constipation. Of the 3850 subjects, 34 had a positive TTG and EMA, yielding a prevalence of 0.8%. (Thirty-one of these 34 had not been previously diagnosed with CD, yielding an undiagnosed-to-diagnosed ratio of 10:1.) When comparing seropositive to seronegative individuals with regard to gastrointestinal symptoms, none of these symptoms were predictive of seropositivity. This null finding was due in part to these symptoms being quite common; more than 80% of all respondents had at least one such symptom. Thus, an aggressive case-finding strategy may closely resemble a de facto mass screening approach.

At present, there is no universally accepted threshold for testing for CD among physicians who have adopted this recommended strategy of case finding. Consensus statements from the United States and Europe broadly agree with the need to test for CD in scenarios such as chronic diarrhea and unexplained iron deficiency.[30–33] However, there is less agreement on whether screening asymptomatic patients in high-prevalence groups (such as first-degree relatives or patients with autoimmune thyroiditis) should be recommended[31–33] or merely offered with the caveat that the benefits of diagnosing asymptomatic patients are unclear.[30] Because a low threshold (ie, a long list of symptoms that would prompt testing) may result in a testing a large proportion of patients seeking health care, it is imperative that physicians using this strategy have a solid understanding of the performance characteristics of serologic tests.

SEROLOGIC AND GENETIC TESTING
Serum Antibody Tests

CD is characterized by the presence of diverse antibodies in the serum that are made against (1) gliadin (conventional gliadin antibodies and deamidated gliadin peptide antibodies), a component of gluten, and (2) connective tissue components (tissue transglutaminase antibodies and endomysial antibodies). Overall, these tests are useful for the diagnosis of CD, although the diagnostic performance may be different for each test.

Antigliadin antibodies

Conventional gliadin antibodies are no longer recommended because of the lower sensitivity and specificity compared with other available serologic tests. However, there is considerable interest on the use of new-generation deamidated gliadin peptide antibodies because these novel tests have improved diagnostic accuracy in comparison with conventional gliadin antibodies.[34] In a recent review, the pooled sensitivity for IgA tissue deamidated gliadin peptide antibodies was 88%, with specificity of 95%.[14] The role of deamidated gliadin peptide antibodies in diagnosing young children is discussed in the section Diagnosis in Children.

Tissue transglutaminase antibodies

The enzyme tissue transglutaminase was recognized as the CD autoantigen.[35] This enzyme has many functions, including deamidation of gliadin peptides.[36] A wide range of kits with different characteristics measure tissue transglutaminase antibodies, most often by quantitative enzyme-linked immunosorbent assay.[37] The substrates could be guinea pig liver (first-generation assays), human red-cell derived, and human recombinant. In general, specificity tends to be higher with human-based assays than with first-generation assays.[38] The pooled sensitivity and specificity for human-based IgA tissue transglutaminase antibodies (TTG) are both 98%.[14] However, sensitivity (and to a lesser degree specificity) may vary among laboratories.[37] Because of its simplicity and overall good diagnostic accuracy, detection of IgA TTG antibodies is the serologic test of choice for the diagnosis of CD.[31,39] False-positive tests are unusual with human substrates, especially at high titers.[33]

Endomysial antibodies

Endomysial antibodies (EMA) have been available for diagnosis of CD for almost 30 years.[40] The antibodies have been measured using an indirect immunofluorescence technique using monkey esophagus, human jejunum, or human umbilical cord as substrate.[41–43] The target antigen is tissue transglutaminase. The pooled sensitivity and specificity for IgA EMA were found to be 95% and 99%, respectively.[14] Specificity of IgA EMA is similar for tests using either monkey esophagus or human umbilical cord substrates.[42] Despite the high specificity of this antibody, there are several test-related issues that may limit its use in clinical practice. It is semiquantitative, time consuming, operator dependent, and expensive. However, IgA EMA testing can be clinically useful if the result of the IgA TTG test is equivocal.[31] A positive IgA EMA test is strong evidence for CD in patients with nonatrophic intestinal lesions (Marsh 1–2).[44] An emerging indication for IgA EMA testing is to support a nonbiopsy-based diagnosis of celiac disease in symptomatic children with high titer of IgA TTG (see later section Diagnosis in Children).[33]

Clinical Use of Serologic Tests

Serologic tests are useful to evaluate patients with suspected CD, and may be helpful in monitoring adherence to the GFD.[39] Among adult patients with chronic abdominal symptoms, IgA TTG and IgA EMA have high accuracy for the diagnosis of CD.[45] The initial serologic test of choice for CD diagnosis is IgA TTG. Sequential testing (IgA TTG–positive followed by IgA EMA) has been an effective strategy for detection of CD in large epidemiologic studies but its accuracy in clinical practice may require further study, especially if the intention is to avoid an intestinal biopsy for confirmation of CD.[46] Testing for CD is accurate only if the patient continues to follow a gluten-containing diet; therefore, it is important to inform patients that they should not start a GFD until the diagnostic process is completed.[39] Indeed, all serologic tests could become negative after gluten withdrawal.[47] False-negative serologic testing should be strongly considered in patients with selective IgA deficiency. In this scenario, cascade testing or, alternatively, concurrent measurement of total IgA should be considered. IgA- deficient patients should be evaluated by measurement of immunoglobulin G (IgG) TTG, IgG deamidated gliadin peptides (DGP), and/or IgG EMA.[14] In addition, a false-negative test result is more likely in young children (<2 years of age) and among patients with nonatrophic lesions.[39] Further assessment is needed when serology tests are negative but clinical suspicion of CD is high; approximately 10% of patients with CD are seronegative. Intestinal biopsy to confirm or exclude CD is indicated in people with (1) a positive serologic result from any TTG, deamidated gliadin antibodies, or EMA test; and (2) seronegative patients if celiac disease is highly suspected and genetic testing is positive. A cascade testing algorithm used at Mayo Clinic for the diagnosis of CD is summarized in **Fig. 1.**

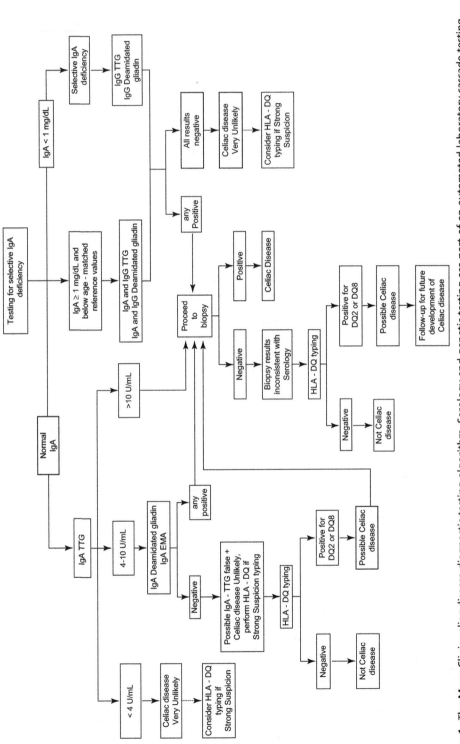

Fig. 1. The Mayo Clinic celiac disease diagnostic testing algorithm. Serology and genetic testing are part of an automated laboratory cascade testing, meaning that a sequence of tests driven by real-time results is used to diagnose celiac disease using a single blood draw. This cascade testing is intended for adults on a gluten-containing diet. (*Courtesy of the Mayo Foundation for Medical Education and Research; with permission.*)

Genetic testing

Almost all patients with CD are positive for either HLA-DQ2 (heterodimer DQA1*05/DQB1*02) or HLA-DQ8 (heterodimer DQA1*03/DQB1*0302).[48] HLA-DQ2 is carried in approximately 95% of patients with CD. Thus the absence of these heterodimers has a high negative predictive value. Approximately 25% to 30% of persons of European ancestry have one of these genotypes,[49,50] so a positive result is of little diagnostic value. Of 1008 European patients with CD, 61 were identified who carry neither the DQ2 nor DQ8 heterodimers, but 57 encoded half of the DQ2 heterodimer.[51] Other non-HLA risk factors have been used to improve identification of high-risk individuals for CD, but its role on clinical evaluation of patients with suspicion of celiac disease will require further study.[52] Routine addition of genetic testing (HLA-DQ testing) to TTG and EMA (or vice versa) does not increase diagnostic performance compared with either testing strategy alone.[53] Thus, HLA-DQ genotyping is not indicated in the initial evaluation of CD. Genetic testing could be useful to exclude the diagnosis of CD (negative genetic testing) in selected cases when diagnosis is uncertain (ie, equivocal small bowel histology).[50] Genetic testing could be especially useful to exclude CD in patients already on a GFD, because this test is not affected by gluten exclusion.

SMALL INTESTINAL BIOPSY

Despite the diagnostic advances afforded by the availability of serologic testing, the histologic finding on small intestinal biopsy remains the gold standard for the diagnosis of CD, although in certain scenarios this may no longer be the case in pediatric patients (see later discussion). Duodenal biopsy for the diagnosis of CD is most commonly performed after a patient is found to have a positive serologic test. However, diagnostic biopsy may also be performed in the seronegative individual with signs and symptoms highly suspicious for CD, as none of the available serologic tests has a sensitivity of 100%.

Biopsy can also be useful in the common (but less than ideal) scenario where a patient has already commenced a GFD before seeking medical care. The serologies in most patients with CD normalize after 6 to 12 months of adherence to the GFD, but the histopathologic changes can persist for far longer; a recent study of patients with CD who underwent serial biopsy found that the median time to mucosal healing was 3.8 years.[54] Moreover, even those patients with confirmed mucosal healing often have persistent intraepithelial lymphocytosis in the context of a normal crypt-to-villous ratio.[55] Therefore, a patient with CD who is already adherent to the diet may have normal serologies but persistent histopathologic evidence of CD. However, it should be recommended not to start a GFD before completion of diagnostic investigations.

Endoscopic findings such as scalloping, fissures, a mosaic appearance, and decreased folds are often seen, but are neither sensitive nor specific findings in CD. In one study of 13 patients with scalloping of the duodenum but who ultimately were found not to have CD, alternative causes included human immunodeficiency virus infection, eosinophilic enteritis, and giardiasis.[56] A study of 129 patients with newly diagnosed CD found that approximately one-third of such patients had an endoscopic appearance that was entirely normal, despite histopathologic evidence of intraepithelial lymphocytosis and villous atrophy.[57]

Despite the imperfect sensitivities of serologic testing and the poor predictive value of a normal endoscopic appearance, many patients with symptoms consistent with CD undergo EGD but do not have a duodenal biopsy during the procedure. In an analysis of the Clinical Outcomes Research Initiative (CORI) national endoscopic database, Harewood and colleagues[58] identified 3992 patients who underwent EGD for the indications of diarrhea, iron deficiency, anemia, and weight loss during the years spanning 2000 to 2003. Of these 3992 patients, all of whom had a normal-appearing duodenum, biopsy was performed in only 438 (11%). In a follow-up study of the CORI database spanning the years 2004 to 2009, the rate of duodenal biopsy during examinations with the same indication improved but remained low, at 43%.[59] In this study, men were less likely than women to undergo biopsy (OR 0.81, 95% CI 0.75–0.88), despite equal seroprevalence rates on screening,[3] and older individuals were less likely than younger patients to undergo biopsy (OR for age ≥70 compared with age 20–49, 0.51; 95% CI, 0.46–0.57), despite the fact that CD can present at any age, including in elderly individuals.[60] The overall low rates of biopsy during EGD for symptoms that may be manifestations of CD indicate that endoscopist-related factors may be contributing in part to the underdiagnosis of CD.

Because the pathologic findings in CD can be patchy and can affect areas of the duodenum with varying degrees of severity, multiple specimens from the duodenum should be submitted during biopsy to determine whether CD is present. Guidelines issued by the American Gastroenterological Association state that 4 to 6 specimens be submitted during duodenal biopsy.[39] This recommendation is based on the investigators' understanding of the patchy nature of the disease, but was subsequently supported by the results of a study of CD patients, in which the sensitivity of biopsy for the diagnosis of CD declined when fewer than 4 specimens were submitted.[61]

In clinical practice in the United States, adherence to the standard of submitting 4 to 6 specimens during duodenal biopsy appears to be poor. An analysis of a national pathology database identified 132,352 patients who underwent duodenal biopsy during EGDs performed in the years spanning 2006 to 2009.[62] Of these 132,352 patients, 4 or more specimens were submitted during duodenal biopsy in only 45,995 (35%). Older patients were less likely than younger patients to have 4 or more specimens submitted (OR for age ≥80 vs age <30, 0.67; 95% CI, 0.57–0.78), and patients with a procedure indication of diarrhea were more likely to have 4 or more specimens submitted than those with anemia (OR 1.20; 95% CI 1.10–1.30). The incremental diagnostic yield of adhering to this standard was high. The proportion of patients with a histologic diagnosis of CD was only 0.7% when fewer than 4 specimens were submitted, compared with 1.8% when 4 or more specimens were submitted. Even when the clinical indication was explicitly noted as suspected CD, adherence to this biopsy standard only occurred in 38.5% of all submissions. As the diagnostic yield for CD more than doubled regardless of the indication for the procedure, the submission of at least 4 specimens during duodenal biopsy would likely substantially increase the rate of CD diagnosis.

Other factors that may affect the diagnosis rate of CD during EGD include failure to biopsy the duodenal bulb[63] and misinterpretation of subtle histopathology.[64] Issues related to histopathologic interpretation of duodenal bulb specimens and of interobserver variability in the histopathologic diagnosis of CD are covered in further detail in the article Histopathology of Celiac Disease elsewhere in this issue by Feir Bao and Govind Bhagat.

Thus, the authors propose that adequate sampling for CD diagnosis should include 4 or more specimens of the duodenum and should include the duodenal bulb.

Because of the limitations associated with duodenal biopsy, some have advocated for diagnostic criteria that include, but do not entirely depend on, biopsy results. Catassi and Fasano[65] proposed a 5-point scoring system that incorporates (1) symptoms of CD (such as diarrhea, weight loss, and iron-deficiency anemia); (2) positive CD serologies at high titer; (3) the presence of a DQ2 or DQ8 haplotype; (4) characteristic histopathologic findings; and (5) a serologic or histologic response to the GFD. The presence of 4 out of the 5 criteria (or 3 out of 4, if gene testing is not performed) would meet diagnostic criteria for CD according to this proposed system, which has not yet been validated prospectively.

This algorithm would allow for patients who have signs and symptoms of CD but have borderline histology, or who refuse biopsy, to be classified as having CD. If this approach is widely adopted, patients meeting the 4 nonhistologic criteria for CD would not require a biopsy. However, any gain in sensitivity in a noninvasive scoring system is done at the cost of specificity. The algorithm would consider patients to have CD if they are not HLA-tested but have symptoms and serologies that improve on a GFD. Given the imperfect specificity of currently available serologies and the known phenomenon of gluten sensitivity in the absence of CD,[66] a significant proportion of such patients may not have a positive HLA-DQ2 or HLA-DQ8, and thus will likely not have CD as currently understood. Thus, an algorithm as described here that allows for a diagnosis of CD in adults without histologic evidence is not likely to be widely adopted by clinicians and investigators in the near future.

DIAGNOSIS IN CHILDREN

It is worth mentioning that the realm of diagnosing CD historically has been solidly in the hands of pediatric gastroenterologists. It was in fact a meeting of the then just-created European Society for Pediatric Gastroenterology that established in 1969 the first diagnostic criteria, subsequently widely followed by adult as well as pediatric gastroenterologists worldwide. Essentially born in Europe with mostly biochemical research around the description of several new congenital disorders of digestion and absorption, pediatric gastroenterology soon emerged and became a powerful force in defining CD and in indicating how to diagnose it.

In the mid to late 1960s, it had become clear that CD could be diagnosed with the peroral jejunal biopsy showing atrophy of the villi, but because there were many causes of that lesion (and at that time especially chronic intestinal infections and milk protein allergy), a strong word of caution was exerted by the medical community not to diagnose CD until it could be proved that gluten was indeed the cause of the mucosal atrophy. Thus not only was a clinical complete remission on GFD considered necessary, but this had to be followed by the documentation of the normalization of the lesion, and finally by its recurrence once gluten was reintroduced into the diet. These criteria were formalized in 1969 by a panel of experts in the then newly formed European Society for Pediatric Gastroenterology (ESPGA, today ESPGHAN: European Society for Pediatric Gastroenterology, Hepatology and Nutrition).

These so-called Interlaken criteria (named after the area in Switzerland where this expert-only gathering took place) did not take into account another important discovery that had been made several years earlier: children with CD possessed antibodies caused by the ingestion of gluten. The first category to be discovered were the antigliadin antibodies, detected and reported by Berger and colleagues[67] in 1964. Seven years later, Seah and colleagues[68] identified for the first time not an antifood protein, but an actual autoantibody in the serum of celiac children: the antireticulins. However, it took several years before their diagnostic utility was fully appreciated, and the real leap forward occurred in 1984 when the EMA were described,[69] which soon dominated the scene owing to their high specificity.

In the late 1980s a large, multicenter Italian study demonstrated that by relying on strict clinical and laboratory criteria, and now also supported by EMA, a correct diagnosis of CD could be reached in 95% of cases by limiting to the one initial biopsy.[70] This plea for a change was soon followed by new diagnostic guidelines published the following year by ESPGHAN.[71] These guidelines have been widely followed worldwide not only in pediatric but also in adult gastroenterology. Even though they were not evidence-based in the strictest sense of the word as used today,[72] such recommendations still stemmed largely from the cited experience[70] and proved very useful, not only in clinical practice but also as a reference for research.

The discovery in 1997 that tissue transglutaminase was the autoantigen in CD led soon to the identification of a very sensitive marker: the TTG. Initially available as derived from guinea pigs (and hence with a good but not perfect sensitivity and specificity), the TTG were later developed from human origin and soon were shown to have extremely high sensitivity and good specificity.[73–75] North American pediatric gastroenterologists, in a plea to improve the poor diagnosis rates and long diagnostic delay (estimated to be higher than 10 years), were quick to understand the potential of TTG in the diagnosis, and in 2005 a panel of experts from NASPGHAN published evidence-based diagnostic recommendations directed at all physicians dealing with children who should be considered as possible CD patients.[32] This guideline provides algorithms that are essentially based on performing first the TTG assay in children at risk (groups at risk are defined on clinical presentations and/or belonging to categories wherein the prevalence of CD is known to be higher), and then proceeding with further workup only on those who have a positive TTG titer, regardless of its value. It is unclear how widely followed these recommendations have been; but certainly we have witnessed a major advance in the diagnosis rates in children over the past few years, in part attributable to an improving awareness of this condition, which has hit the media with a great impact.

Anti–Deamidated Gliadin Peptides

In pediatric age groups, there is evidence for a special role of the relatively new antibodies: the DGP. Antibodies from patients with CD have enhanced binding to DGP in comparison with controls.[76] The deamidation of gliadin peptides occurs via a reaction catalyzed by tissue transglutaminase. In 2004, antibodies against the DGP were shown to be accurate indicators for CD.[77] Thus, in recent years many studies have been done to discern what role these antibodies can play in the disease diagnosis and follow-up in the pediatric population. In IgA-deficient subjects (ie, patients having less than 20 mg/dL of total IgA in their serum), DGP IgG has sensitivity and specificity similar to that of TTG IgG, so they have been proposed as a useful test in such patients.[78,79]

Even in patients with normal total IgA levels, TTG IgA and EMA are often negative in children with CD who are younger than 2 years. In the past, antigliadin antibodies were used as a nonspecific marker of increased intestinal permeability to food proteins in young children, but because of the low specificity for CD (<80%) their use has been abandoned. However, the newer DGP do not suffer from such poor specificity and, most importantly for pediatricians dealing with very young children, DGP has a high sensitivity in this patient population. Barbato and colleagues[80] showed this in a study of 11 children younger than 2 years who had normal values of TTG and EMA but positive levels of DGP and subsequent histologic findings of CD on endoscopy. To further support the use of DGP in young children, Monzani and colleagues[81] showed that DGP IgA and IgG had sensitivity levels of 100% in children younger than 3 years. Similar results were also recently obtained by Mubarak and colleagues[82] in an investigation of 212 children with suspected CD: when the analysis was restricted to the 41 children younger than 2 years, the DGP IgG had a diagnostic accuracy of 100%.

However, the peculiar place occupied by DGP in the pediatric age group goes beyond their important role in screening: in fact, DGP appears to be especially useful in monitoring dietary compliance. In 2007, Liu and colleagues[83] showed that after initiation of the GFD, these antibodies became undetectable sooner than TTG, thus opening the way to further investigate their usefulness in this regard. Monzani and colleagues[81] followed a population of 28 children and showed that DGP had a higher sensitivity than TTG IgA for monitoring compliance to the GFD; in 106 children on a GFD for more than 1 year, sensitivity to detect dietary lapses was 60% for DGP IgA and 76% for DGP IgA + IgG, whereas TTG IgA sensitivity was much lower, at 24%. Thus, while both IgA and IgG DGPs possessed higher sensitivity than TTG IgA, the combination of DGP IgA and DGP IgG performed better. Nachman and colleagues[84] used a long-term prospective study to evaluate the predictive value of antibodies in monitoring compliance to the GFD in adults. The study was on 53 adults recently diagnosed with CD, and compared a complete set of antibodies including TTG IgA, EMA, DGP IgA, and assays combining up to 4 different antibodies. The results showed that DGP IgA and TTG IgA were the most appropriate and consistent for monitoring compliance.

In addition to screening young children and monitoring dietary compliance both in children and in adults, DGP may play a role in detection of early cases of CD, defined as individuals with positive celiac autoantibodies who show mucosal changes of only Marsh 1 or 2 (ie, no villous atrophy) but who subsequently develop villous atrophy (Marsh 3) when continuing to eat gluten. In a study on 42 adults proven to have early-stage CD despite normal small bowel mucosal morphology (Marsh 1–2), and in 20 subjects with villous atrophy (Marsh 3), Kurppa and colleagues[85] found that sensitivity to detect early-stage CD was 79% for DGP versus 64% for TTG.

In summary, in children the present evidence shows that TTG IgA and DGP IgA and IgG have superb and similar abilities to detect celiac disease, and that DGP IgG is also as good as TTG IgG in detecting IgA-deficient CD patients. In addition, DGP appears to have a unique and superior role in screening for very young children with CD, and may be superior to TTG in carefully monitoring dietary compliance in diagnosed patients.

Diagnosis Without a Biopsy

Increased awareness and the 2005 NASPGHAN guidelines certainly allowed an improved diagnosis rate in North America, despite recent evidence of still inadequate use of a correct diagnostic approach by practicing gastroenterologists.[86] Could then these guidelines be simplified? Studies from both sides of the Atlantic began raising the possibility that an accurate selection of patients might allow avoiding the biopsy altogether. In fact, it was shown that a good correlation existed between intensity of the intestinal damage and levels of serum TTG,[87] and that selecting patients with elevated titers of TTG could result in an extremely high positive predictive value, hence predicting the possibility of avoiding the intestinal biopsy.[88–91]

In addition, great emphasis has been placed by investigators on the diagnostic dilemma for patients presenting only minor or no changes of duodenal mucosa at histologic analysis.[92,93] Do these patients have CD or not? Can we consider them as potential CD patients carrying a risk of developing the full-blown disease at a later stage? In essence, do they need to adhere to a GFD? Numerous speculations and proposed algorithms and scores have appeared,[65,94] and certainly the issue is still evolving as advances are made. The rapid evolution of diagnostic criteria for CD is best exemplified by a simple analysis of articles listed in Medline (Pubmed.org): a search for "celiac disease diagnosis" in a 180-day period in 2011/2012 revealed 176 entries: nearly 1 article published every day on the subject!

For these reasons, ESPGHAN convened a panel that was charged with the task of providing new, strictly evidence-based recommendations for the diagnosis of CD in children. Their conclusions have been recently published,[33] 22 years after the historical article of 1990, and are expected to set the new, worldwide standard for such diagnosis. In brief, a panel of 17 experts defined CD and developed new diagnostic criteria based on the Delphi process. Two groups of patients were defined with different diagnostic approaches to diagnosing CD: children with symptoms suggestive of CD (group 1) and asymptomatic children at increased risk for CD (group 2). In group 1, the guideline suggests that diagnosis of CD is based on symptoms, positive serology, and histology that is consistent with CD. If TTG IgA is high (this is defined as more than 10 times the upper limit of normal), and only when there is also additional evidence of a compatible HLA haplotype and of a positive titer of serum EMA, CD can be diagnosed without a duodenal biopsy. In group 2, the diagnosis of CD would be based on positive serology and histology, hence in all cases with the documentation of a positive biopsy.

Within weeks after publication of these guidelines, a study whose results criticize them had already appeared.[95] These investigators analyzed retrospectively 145 consecutive CD patients with positive TTG who had an intestinal biopsy. The positive predictive value for different cutoff points of TTG levels for the diagnosis of CD was assessed, and a simulation was performed in a setting of routine clinical practice so as to calculate the posttest probability of celiac disease. No cutoff level was found to be associated with a positive predictive value of 100%. The highest positive predictive value (98.6%) was associated with a cutoff of 80 U/mL (11.4 times upper limit of normal). Furthermore, in the frequent clinical situations carrying a pretest probability of less than 10%, the posttest probability was not superior to 90% even with the highest levels of TTG. Thus, the need for a confirmatory intestinal biopsy may still be present.

In conclusion, it must be noted that the new ESPGHAN evidence-based guideline does not recommend skipping the biopsy in the selected aforementioned cases, but simply allows the physician to do so at his or her discretion. As in all cases in medicine, the diagnosis is essentially a contract that must be stipulated in each individual case between the doctor and the patient, and is based on one side on the physician's experience, knowledge of the literature, and diagnostic acumen; and on the other on the understanding and fully informed consent of the patient's family, given without reservations. No guidelines, no matter how largely evidence based, can possibly ever replace such mutual trust.

REFERENCES

1. Murray JA, Van Dyke C, Plevak MF, et al. Trends in the identification and clinical features of celiac disease in a North American community, 1950-2001. Clin Gastroenterol Hepatol 2003;1:19–27.
2. Green PH, Neugut AI, Naiyer AJ, et al. Economic benefits of increased diagnosis of celiac disease in a national managed care population in the United States. J Insur Med 2008;40:218–28.
3. Fasano A, Berti I, Gerarduzzi T, et al. Prevalence of celiac disease in at-risk and not-at-risk groups in the United States: a large multicenter study. Arch Intern Med 2003;163:286–92.
4. Rubio-Tapia A, Kyle RA, Kaplan EL, et al. Increased prevalence and mortality in undiagnosed celiac disease. Gastroenterology 2009;137:88–93.
5. Katz KD, Rashtak S, Lahr BD, et al. Screening for celiac disease in a North American population: sequential serology and gastrointestinal symptoms. Am J Gastroenterol 2011;106:1333–9.
6. Catassi C, Kryszak D, Bhatti B, et al. Natural history of celiac disease autoimmunity in a USA cohort followed since 1974. Ann Med 2010;42:530–8.
7. Catassi C, Fabiani E, Ratsch IM, et al. The coeliac iceberg in Italy. A multicentre antigliadin antibodies screening for coeliac disease in school-age subjects. Acta Paediatr Suppl 1996;412:29–35.

8. Virta LJ, Kaukinen K, Collin P. Incidence and prevalence of diagnosed coeliac disease in Finland: results of effective case finding in adults. Scand J Gastroenterol 2009;44:933–8.

9. Fasano A. Should we screen for coeliac disease? Yes. BMJ 2009;339:b3592.

10. Ludvigsson JF, Montgomery SM, Ekbom A, et al. Small-intestinal histopathology and mortality risk in celiac disease. JAMA 2009;302:1171–8.

11. Hershcovici T, Leshno M, Goldin E, et al. Cost effectiveness of mass screening for coeliac disease is determined by time-delay to diagnosis and quality of life on a gluten-free diet. Aliment Pharmacol Ther 2010;31:901–10.

12. Shamir R, Hernell O, Leshno M. Cost-effectiveness analysis of screening for celiac disease in the adult population. Med Decis Making 2006;26:282–93.

13. Long KH, Rubio-Tapia A, Wagie AE, et al. The economics of coeliac disease: a population-based study. Aliment Pharmacol Ther 2010;32:261–9.

14. Leffler DA, Schuppan D. Update on serologic testing in celiac disease. Am J Gastroenterol 2010;105:2520–4.

15. Metzger MH, Heier M, Maki M, et al. Mortality excess in individuals with elevated IgA anti-transglutaminase antibodies: the KORA/MONICA Augsburg cohort study 1989-1998. Eur J Epidemiol 2006;21:359–65.

16. Canavan C, Logan RF, Khaw KT, et al. No difference in mortality in undetected coeliac disease compared with the general population: a UK cohort study. Aliment Pharmacol Ther 2011;34:1012–9.

17. Lohi S, Maki M, Rissanen H, et al. Prognosis of unrecognized coeliac disease as regards mortality: a population-based cohort study. Ann Med 2009;41:508–15.

18. Johnston SD, Watson RG, McMillan SA, et al. Coeliac disease detected by screening is not silent–simply unrecognized. QJM 1998;91:853–60.

19. Godfrey JD, Brantner TL, Brinjikji W, et al. Morbidity and mortality among older individuals with undiagnosed celiac disease. Gastroenterology 2010;139:763–9.

20. Tio M, Cox MR, Eslick GD. Meta-analysis: coeliac disease and the risk of all-cause mortality, any malignancy and lymphoid malignancy. Aliment Pharmacol Ther 2012;35:540–51.

21. Sharaiha RZ, Lebwohl B, Reimers L, et al. Increasing incidence of enteropathy-associated T-cell lymphoma in the United States, 1973-2008. Cancer 2011. [Epub ahead of print]. http://dx.doi.org/10.1002/cncr.26700.

22. Vilppula A, Kaukinen K, Luostarinen L, et al. Clinical benefit of gluten-free diet in screen-detected older celiac disease patients. BMC Gastroenterol 2011;11:136.

23. Catassi C, Kryszak D, Louis-Jacques O, et al. Detection of celiac disease in primary care: a multicenter case-finding study in North America. Am J Gastroenterol 2007;102:1454–60.

24. Green PH, Cellier C. Celiac disease. N Engl J Med 2007;357:1731–43.

25. Chin RL, Sander HW, Brannagan TH, et al. Celiac neuropathy. Neurology 2003; 60:1581–5.

26. Gabrielli M, Cremonini F, Fiore G, et al. Association between migraine and celiac disease: results from a preliminary case-control and therapeutic study. Am J Gastroenterol 2003;98:625–9.

27. Nachman F, Vazquez H, Gonzalez A, et al. Gastroesophageal reflux symptoms in patients with celiac disease and the effects of a gluten-free diet. Clin Gastroenterol Hepatol 2011;9:214–9.

28. Meyer D, Stavropolous S, Diamond B, et al. Osteoporosis in a North American adult population with celiac disease. Am J Gastroenterol 2001;96:112–9.

29. Brar P, Kwon GY, Holleran S, et al. Change in lipid profile in celiac disease: beneficial effect of gluten-free diet. Am J Med 2006;119:786–90.

30. NIH Consensus Development Conference on Celiac Disease. NIH Consens State Sci Statements 2004;21:1–23.

31. NICE clinical guideline CG86: Coeliac disease: recognition and assessment of coeliac disease. (Available at: www.nice.org.uk/CG86). Accessed August 9, 2012.

32. Hill ID, Dirks MH, Liptak GS, et al. Guideline for the diagnosis and treatment of celiac disease in children: recommendations of the North American Society for Pediatric Gastroenterology, Hepatology and Nutrition. J Pediatr Gastroenterol Nutr 2005;40:1–19.

33. Husby S, Koletzko S, Korponay-Szabo IR, et al. European Society for Pediatric Gastroenterology, Hepatology, and Nutrition guidelines for the diagnosis of coeliac disease. J Pediatr Gastroenterol Nutr 2012;54:136–60.

34. Rashtak S, Ettore MW, Homburger HA, et al. Comparative usefulness of deamidated gliadin antibodies in the diagnosis of celiac disease. Clin Gastroenterol Hepatol 2008;6:426–32 [quiz: 370].

35. Dieterich W, Ehnis T, Bauer M, et al. Identification of tissue transglutaminase as the autoantigen of celiac disease. Nat Med 1997;3:797–801.

36. Schuppan D, Junker Y, Barisani D. Celiac disease: from pathogenesis to novel therapies. Gastroenterology 2009;137:1912–33.

37. Li M, Yu L, Tiberti C, et al. A report on the International Transglutaminase Autoantibody Workshop for Celiac Disease. Am J Gastroenterol 2009;104:154–63.

38. Sblattero D, Berti I, Trevisiol C, et al. Human recombinant tissue transglutaminase ELISA: an innovative diagnostic assay for celiac disease. Am J Gastroenterol 2000;95:1253–7.

39. Rostom A, Murray JA, Kagnoff MF. American Gastroenterological Association (AGA) Institute technical review on the diagnosis and management of celiac disease. Gastroenterology 2006;131:1981–2002.

40. Chorzelski TP, Sulej J, Tchorzewska H, et al. IgA class endomysium antibodies in dermatitis herpetiformis and coeliac disease. Ann N Y Acad Sci 1983;420:325–34.

41. Karpati S, Stolz W, Meurer M, et al. Extracellular binding sites of IgA anti-jejunal antibodies on normal small bowel detected by indirect immunoelectronmicroscopy. J Invest Dermatol 1991;96:228–33.

42. Ladinser B, Rossipal E, Pittschieler K. Endomysium antibodies in coeliac disease: an improved method. Gut 1994;35:776–8.

43. Volta U, Molinaro N, Fratangelo D, et al. IgA antibodies to jejunum. Specific immunity directed against target organ of gluten-sensitive enteropathy. Dig Dis Sci 1994;39:1924–9.

44. Kurppa K, Collin P, Viljamaa M, et al. Diagnosing mild enteropathy celiac disease: a randomized, controlled clinical study. Gastroenterology 2009;136:816–23.

45. van der Windt DA, Jellema P, Mulder CJ, et al. Diagnostic testing for celiac disease among patients with abdominal symptoms: a systematic review. JAMA 2010;303:1738–46.

46. Walker MM, Murray JA, Ronkainen J, et al. Detection of celiac disease and lymphocytic enteropathy by parallel serology and histopathology in a population-based study. Gastroenterology 2010;139:112–9.

47. Midhagen G, Aberg AK, Olcen P, et al. Antibody levels in adult patients with coeliac disease during gluten-free diet: a rapid initial decrease of clinical importance. J Intern Med 2004;256:519–24.

48. Sollid LM. Molecular basis of celiac disease. Annu Rev Immunol 2000;18:53–81.

49. Sollid LM, Markussen G, Ek J, et al. Evidence for a primary association of celiac disease to a particular HLA-DQ alpha/beta heterodimer. J Exp Med 1989;169: 345–50.

50. Kaukinen K, Partanen J, Maki M, et al. HLA-DQ typing in the diagnosis of celiac disease. Am J Gastroenterol 2002;97:695–9.
51. Karell K, Louka AS, Moodie SJ, et al. HLA types in celiac disease patients not carrying the DQA1*05-DQB1*02 (DQ2) heterodimer: results from the European Genetics Cluster on Celiac Disease. Hum Immunol 2003;64:469–77.
52. Romanos J, van Diemen CC, Nolte IM, et al. Analysis of HLA and non-HLA alleles can identify individuals at high risk for celiac disease. Gastroenterology 2009; 137:834–40, 840.e1–3.
53. Hadithi M, von Blomberg BM, Crusius JB, et al. Accuracy of serologic tests and HLA-DQ typing for diagnosing celiac disease. Ann Intern Med 2007;147: 294–302.
54. Rubio-Tapia A, Rahim MW, See JA, et al. Mucosal recovery and mortality in adults with celiac disease after treatment with a gluten-free diet. Am J Gastroenterol 2010;105:1412–20.
55. Iltanen S, Holm K, Partanen J, et al. Increased density of jejunal gammadelta+ T cells in patients having normal mucosa—marker of operative autoimmune mechanisms? Autoimmunity 1999;29:179–87.
56. Shah VH, Rotterdam H, Kotler DP, et al. All that scallops is not celiac disease. Gastrointest Endosc 2000;51:717–20.
57. Dickey W, Hughes D. Disappointing sensitivity of endoscopic markers for villous atrophy in a high-risk population: implications for celiac disease diagnosis during routine endoscopy. Am J Gastroenterol 2001;96:2126–8.
58. Harewood GC, Holub JL, Lieberman DA. Variation in small bowel biopsy performance among diverse endoscopy settings: results from a national endoscopic database. Am J Gastroenterol 2004;99:1790–4.
59. Lebwohl B, Tennyson C, Holub JL, et al. Gender and racial disparities in duodenal biopsy for the diagnosis of celiac disease. Am J Gastroenterol 2011; 106:S82–3.
60. Mukherjee R, Egbuna I, Brar P, et al. Celiac disease: similar presentations in the elderly and young adults. Dig Dis Sci 2010;55:3147–53.
61. Pais WP, Duerksen DR, Pettigrew NM, et al. How many duodenal biopsy specimens are required to make a diagnosis of celiac disease? Gastrointest Endosc 2008;67:1082–7.
62. Lebwohl B, Kapel RC, Neugut AI, et al. Adherence to biopsy guidelines increases celiac disease diagnosis. Gastrointest Endosc 2011;74:103–9.
63. Gonzalez S, Gupta A, Cheng J, et al. Prospective study of the role of duodenal bulb biopsies in the diagnosis of celiac disease. Gastrointest Endosc 2010;72: 758–65.
64. Arguelles-Grande C, Tennyson CA, Lewis SK, et al. Variability in small bowel histopathology reporting between different pathology practice settings: impact on the diagnosis of coeliac disease. J Clin Pathol 2012;65(3):242–7 [Epub 2011 Nov 12].
65. Catassi C, Fasano A. Celiac disease diagnosis: simple rules are better than complicated algorithms. Am J Med 2010;123:691–3.
66. Verdu EF, Armstrong D, Murray JA. Between celiac disease and irritable bowel syndrome: the "no man's land" of gluten sensitivity. Am J Gastroenterol 2009; 104:1587–94.
67. Berger E, Buergin-Wolff A, Freudenberg E. Diagnostic value of the demonstration of gliadin antibodies in celiac disease. Klin Wochenschr 1964;42:788–90 [in German].
68. Seah PP, Fry L, Rossiter MA, et al. Anti-reticulin antibodies in childhood coeliac disease. Lancet 1971;2:681–2.

69. Chorzelski TP, Beutner EH, Sulej J, et al. IgA anti-endomysium antibody. A new immunological marker of dermatitis herpetiformis and coeliac disease. Br J Dermatol 1984;111:395–402.

70. Guandalini S, Ventura A, Ansaldi N, et al. Diagnosis of coeliac disease: time for a change? Arch Dis Child 1989;64:1320–4 [discussion: 4–5].

71. Walker-Smith JA, Guandalini S, Schmitz J, et al. Revised criteria for diagnosis of coeliac disease. Report of a Working Group of ESPGAN. Arch Dis Child 1990;65: 909–11.

72. Schoenfeld P, Guyatt G, Hamilton F, et al. An evidence-based approach to gastroenterology diagnosis. Gastroenterology 1999;116:1230–7.

73. Wong RC, Wilson RJ, Steele RH, et al. A comparison of 13 guinea pig and human anti-tissue transglutaminase antibody ELISA kits. J Clin Pathol 2002;55:488–94.

74. Hill PG, McMillan SA. Anti-tissue transglutaminase antibodies and their role in the investigation of coeliac disease. Ann Clin Biochem 2006;43:105–17.

75. Collin P, Kaukinen K, Vogelsang H, et al. Antiendomysial and antihuman recombinant tissue transglutaminase antibodies in the diagnosis of coeliac disease: a biopsy-proven European multicentre study. Eur J Gastroenterol Hepatol 2005;17:85–91.

76. Aleanzi M, Demonte AM, Esper C, et al. Celiac disease: antibody recognition against native and selectively deamidated gliadin peptides. Clin Chem 2001; 47:2023–8.

77. Schwertz E, Kahlenberg F, Sack U, et al. Serologic assay based on gliadin-related nonapeptides as a highly sensitive and specific diagnostic aid in celiac disease. Clin Chem 2004;50:2370–5.

78. Vermeersch P, Geboes K, Marien G, et al. Diagnostic performance of IgG anti-deamidated gliadin peptide antibody assays is comparable to IgA anti-TTG in celiac disease. Clin Chim Acta 2010;411:931–5.

79. Villalta D, Tonutti E, Prause C, et al. IgG antibodies against deamidated gliadin peptides for diagnosis of celiac disease in patients with IgA deficiency. Clin Chem 2010;56:464–8.

80. Barbato M, Maiella G, Di Camillo C, et al. The anti-deamidated gliadin peptide antibodies unmask celiac disease in small children with chronic diarrhoea. Dig Liver Dis 2011;43:465–9.

81. Monzani A, Rapa A, Fonio P, et al. Use of deamidated gliadin peptide antibodies to monitor diet compliance in childhood celiac disease. J Pediatr Gastroenterol Nutr 2011;53:55–60.

82. Mubarak A, Gmelig-Meyling FH, Wolters VM, et al. Immunoglobulin G antibodies against deamidated-gliadin-peptides outperform anti-endomysium and tissue transglutaminase antibodies in children <2 years age. APMIS 2011;119:894–900.

83. Liu E, Li M, Emery L, et al. Natural history of antibodies to deamidated gliadin peptides and transglutaminase in early childhood celiac disease. J Pediatr Gastroenterol Nutr 2007;45:293–300.

84. Nachman F, Sugai E, Vazquez H, et al. Serological tests for celiac disease as indicators of long-term compliance with the gluten-free diet. Eur J Gastroenterol Hepatol 2011;23:473–80.

85. Kurppa K, Lindfors K, Collin P, et al. Antibodies against deamidated gliadin peptides in early-stage celiac disease. J Clin Gastroenterol 2011;45:673–8.

86. Parakkal D, Du H, Semer R, et al. Do gastroenterologists adhere to diagnostic and treatment guidelines for celiac disease? J Clin Gastroenterol 2012;46:e12–20.

87. Diamanti A, Colistro F, Calce A, et al. Clinical value of immunoglobulin A antitransglutaminase assay in the diagnosis of celiac disease. Pediatrics 2006;118: e1696–700.

88. Barker CC, Mitton C, Jevon G, et al. Can tissue transglutaminase antibody titers replace small-bowel biopsy to diagnose celiac disease in select pediatric populations? Pediatrics 2005;115:1341–6.
89. Alessio M, Tonutti E, Brusca I, et al. Correlation between IgA tissue transglutaminase antibody ratio and histological finding in celiac disease: a multicentre study. J Pediatr Gastroenterol Nutr 2012;55(1):44–9.
90. Basso D, Guariso G, Bozzato D, et al. New screening tests enrich anti-transglutaminase results and support a highly sensitive two-test based strategy for celiac disease diagnosis. Clin Chim Acta 2011;412:1662–7.
91. Sugai E, Moreno ML, Hwang HJ, et al. Celiac disease serology in patients with different pretest probabilities: is biopsy avoidable? World J Gastroenterol 2010; 16:3144–52.
92. Kurppa K, Ashorn M, Iltanen S, et al. Celiac disease without villous atrophy in children: a prospective study. J Pediatr 2010;157:373–80, 380.e1.
93. Tosco A, Salvati VM, Auricchio R, et al. Natural history of potential celiac disease in children. Clin Gastroenterol Hepatol 2011;9:320–5 [quiz: e36].
94. Rozenberg O, Lerner A, Pacht A, et al. A new algorithm for the diagnosis of celiac disease. Cell Mol Immunol 2011;8:146–9.
95. Fernandez-Banares F, Alsina M, Modolell I, et al. Are positive serum-IgA-tissue-transglutaminase antibodies enough to diagnose coeliac disease without a small bowel biopsy? Post-test probability of coeliac disease. J Crohns Colitis 2012;6: 861–6.

Histopathology of Celiac Disease

Fei Bao, MD[a],*, Govind Bhagat, MBBS[b],*

KEYWORDS

- Small bowel biopsy • Histopathology • Villous atrophy • Intraepithelial lymphocytes
- Classification • Standardized pathology report

KEY POINTS

- Histopathologic evaluation of celiac disease.
- Site and number of small bowel biopsies.
- Histopathologic features of celiac disease and differential diagnostic considerations.
- Comparison of the old and new classifications of celiac disease.
- Benefit of standardized pathology reports.

DIAGNOSTIC CRITERIA

Histopathologic abnormalities of the small bowel mucosa were first described by Paulley in surgical resection specimens of intestines in 1954.[1] Villous atrophy was a characteristic feature observed in patients with celiac disease (CD), which is now a recognized component of the histologic triad for diagnosing CD. In earlier times, the histopathologic diagnosis of CD was based exclusively on detecting villous atrophy in small bowel biopsies.[2] The recognition of milder degrees of injury in the small bowel mucosa of patients with CD was an important step forward in expanding the histopathologic manifestations of CD. In the 1990s, Marsh[3] described and classified the histologic patterns of small intestinal mucosal injury, the spectrum ranging from normal villous architecture with increased intraepithelial lymphocytes (IELs) as the sole abnormality to total villous atrophy with crypt hyperplasia and increased lamina propria inflammation. The Marsh classification was composed of 4 categories (types 1–4) representing progressive states of mucosal injury, which was modified by Oberhuber in 1999.[4] The Oberhuber classification subdivided the type 3 lesion (flat mucosa) into 3 groups based on the severity of villous atrophy; mild to moderate (partial) villous atrophy (type 3A), marked (subtotal) villous atrophy (type 3B) and completely flat mucosa (total) villous atrophy (type 3C). The modified Marsh-Oberhuber classification is currently used by many pathologists.

The authors have no relevant financial interest.

[a] Department of Pathology and Cell Biology, Columbia University Medical Center and New York Presbyterian Hospital, VC14-238 C, 630 West 168th Street, New York, NY 10032, USA;
[b] Department of Pathology and Cell Biology, Columbia University Medical Center and New York Presbyterian Hospital, VC-14-228, 630 West 168th Street, New York, NY 10032, USA
* Corresponding authors.
E-mail addresses: fb2266@columbia.edu; gb96@columbia.edu

In recent years, the diagnostic approach to CD has changed, because of a better understanding of the clinical manifestations of CD and the availability of more sensitive and specific serologic tests, as well as high-resolution HLA typing for disease susceptibility alleles.[5–8] Most importantly, the presence of total villous atrophy is no longer necessary for diagnosing CD, provided the established spectrum of histopathologic features of CD is present.[9] Nevertheless, small bowel mucosal biopsy remains the gold standard for diagnosing CD. All serologic tests and small bowel biopsies need to be performed while the patient is on a gluten-containing diet. According to the US National Institutes of Health consensus statement,[5] serologic testing is recommended as the first step in pursuing a diagnosis of CD. Duodenal biopsy is recommended in individuals with a positive celiac antibody test, when serologic results are nondiagnostic and in individuals at risk for CD who have suggestive clinical symptoms, such as first-degree relatives of CD and patients with iron-deficient anemia, cryptogenic hypertransaminitis, and CD-associated autoimmune disorders. With positive serology and a biopsy showing characteristic findings of intraepithelial lymphocytosis, crypt hyperplasia, and villous atrophy, a presumptive diagnosis of CD can be made. Definitive diagnosis requires symptom resolution on commencing a gluten-free diet (GFD). A repeat biopsy to show normalized histology after a GFD is no longer required for diagnosing CD, although it is often used to document healing.

SITE AND NUMBER OF SMALL BOWEL BIOPSIES

Although small bowel biopsy remains the gold standard for diagnosing CD, there is a wide spectrum of histologic abnormalities, which can make interpretation problematic for pathologists. Endoscopic and pathologic findings have revealed that the mucosal damage is most severe in the proximal small intestine, including the duodenum and upper jejunum, and diminishes distally.[10] However, CD is a patchy disease, and the patchy and irregular mucosal lesions are just as prevalent as continuous and diffuse lesions.[11–13] Many studies have advocated obtaining multiple biopsies from different regions of the proximal small intestine, but there are no uniform, agreed-on recommendations or guidelines for the number (or site) of biopsies required for diagnosis. A recent large-scale retrospective study conducted in the United States showed that the probability of a new diagnosis of CD was doubled when 4 or more specimens were submitted for histopathologic assessment.[12] Another retrospective study from Canada showed that the diagnosis of untreated CD was confirmed in 90% when 2 duodenal biopsies were obtained, the detection of CD was increased to 95% when increasing the number of biopsies to 3, and 100% detection was achieved when 4 biopsies were obtained.[13] Inadequate sampling may lead to a false-negative diagnosis, and poorly oriented biopsy specimens can cause both underinterpretation and overinterpretation of the histologic abnormalities. Superficial biopsy samples lacking the muscularis mucosa can cause separation of the villous bases, resulting in shorter and thicker villi that can be misinterpreted as villous atrophy and favor a diagnosis of CD.[14] Likewise, an erroneous diagnosis of increased IELs can be rendered when only detached villi are present for review. Historically, biopsies were taken from the jejunum to diagnose CD.[15,16] Studies since the mid-1990s have shown that biopsies from the second part of the duodenum are sufficient for diagnosis without loss of sensitivity or specificity.[17,18] Biopsies from the duodenal bulb should be interpreted with caution because this area is exposed to gastric acid and is prone to peptic injury and Brunner glands can also be prominent in the bulb. The villi in this location are typically shorter in length,[19] and they may also have a bifid appearance. However, the duodenal bulb is also the most sensitive site to detect mucosal injury induced by gluten, because the duodenal bulb is the first to be exposed to partially digested food admixed with acid and pepsin and is the first contact point of gluten with the small bowel mucosa. Hence, it is possibly the site of earliest injury. The severity of mucosal damage is believed to follow a proximal to distal gradient. While, healing of the small bowel mucosa proceeds in a distal to proximal direction.[14] Many investigators have shown that CD-related histologic lesions are present in the bulb mucosa, and importantly, isolated mucosal abnormalities at this site can be seen in up to 10% of adult and pediatric CD cases.[20–22] Hence, in practice, it seems reasonable to suggest that 4 to 6 endoscopic biopsy specimens be taken from the duodenum, with at least 2 samples from the bulb region.

HISTOPATHOLOGIC EVALUATION OF CD

Histopathologic evaluation of small bowel biopsies should be performed on well-oriented biopsy pieces that contain 3 to 4 consecutive villous-crypt units visualized in their entirety and arranged parallel to each other. The normal ratio of villous height to crypt depth ranges from 3:1 to 5:1,[23] and a ratio of 2:1 has been suggested to be normal for the duodenal bulb and in children.[24] Scattered IELs are present normally, which are more prominent along the lateral edge of villi, decreasing in number from the villous base toward the tip, the so-called decrescendo pattern,[25] shown in **Fig. 1**. Biopsies from patients with CD displaying normal villous and crypt architecture lack this pattern as a result of increased density of lymphocytes at the proximal

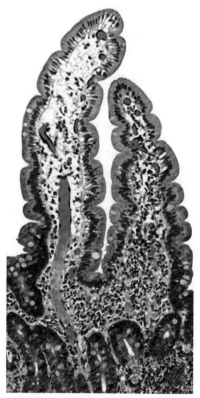

Fig. 1. Normal duodenal mucosa, with a normal villous/crypt ratio (>3:1) and scattered IELs, showing the normal decrescendo pattern (hematoxylin-eosin, ×100).

portions of villi, especially the villous tips, causing an even distribution of IELs along the villous length or an inversion of the normal pattern. The presence of diffuse and uniform infiltration of IELs is the most sensitive morphologic feature of CD, with 1 study showing that 75% of those with proven CD showed this feature compared with 4% of nonceliacs and 0% of controls.[26] Therefore, a practical approach is to scan the villi and look for loss of the normal decrescendo pattern and the presence of diffuse infiltration or a top-heavy pattern of IELs. However, loss of the decrescendo pattern, although more sensitive, is not specific for CD.[27,28] The upper limit of normal IEL numbers was previously considered to be 40 lymphocytes/100 epithelial cells, which was derived from older studies assessing jejunal biopsy samples, and was used as a diagnostic criterion in the Marsh-Oberhuber classification.[4] More recent studies have shown that the upper limit of normal for duodenal IELs is closer to 25 IELs/100 epithelial cells.[29] Counts between 25 and 29 IELs/100 epithelial cells are considered a borderline increase, whereas a count of 30 or more represents a definite increase in IELs that increases the likelihood of CD.[30] A simpler method, whereby villous tip IELs are counted, has been proposed by some investigators. IELs are counted in 20 villous tip enterocytes in 5 randomly selected villi. The upper limit of normal for IELs is 5/20 enterocytes, with counts of 6 or more representing an increase in IELs. It is a fast and simple alternative to the more cumbersome method of counting IELs along 100 or 500 enterocytes and correlates well with the traditional methods.[28] Immunohistochemistry for CD3 is helpful to highlight the distribution pattern of IELs. Although there are a variety of ways for counting IELs, absolute counts are time-consuming and impractical for routine practice. There is little need for counting IELs when there is diffuse marked intraepithelial lymphocytosis. However, counting IELs with or without the aid of an immunohistochemical stain for CD3 is helpful in cases with patchy or mild increases in IELs. Overall, the distribution pattern of IELs (loss of normal decrescendo pattern) may be more valuable than the counts. Immunophenotypic studies have shown that the increased IELs represent an expansion of both, cytotoxic $\alpha\beta$ T cells and $\gamma\delta$ T cells; the former predominate and 60% to 70% express CD8, whereas the latter are mostly CD8–. The $\gamma\delta$ T cells comprise 1% to 10% of IELs in normal small intestinal mucosa, but increase in patients with CD, in whom they can represent up to 15%–30% of all IELs.[31,32]

Microscopic examination of the small bowel biopsies should be performed in a sequential algorithmic manner, ensuring inspection and evaluation, not only of the mucosa and submucosa (when present) but also the luminal aspect, to identify adherent or free-floating infectious micro-organisms, foreign objects, and so forth.[33] The histopathologic findings in the different compartments of small bowel biopsies from patients with CD are a reflection of the pathogenetic mechanisms of this disease, which is mediated by CD4+ T cells, responding to gliadin peptides presented by antigen-presenting cells bearing the HLA DQ2 or DQ8 alleles, as well as activation of intraepithelial cytotoxic CD8+ T cells.[34–37] Activation of the adaptive and innate immune response pathways leads to the production of various cytokines and antibodies against tissue transglutaminase, as well as antigliadin, antireticulin, and antiendomysial antibodies. At the histologic level, this situation is manifested by expansion of the lamina propria by a mixed lymphocytic and plasma cell infiltrate accompanied by variable numbers of eosinophils, neutrophils, and macrophages intraepithelial lymphocytes and epithelial damage.

OLD AND NEW CLASSIFICATIONS OF CD

Michael Marsh introduced a grading scheme to classify the morphologic spectrum of gluten-sensitive enteropathy in 1992, based on his studies of a variety of small intestinal disorders and investigation of the intestinal response to gluten challenge. Oberhuber[4] modified some of the parameters, and published a modified scheme in 1999. The trend toward lower cutoff numbers of IELs is reflected by the incorporation of 30 IELs per 100 enterocytes into the revised Marsh-Oberhuber classification scheme.[9] The Marsh-Oberhuber classification describes 4 progressive states of small intestinal mucosal injury (**Table 1**). This classification is used by some pathologists to evaluate the duodenal mucosal lesions in patients with CD. However, this classification scheme has been shown to be less reproducible, leading to significant intraobserver and interobserver variation. The type 1 and 2 mucosal alterations are often not recognized by non-specialist pathologists, and a high degree of interobserver variability has been noted for type 3a and 3b lesions, even among expert gastrointestinal pathologists. A new histologic classification has recently been proposed by Corazza and Villanacci (see **Table 1**),[38] who have suggested dividing the mucosal lesions of CD into 2 categories: nonatrophic lesion (grade A, shown in **Fig. 2**A) and atrophic lesion (grade B). Grade A incorporates the type 1 (infiltrative) and type 2 (hyperplastic) lesions of The Marsh-Oberhuber classification. Grade B lesions are further subdivided into B1 (shown in **Fig. 2**B) and B2 (shown in **Fig. 2**C) based on the presence or absence of villi. Marsh-Oberhuber type 3A and 3B lesions are grouped into a single grade as grade B1; type 3C (flat mucosa) lesion is classified as grade B2. The type 4 (atrophic) lesion has been removed from their classification, based on the evidence that it is a rare pattern and it is usually found in patients with refractory sprue, ulcerative jejunoileitis, and enteropathy-associated T-cell lymphoma (EATL),[10] which have all been shown to be characterized by aberrant clonal T-cell expansions by immunohistochemical studies and molecular analysis.[39–41] The new 3-tiered classification is simpler and has been shown to result in better interobserver agreement compared to the more detailed Marsh-Oberhuber classification.[42] Its use may contribute to

Table 1
Old and new classifications for pathologic evaluation of mucosal changes associated with CD

Marsh-Oberhuber Classification		Corazza-Villanacci Classification	
Type 1	Normal villous and crypt architecture with ≥30 IELs/100 enterocytes	Grade A	Nonatrophic, with normal villous architecture with or without crypt hyperplasia and ≥25 IELs/100 enterocytes
Type 2	Normal villous architecture, crypt hyperplasia, and ≥30 IELs/100 enterocytes		
Type 3a	Partial villous atrophy with villous/crypt ratio of <3:1 or 2:1, crypt hyperplasia, and ≥30 IELs/100 enterocytes	Grade B1	Atrophic, with villous/crypt ratio <3:1, 2:1, or 1:1, villi still detectable and ≥25 IELs/100 enterocytes
Type 3b	Subtotal villous atrophy with villous/crypt ratio of <1:1, crypt hyperplasia and ≥30 IELs/100 enterocytes		
Type 3c	Total villous atrophy (flat mucosa) with marked crypt hyperplasia and ≥30 IELs/100 enterocytes	Grade B2	Atrophic and completely flat mucosa, villi no longer detectable, and ≥25 IELs/100 enterocytes
Type 4	Atrophic hypoplastic lesion (flat mucosa) with only a few crypts and near normal IEL counts	Deleted	

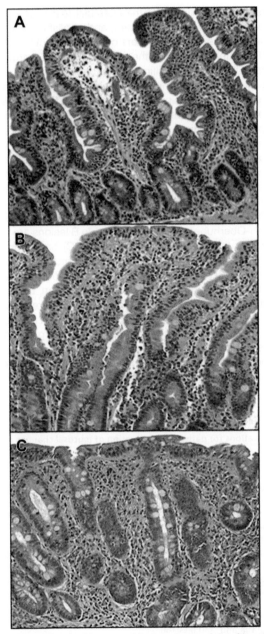

Fig. 2. Different grades of duodenal mucosal lesions in CD. (*A*) Infiltrative type (type 1) or nonatrophic lesion (grade A), showing normal crypt and villous architecture and increased numbers of IELs (IELs, hematoxylin-eosin, ×100). (*B*) Destructive type (type 3b) or atrophic lesion (grade B1), showing moderate villous atrophy and a diffuse increase in IELs (hematoxylin-eosin, ×100). (*C*) Flat lesion (type 3c or grade B2), manifesting total villous atrophy and diffuse increase in IELs (hematoxylin-eosin, ×100).

more uniform diagnostic reporting in cases of CD and enhance communication between pathologists and clinicians. However, clinicopathologic studies are needed to validate the new classification. **Table 1** compares the old and new classifications.

CORRELATION OF MUCOSAL DAMAGE WITH SEROLOGIC ABNORMALITIES

The symptoms of patients with CD were suggested to be related to the length of small bowel injury, but not to the histopathologic severity of the intestinal mucosal lesion sampled by proximal small bowel endoscopic biopsies per se.[10,25] This hypothesis is debatable and recent investigations based on videocapsule studies have argued against this supposition. However, the degree of mucosal damage has been shown to correlate with the presence and titers of both tissue transglutaminase antibodies (tTGA) and endomysium antibodies (EMA). Studies have shown that EMA seropositivity correlates with more severe villous atrophy, but not with the presence of gastrointestinal symptoms or the clinical mode of disease presentation.[43] One study has also shown that IgA tTGA levels of 100 units or greater occur almost exclusively in adults and children manifesting severe degrees of villous atrophy (Marsh 3 lesions).[44] Celiac patients with lesser degrees of villous atrophy are less likely to have positive serologies, especially cases with minimal histologic alterations or those with normal villous architecture and intraepithelial lymphocytosis as the sole abnormality.[9] Normalization of architectural changes of the duodenal mucosa can be variable and may take from 6 to 24 months after the induction of GFD; recovery may remain incomplete in some adult patients for longer periods.[45] Studies have shown that in celiac patients adhering to strict GFD for more than 1 year, up to 75% had remission of symptoms and biopsies showed normal villous architecture, but 50% to 70% still had increased IELs.[46,47] Follow-up by serology with a normal tTGA level does not predict recovery of villous atrophy in celiac patients on a GFD. One study reported that 16 of 48 (33%) patients with CD on a GFD had persistent villous atrophy, and 7 of these 16 patients (44%) had normal tTGA levels.[48]

SERONEGATIVE CD

Seronegative CD is believed to account for up to 15% of all celiac patients.[43] Seronegative CD poses a clinical challenge and requires integration of clinical, genetic, and histopathologic findings because these individuals lack serum autoantibodies.[49] These individuals are more likely to have either normal villous architecture with increased IELs or mild degrees of villous atrophy, and they likely lack a humoral response to the autoantigen (tissue transglutaminase) or gliadin.[50] The sensitivity of serum anti-EMA or tTGA antibody-based tests is low in these cases, reportedly 31% to 70% for CD with mild villous atrophy.[51,52] Newer tests for antibodies against deamidated gliadin peptides can detect 20% to 30% of patients who are seronegative for IgA tTGA.[53] Hence, more sensitive tests for detection of serum autoantibodies are needed in cases manifesting limited mucosal inflammation. Detection of mucosal IgA-tissue transglutaminase immune deposits has been proposed as one of the most sensitive approaches to identify CD with minimal or no villous atrophy. Presence of these deposits in the lamina propria suggests activation of the local mucosal antibody response in the absence of a systemic humoral response. The sensitivity and specificity of this method is reported to be 93%.[54] Evaluation of the number and pattern of IELs at the villous tips and detecting increased intraepithelial γ/δ T cells in biopsy samples by immunohistochemistry and flow cytometry can also help in diagnosing cases of CD with mild enteropathy lacking serologic abnormalities.[55]

DIFFERENTIAL DIAGNOSIS

Differential diagnosis of CD includes a variety of disorders that manifest villous atrophy or increased IELs. Intraepithelial lymphocytosis is a characteristic histologic feature of CD; however, in the absence of villous atrophy it is a nonspecific finding. In some series, up to 2.5% of duodenal biopsies show increased IELs ($\geq$ 25 IELs/per 100 enterocytes) in the absence of villous architectural changes.[56] Common causes for increased IELs with normal villous architecture are listed in **Table 2**. *Helicobacter pylori*-associated gastroduodenitis (the leading cause),[57] non-gluten food hypersensitivity, including cow's milk, soy protein, fish, rice, and chicken hypersensitivity, medication (primarily nonsteroidal antiinflammatory drugs [NSAIDs]) induced injury, and other infectious and immune disorders. The prevalence of CD as the etiology for cases that display increased IELs and architecturally normal duodenal biopsies is only about 10% to 20%.[58,59] A major challenge facing both clinicians and pathologists is to diagnose CD when Marsh type 1 or grade A lesions (according to the Corazza-Villanacci classification) are present. The specificity of histopathologic findings in the small bowel biopsy is greater when villous atrophy (partial, subtotal, or total) is present. However, other entities such as tropical sprue (TS), autoimmune enteropathy (AE), common variable immunodeficiency (CVID), collagenous sprue (CS), bacterial overgrowth, inflammatory bowel disease, and drug-induced mucosal injury, among other disorders listed in **Table 2**, can all cause villous atrophy with or without a concomitant increase in IELs. We briefly discuss some small intestinal disorders that can be challenging to differentiate from CD based on histopathologic criteria, including a few that might present as overlap disorders with CD.

TS affects residents of or visitors to the tropics, including the Caribbean countries, as well as South America, West Africa, and Asia.[60] The histologic findings are similar to those of CD. In contrast to the predominance of proximal small intestinal injuries, the

Table 2
Differential diagnosis of CD with or without villous atrophy

Normal Villous Architecture and Increased IELs	Villous Atrophy With/Without Increased IELs
Food hypersensitivity (eg, cow's milk, soy, fish, eggs, rice, and chicken)	Infections (tropical sprue, *Giardia*, Whipple disease, *Mycobacterium avium complex*)
Peptic ulcer disease	Refractory sprue
Helicobacter pylori-associated gastroduodenitis	Collagenous sprue
Drugs (NSAIDs, proton pump inhibitor)	Autoimmune enteropathy, immune-mediated enteropathy
Infections (eg, viral enteritis, *Giardia*, *Cryptosporidium*)	Immunodeficiency (common variable immune deficiency)
Immune dysregulation (rheumatoid arthritis, Hashimoto thyroiditis, SLE, multiple sclerosis, autoimmune enteropathy)	Graft-versus-host disease
	Inflammatory bowel disease (Crohn disease)
Immunodeficiency (common variable immune deficiency)	Drugs (mycophenolate mofetil, colchicine, olmesartan)
Graft-versus-host disease	Chemoradiation therapy, immunomodulatory drug therapy (anti-CTLA4 antibody)
Inflammatory bowel disease	Eosinophilic gastroenteritis
Bacterial overgrowth, blind loop syndrome	Bacterial overgrowth
Lymphocytic and collagenous colitis	EATL
Irritable bowel syndrome	Nutritional deficiency

Abbreviations: CTLA4, cytotoxic T-lymphocyte antigen 4; NSAIDs, nonsteroidal antiinflammatory drugs; SLE, systemic lupus erythematosus.

changes of TS are equally prominent in the ileum and in the proximal jejunum.[61] This distribution may explain the more common association of TS with megaloblastic anemia caused by vitamin B_{12} and folate deficiency. Although no definite causal organisms have been identified, much evidence points to an infectious cause, and broad-spectrum antibiotic therapy usually results in rapid recovery of TS.[62]

AE comprises a rare group of immune-mediated disorders involving the intestines, which occur primarily in young children and infants but can also affect adults in some instances. In young males, an X-linked, severe form of the disorder is associated with immune dysregulation and polyendocrinopathy (IPEX) caused by a germ line mutation in the FOXP3 gene located on the X chromosome.[63] The disease commonly affects the small bowel, with involvement of the stomach and colon described in some cases. Histopathologic changes in AE show some similarities with CD. The small bowel biopsies show variable, sometimes total, villous atrophy and crypt hyperplasia with dense lymphoplasmacytic infiltrate in the lamina propria, and neutrophils with crypt abscesses can be seen in severe cases.[64–66] Although IELs may be seen in the intestinal epithelium, they are more often seen in the crypts; unlike CD, marked surface intraepithelial lymphocytosis is usually not present.[65] One of the hallmarks of AE is the presence of antienterocyte antibodies and some patients may also have antigoblet cell, antiparietal cell, and antismooth muscle antibodies. Antigliadin and antireticulin antibodies have also been described in AE.[66] Patients with antigoblet cell antibodies, in some instances, show absence or reduced numbers of goblet cells, endocrine cells, and Paneth cells on biopsy. It has been shown that antigoblet cell antibodies are not specific for this disorder, because they can be detected in a variety of intestinal disorders and even in normal individuals. Patients with AE present with protracted secretory diarrhea and weight loss, unresponsive to a GFD or total parental nutrition. Steroids and immunosuppressive therapy have been used with efficacy. Cases of overlap AE and CD have been described, based on the presence of antienterocyte antibodies and lack of appropriate response to a GFD, often requiring immunomodulatory drug therapy.[67] However, further studies are required to determine the frequency of antienterocyte antibodies in patients with CD to determine whether the presence of such antibodies signifies a distinct subset of patients with unique features.

CVID is the most common primary immunodeficiency disorder after isolated IgA deficiency, which is characterized by a failure of terminal B-cell maturation into plasma cells, leading to decreased serum immunoglobulin levels.[68] Patients with CVID are prone to infections, especially giardiasis and bacterial overgrowth, and they have chronic gastrointestinal complaints, including diarrhea and malabsorption.[68,69] Small bowel biopsies show a wide range of histologic changes, from increased IELs with variable degree of villous atrophy resembling CD, to nodular lymphoid hyperplasia, acute duodenitis (neutrophilic infiltration), and low-grade lymphoma in some cases.[70] A characteristic feature of CVID is the absence or rarity of plasma cells in the lamina propria, hence an immunohistochemical stain for CD138 is helpful in diagnosis. CVID can superficially resemble CD, and studies have also described CD in patients with CVID.[71,72] AE has also been described in several patients with CVID,[68,73] and antienterocyte antibodies have been reported in patients with CVID.[67,74] We have also encountered such patients, whose duodenal biopsies show histologic features of both CVID and AE (shown in **Fig. 3**).

CS is a rare type of small bowel enteropathy associated with chronic diarrhea and severe malabsorption, typically affecting middle-aged or elderly women.[75,76] Histologically, CS is characterized by villous atrophy, crypt hyperplasia, and a thick subepithelial collagen band (usually >10 μm), which entraps small capillaries and cellular

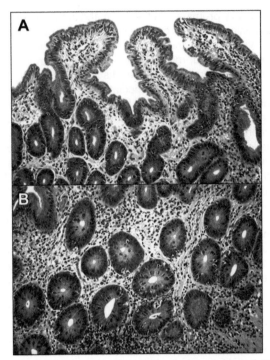

Fig. 3. Histopathologic findings in a patient with combined AE and CVID. (*A*) Duodenal biopsy shows moderate villous atrophy, surface intraepithelial lymphocytosis, and absence of goblet cells and Paneth cells (hematoxylin-eosin, ×200). (*B*) Duodenal biopsy shows absence of plasma cells, and increased apoptosis as well as mitotic figures in the deep crypt epithelium (hematoxylin-eosin, ×200).

elements in the lamina propria,[77] shown in **Fig. 4**. Cases of CS have been reported in individuals with CD, TS, and CVID, and have also been described as a manifestation of malignancy-related paraneoplastic syndromes.[75] Recent studies have highlighted a significant association of CS with CD (40%–86%), including patients with refractory CD.[39,75,78] However, a clear etiology of this disorder in some cases remains undetermined. Patients with CS were believed to have a uniformly poor prognosis with high morbidity (caused by severe malnutrition) and mortality, but more recent studies, from our institution and others, have shown that with current therapeutic management strategies, including active monitoring for adherence to a GFD and use of immunomodulatory drugs, patients with CS can have good clinical outcomes.[75,76]

A recent study has described cases of unspecified immune-mediated enteropathy as a common cause of nonceliac enteropathy manifesting villous atrophy.[79] Most patients had chronic diarrhea, abdominal pain, and weight loss. A second autoimmune disease was present in half (5 of 10 patients), and 5 of 9 (55.6%) patients tested were found to have low serum gammaglobulin levels, but none had antienterocyte antibodies. Most of the reported patients responded to immunosuppressive therapy, although a minority resolved spontaneously. However, the cause and pathogenesis of this condition are unknown at present and warrant further investigation.

As the recognition of milder degrees of mucosal injury and spectrum of histopathologic changes associated with CD has broadened, so has the list of differential diagnostic considerations. Because of the now better-appreciated complex nature and

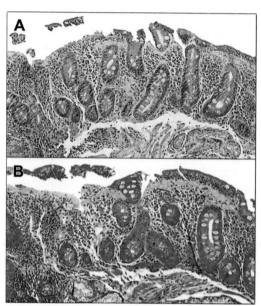

Fig. 4. Representative example of a case of CS associated with CD. (*A*) Thickened subepithelial basement membrane and fibrosis, epithelial denudation, and patchy intraepithelial lymphocytosis (hematoxylin-eosin, ×100). (*B*) Trichrome stain highlights a moderate degree of subepithelial fibrosis (Trichrome, ×100).

atypical presentation of CD, communication between pathologists and clinicians is of paramount importance to correctly interpret the clinical, histologic, and laboratory data. This communication is imperative, because a diagnosis of CD has a significant social impact and is associated with profound changes in an individual's lifestyle. An open dialogue between the pathologist and treating physician better enables inclusion or exclusion of CD as a cause of the patient's symptoms and engenders a clinically relevant discussion regarding important histopathologic findings and the possible differential diagnoses. The final diagnosis of CD should be made by an adult or pediatric gastroenterologist, factoring all the data including the histopathologic findings.

TEMPLATED PATHOLOGY REPORTING

A checklist-based, templated pathology report can be beneficial to ensure capturing and reporting of all relevant histopathologic features.[33] Such reports should include:

1. Site and number of biopsy specimens, with a comment on specimen orientation
2. Villous/crypt ratio
3. Presence and degree of villous atrophy
4. Increase in IELs (use of immunohistochemistry for CD3 in equivocal cases)
5. Presence/absence of surface epithelium damage
6. Presence of subepithelial collagen
7. Lamina propria inflammation (type and degree)
8. Other: clinical information and serology results, differential diagnoses deemed relevant, and histopathologic impression, consistent with or suggestive of CD. Classification of the lesion using the Marsh-Oberhuber or Corazza and Villanacci classification might be useful for comparison of cases from other institutes and for investigative work.

Use of such standardized reporting might not only help decrease the interobserver variability among pathologists with regard to reporting small bowel histopathology, as it ensures description of all histologic parameters, but may also increase the diagnosis of CD in the community.[80]

SUMMARY

CD is a common immune-mediated disorder affecting individuals worldwide that seems to be increasing in prevalence, as a result of a better understanding of the clinical manifestations associated with the disease, availability of more sensitive and specific serologic tests, and a better recognition of the histopathologic spectrum of CD. Small bowel biopsy remains the gold standard for diagnosing CD. Because of the changing presentation of disease and the recognition of many potential histopathologic mimics, communication between pathologists and gastroenterologists is essential for appropriate interpretation of small bowel biopsy specimens. Clinical, histopathologic, and laboratory data need to be assessed for appropriate diagnosis. This review provides helpful hints for the diagnostic assessment and reporting of CD histopathology, as well as an update on the extant classification schemes, with the hope of improving the rate of CD diagnosis among pathologists and gastroenterologists.

REFERENCES

1. Paulley JW. Observation on the aetiology of idiopathic steatorrhoea; jejunal and lymph-node biopsies. Br Med J 1954;2(4900):1318–21.
2. Shiner M. Duodenal biopsy. Lancet 1956;270(6906):17–9.
3. Marsh MN. Gluten, major histocompatibility complex and the small intestine: a molecular and immunobiologic approach to the spectrum of gluten sensitivity (celiac sprue). Gastroenterology 1992;102(1):330–54.
4. Oberhuber G, Granditsch G, Vogelsang H. The histopathology of celiac disease: time for a standardized report scheme for pathologists. Eur J Gastroenterol Hepatol 1999;11(10):1185–94.
5. NIH Consensus Development Conference on Celiac Disease. NIH Consens State Sci Statements 2004;21(1):1–23.
6. Rostom A, Murray JA, Kagnoff MF. American Gastroenterological Association (AGA) Institute technical review on the diagnosis and management of celiac disease. Gastroenterology 2006;131(6):1981–2002.
7. Ensari A. Gluten-sensitive enteropathy (celiac disease): controversies in diagnosis and classification. Arch Pathol Lab Med 2010;134(6):826–36.
8. Volta U, Villanacci V. Celiac disease: diagnostic criteria in progress. Cell Mol Immunol 2011;8(2):96–102.
9. Green PH, Rostami K, Marsh MN. Diagnosis of coeliac disease. Best Pract Res Clin Gastroenterol 2005;19(3):389–400.
10. Marsh MN, Crowe PT. Morphology of the mucosal lesion in gluten sensitivity. Baillieres Clin Gastroenterol 1995;9(2):273–93.
11. Hopper AD, Cross SS, Sanders DS. Patchy villous atrophy in adult patients with suspected gluten-sensitive enteropathy: is a multiple duodenal biopsy strategy appropriate? Endoscopy 2008;40(3):219–24.
12. Lebwohl B, Kapel RC, Neugut AI, et al. Adherence to biopsy guidelines increases celiac disease diagnosis. Gastrointest Endosc 2011;74(1):103–9.
13. Pais WP, Duerksen DR, Pettigrew NM, et al. How many duodenal biopsy specimens are required to make a diagnosis of celiac disease? Gastrointest Endosc 2008;67(7):1082–7.

14. Dickson BC, Streutker CJ, Chetty R. Coeliac disease: an update for pathologists. J Clin Pathol 2006;59(10):1008–16.
15. McNeish AS, Harms HK, Rey J, et al. The diagnosis of coeliac disease. A commentary on the current practices of members of the European Society for Paediatric Gastroenterology and Nutrition (ESPGAN). Arch Dis Child 1979; 54(10):783–6.
16. Goulet OJ, Brousse N, Canioni D, et al. Syndrome of intractable diarrhoea with persistent villous atrophy in early childhood: a clinicopathological survey of 47 cases. J Pediatr Gastroenterol Nutr 1998;26(2):151–61.
17. Granot E, Goodman-Weill M, Pizov G, et al. Histological comparison of suction capsule and endoscopic small intestinal mucosal biopsies in children. J Pediatr Gastroenterol Nutr 1993;16(4):397–401.
18. Meijer JW, Wahab PJ, Mulder CJ. Small intestinal biopsies in celiac disease: duodenal or jejunal? Virchows Arch 2003;442(2):124–8.
19. Rubin CE, Brandborg LL, Phelps PC, et al. Studies of celiac disease. I. The apparent identical and specific nature of the duodenal and proximal jejunal lesion in celiac disease and idiopathic sprue. Gastroenterology 1960;38:28–49.
20. Bonamico M, Thanasi E, Mariani P, et al. Duodenal bulb biopsies in celiac disease: a multicenter study. J Pediatr Gastroenterol Nutr 2008;47(5):618–22.
21. Gonzalez S, Gupta A, Cheng J, et al. Prospective study of the role of duodenal bulb biopsies in the diagnosis of celiac disease. Gastrointest Endosc 2010; 72(4):758–65.
22. Rashid M, MacDonald A. Importance of duodenal bulb biopsies in children for diagnosis of celiac disease in clinical practice. BMC Gastroenterol 2009;9(10): 78–85.
23. Segal GH, Petras RE. Small intestine. In: Sterberg SS, editor. Histology for pathologists. 2nd edition. Philadelphia: Lippincott-Raven; 1997. p. 495–518.
24. Philips AD. The small intestinal mucosa. In: Whitehead R, editor. Gastrointestinal and oesophageal pathology. New York: Churchill Livingstone; 1989. p. 29–39.
25. Goldstein NS. Proximal small-bowel mucosal villous intraepithelial lymphocytes. Histopathology 2004;44(3):199–205.
26. Goldstein NS, Underhill J. Morphologic features suggestive of gluten sensitivity in architecturally normal duodenal biopsy specimens. Am J Clin Pathol 2001;116(1): 63–71.
27. Järvinen TT, Collin P, Rasmussen M, et al. Villous tip intraepithelial lymphocytes as markers of early-stage coeliac disease. Scand J Gastroenterol 2004;39(5): 428–33.
28. Biagi F, Luinetti O, Campanella J, et al. Intraepithelial lymphocytes in the villous tip: do they indicate potential coeliac disease? J Clin Pathol 2004;57(8):835–9.
29. Hayat M, Cairns A, Dixon MF, et al. Quantitation of intraepithelial lymphocytes in human duodenum: what is normal? J Clin Pathol 2002;55(5):393–4.
30. Veress B, Franzén L, Bodin L, et al. Duodenal intraepithelial lymphocyte-count revisited. Scand J Gastroenterol 2004;39(2):138–44.
31. Mäki M, Holm K, Collin P, et al. Increase in gamma/delta T cell receptor bearing lymphocytes in normal small bowel mucosa in latent coeliac disease. Gut 1991; 32(11):1412–4.
32. Halstensen TS, Scott H, Brandtzaeg P. Intraepithelial T cells of the TcR gamma/ delta+ CD8- and V delta 1/J delta 1+ phenotypes are increased in coeliac disease. Scand J Immunol 1989;30(6):665–72.
33. Bao F, Green PH, Bhagat G. An update on celiac disease histopathology and the road ahead. Arch Pathol Lab Med 2012;136(7):735–45.

34. Volta U, Molinaro N, Fusconi M, et al. IgA antiendomysial antibody test. A step forward in celiac disease screening. Dig Dis Sci 1991;36(6):752–6.
35. Lerner A, Kumar V, Iancu TC. Immunological diagnosis of childhood coeliac disease: comparison between antigliadin, antireticulin and antiendomysial antibodies. Clin Exp Immunol 1994;95(1):78–82.
36. Sollid LM, Molberg O, McAdam S, et al. Autoantibodies in coeliac disease: tissue transglutaminase–guilt by association? Gut 1997;41(6):851–2.
37. Dieterich W, Laag E, Schöpper H, et al. Autoantibodies to tissue transglutaminase as predictors of celiac disease. Gastroenterology 1998;115(6):1317–21.
38. Corazza GR, Villanacci V. Coeliac disease. J Clin Pathol 2005;58(6):573–4.
39. Cellier C, Delabesse E, Helmer C, et al. Refractory sprue, coeliac disease, and enteropathy-associated T-cell lymphoma. French Coeliac Disease Study Group. Lancet 2000;356(9225):203–8.
40. Bagdi E, Diss TC, Munson P, et al. Mucosal intra-epithelial lymphocytes in enteropathy-associated T-cell lymphoma, ulcerative jejunitis, and refractory celiac disease constitute a neoplastic population. Blood 1999;94(1):260–4.
41. Farstad IN, Lundin KE. Gastrointestinal intraepithelial lymphocytes and T cell lymphomas. Gut 2003;52(2):163–4.
42. Corazza GR, Villanacci V, Zambelli C, et al. Comparison of the interobserver reproducibility with different histologic criteria used in celiac disease. Clin Gastroenterol Hepatol 2007;5(7):838–43.
43. Abrams JA, Diamond B, Rotterdam H, et al. Seronegative celiac disease: increased prevalence with lesser degrees of villous atrophy. Dig Dis Sci 2004; 49(4):546–50.
44. Donaldson MR, Book LS, Leiferman KM, et al. Strongly positive tissue transglutaminase antibodies are associated with Marsh 3 histopathology in adult and pediatric celiac disease. J Clin Gastroenterol 2008;42(3):256–60.
45. Wahab PJ, Meijer JW, Mulder CJ. Histologic follow-up of people with celiac disease on a gluten-free diet: slow and incomplete recovery. Am J Clin Pathol 2002;118(3):459–63.
46. Lanzini A, Lanzarotto F, Villanacci V, et al. Complete recovery of intestinal mucosa occurs very rarely in adult coeliac patients despite adherence to gluten-free diet. Aliment Pharmacol Ther 2009;29(12):1299–308.
47. Rubio-Tapia A, Rahim MW, See JA, et al. Mucosal recovery and mortality in adults with celiac disease after treatment with a gluten-free diet. Am J Gastroenterol 2010;105(6):1412–20.
48. Hopper AD, Hadjivassiliou M, Hurlstone DP, et al. What is the role of serologic testing in celiac disease? A prospective, biopsy-confirmed study with economic analysis. Clin Gastroenterol Hepatol 2008;6(3):314–20.
49. Catassi C, Fasano A. Celiac disease diagnosis: simple rules are better than complicated algorithms. Am J Med 2010;123(8):691–3.
50. Murray JA. It's not time to put away the biopsy forceps. Am J Gastroenterol 1999; 94(4):869–71.
51. Rostami K, Kerckhaert J, Tiemessen R, et al. Sensitivity of antiendomysium and antigliadin antibodies in untreated celiac disease: disappointing in clinical practice. Am J Gastroenterol 1999;94(4):888–94.
52. Salmi TT, Collin P, Reunala T, et al. Diagnostic methods beyond conventional histology in coeliac disease diagnosis. Dig Liver Dis 2010;42(1):28–32.
53. Sugai E, Hwang HJ, Vázquez H, et al. New serology assays can detect gluten sensitivity among enteropathy patients seronegative for anti-tissue transglutaminase. Clin Chem 2010;56(4):661–5.

54. Salmi TT, Collin P, Järvinen O, et al. Immunoglobulin A autoantibodies against transglutaminase 2 in the small intestinal mucosa predict forthcoming coeliac disease. Aliment Pharmacol Ther 2006;24(3):541–52.
55. Collin P, Kaukinen K, Mäki M. Duodenal intraepithelial lymphocytosis: celiac disease or not? Am J Gastroenterol 2009;104(7):1847 [author reply: 1848].
56. Brown I, Mino-Kenudson M, Deshpande V, et al. Intraepithelial lymphocytosis in architecturally preserved proximal small intestinal mucosa: an increasing diagnostic problem with a wide differential diagnosis. Arch Pathol Lab Med 2006; 130(7):1020–5.
57. Memeo L, Jhang J, Hibshoosh H, et al. Duodenal intraepithelial lymphocytosis with normal villous architecture: common occurrence in *H. pylori* gastritis. Mod Pathol 2005;18(8):1134–44.
58. Kakar S, Nehra V, Murray JA, et al. Significance of intraepithelial lymphocytosis in small bowel biopsy samples with normal mucosal architecture. Am J Gastroenterol 2003;98(9):2027–33.
59. Mahadeva S, Wyatt JI, Howdle PD. Is a raised intraepithelial lymphocyte count with normal duodenal villous architecture clinically relevant? J Clin Pathol 2002; 55(6):424–8.
60. Day DW, Jass JR, Price AB, et al. Morson and Dawson's gastrointestinal pathology. Malden (MA): Blackwell; 2003.
61. Wheby MS, Swanson VL, Bayless TM. Comparison of ileal and jejunal biopsies in tropical sprue. Am J Clin Nutr 1971;24(1):117–23.
62. Walker MM. What is tropical sprue? J Gastroenterol Hepatol 2003;18:887–90.
63. Le Bras S, Geha RS. IPEX and the role of Foxp3 in the development and function of human Tregs. J Clin Invest 2006;116(6):1473–5.
64. Montalto M, D'Onofrio F, Santoro L, et al. Autoimmune enteropathy in children and adults. Scand J Gastroenterol 2009;44(9):1029–36.
65. Russo PA, Brochu P, Seidman EG, et al. Autoimmune enteropathy. Pediatr Dev Pathol 1999;2(1):65–71.
66. Corazza GR, Biagi F, Volta U, et al. Autoimmune enteropathy and villous atrophy in adults. Lancet 1997;350(9071):106–9.
67. Akram S, Murray JA, Pardi DS, et al. Adult autoimmune enteropathy: Mayo Clinic Rochester experience. Clin Gastroenterol Hepatol 2007;5(11):1282–90.
68. Washington K, Stenzel TT, Buckley RH, et al. Gastrointestinal pathology in patients with common variable immunodeficiency and X-linked agammaglobulinemia. Am J Surg Pathol 1996;20(10):1240–52.
69. Ament ME, Ochs HD, Davis SD. Structure and function of the gastrointestinal tract in primary immunodeficiency syndromes. A study of 39 patients. Medicine (Baltimore) 1973;52(3):227–48.
70. Malamut G, Verkarre V, Suarez F, et al. The enteropathy associated with common variable immunodeficiency: the delineated frontiers with celiac disease. Am J Gastroenterol 2010;105(10):2262–75.
71. Chahal P, Weiler CR, Murray JA. Common variable immune deficiency and gastrointestinal tract. Gastroenterology 2005;128(Suppl):A-502, T1552.
72. Bili H, Nizou C, Nizou JY, et al. Common variable immunodeficiency and total villous atrophy regressive after gluten-free diet. Rev Med Interne 1997;18(9): 724–6.
73. Teahon K, Webster AD, Price AB, et al. Studies on the enteropathy associated with primary hypogammaglobulinaemia. Gut 1994;35(9):1244–9.
74. Catassi C, Mirakian R, Natalini G, et al. Unresponsive enteropathy associated with circulating enterocyte autoantibodies in a boy with common variable

hypogammaglobulinemia and type I diabetes. J Pediatr Gastroenterol Nutr 1988; 7(4):608–13.

75. Vakiani E, Arguelles-Grande C, Mansukhani MM, et al. Collagenous sprue is not always associated with dismal outcomes: a clinicopathological study of 19 patients. Mod Pathol 2010;23(1):12–26.

76. Maguire AA, Greenson JK, Lauwers GY, et al. Collagenous sprue: a clinicopathologic study of 12 cases. Am J Surg Pathol 2009;33(10):1440–9.

77. Zhao X, Johnson RL. Collagenous sprue: a rare, severe small-bowel malabsorptive disorder. Arch Pathol Lab Med 2011;135(6):803–9.

78. Robert ME, Ament ME, Weinstein WM. The histologic spectrum and clinical outcome of refractory and unclassified sprue. Am J Surg Pathol 2000;24(5): 676–87.

79. Pallav K, Leffler DA, Tariq S, et al. Noncoeliac enteropathy: the differential diagnosis of villous atrophy in contemporary clinical practice. Aliment Pharmacol Ther 2012;35(3):380–90.

80. Arguelles-Grande C, Tennyson CA, Lewis SK, et al. Variability in small bowel histopathology reporting between different pathology practice settings: impact on the diagnosis of coeliac disease. J Clin Pathol 2012;65(3):242–7.

Management of Celiac Disease

Ikram Nasr, MD[a],*, Daniel A. Leffler, MD[b], Paul J. Ciclitira, MD[c]

KEYWORDS

- Gluten-free diet • Small bowel biopsy • Follow-up • Complications • Osteoporosis

KEY POINTS

- Celiac disease (CD) is an enteropathy-induced immune response that occurs on exposure to toxic gluten in the diet and is reversible once gluten is withdrawn.
- A gluten-free diet is the preferred treatment for CD and leads to reversal of villous atrophy.
- Counseling, nutritional support, and follow-up are vital aspects in CD management.
- The pickup rate of CD has improved with the availability of serologic tests, and this has led to a reduction in morbidity in treated CD cases.
- Managing CD can potentially prevent or cure some of the associated conditions, such as neurologic complications, nutritional deficiencies, and osteoporosis.

INTRODUCTION

Celiac disease (CD) is an abnormal immune response to ingestion of gluten, which results in small intestine inflammation. The clinical and histologic manifestations of this process are potentially reversible when gluten is excluded from the diet. *Gluten* is a generic term used to collectively describe all the cereal proteins that are toxic to individuals with CD.[1] Wheat, barley, and rye have all been shown to cause intestinal inflammation in patients with CD. The classical presentation historically referred to a disease occurring in children younger than 2 years characterized by symptoms of malabsorption and poor growth.[2,3] These events typically occur after gluten is introduced into the diet. A trend is being seen toward fewer patients presenting with symptomatic CD characterized by diarrhea, with a significant shift toward more patients presenting as asymptomatic adults with CD detected at screening.[4]

CD can be associated with other conditions, such as autoimmune disorders and malignancy. The morbidity and mortality of patients with untreated CD is higher compared with those of healthy individuals. Rubio-Tapia and colleagues[5] studied 9133 healthy young adults at Warren Air Force Base (sera were collected between

[a] Department of Gastroenterology, Guy's and St Thomas' Hospitals NHS Trust, Westminster Bridge Road, London SE1 7EH, UK; [b] Division of Gastroenterology, Beth Israel Deaconess Medical Center, 330 Brookline Avenue, Rabb 420, Boston, MA 02215, USA; [c] Division of Diabetes and Nutrition, Department of Gastroenterology, Rayne Institute, St Thomas' Hospitals NHS Trust, Westminster Bridge Road, London SE1 7EH, UK
* Corresponding author.
E-mail address: ikram.nasr@gstt.nhs.uk

Gastrointest Endoscopy Clin N Am 22 (2012) 695–704
http://dx.doi.org/10.1016/j.giec.2012.07.012
1052-5157/12/$ – see front matter © 2012 Published by Elsevier Inc.

giendo.theclinics.com

1948 and 1954) and 12,768 gender-matched subjects from 2 recent cohorts from Olmsted County, Minnesota, with either similar years of birth (n = 5558) or age at sampling (n = 7210) to that of the Air Force cohort. Sera were tested for tissue trans-glutaminase and, if abnormal, for endomysial antibodies. Survival was measured during a follow-up period of 45 years in the Air Force cohort. The prevalence of undi-agnosed CD was 0.2%. During 45 years of follow-up in the older cohort, all-cause mortality was nearly 4-fold greater in persons with undiagnosed CD than among those who were seronegative.

The standard treatment for CD is adhering to a gluten-free diet (GFD), which involves avoiding substances containing toxic gluten, such as wheat, rye, and barley products.[6] Evidence has shown the long-term safety of oats as part of a GFD in patients with CD.[7] However, 5% to 10% may experience a response, because some people have small intestinal T cells that react to oat avenins.[8]

It is equally important to educate patients about the disease diagnosis and prog-nosis, which increases their knowledge about their condition and improves their adherence to the GFD. Patients should be counseled by a dietitian knowledgeable about the condition. Morbidities associated with CD must be addressed and managed when necessary, and preventative measures should also be taken, as detailed in the following sections.

DIETARY TREATMENT
Gluten Exclusion

The cornerstone of therapy is lifelong adherence to a GFD, which involves the exclu-sion of foods containing wheat, rye, and barley. Gluten-free foods by definition should not contain more than 20 mg/kg of gluten.[9] In one study, as little as 50 mg/d was suffi-cient to cause mucosal damage after 3 months.[10] Ingestion of oats is generally safe in CD, but because oats are often contaminated with toxic gluten from wheat and other grains, only oats from a dedicated gluten free source are recommended for inclusion in the GFD. Evidence suggests that oats are not harmful to most individuals with CD.[7,11–14] However, most commercially available oat flour is contaminated with 10% to 15% wheat.

Avoiding cereals containing toxic gluten is a formidable task, because these are found in bread, biscuits, cakes, pastries, breakfast cereals, pasta, beer, and most soups, sauces, and puddings.

Gluten elimination leads to some lifestyle restrictions. As a result, compliance with a strict GFD is limited.[15] Noncompliance is especially likely in patients who are less symptomatic or have better tolerance to gluten. The most common reasons for a lack of response are poor compliance or inadvertent gluten ingestion (**Box 1**).[16,17]

All patients should see a dietician with experience in CD. The dietician should provide formal education about following a GFD. Attention should be given to food labeling and potential pitfalls, and counseling should be provided on weight manage-ment.[18,19] Written information ideally should be provided, and referral to a support group is helpful because it provides individual with CD access to emotional and psychological support and information on the latest GFD products. Through these support groups, patients can share their experiences and develop the sense of not being alone in dealing with this disease. Ideally, a second appointment should be offered after 3 to 6 months to check and answer any questions that have arisen and assess adherence. Further details regarding dietary assessment are discussed in a separate article elsewhere in this issue ("Dietary Assessment in Celiac Disease").

Patients may supplement their diet with commercial gluten-free products. Many gluten-free flours and bread mixes are based on purified wheat starch from which

Box 1
Common sources of hidden gluten

- Sausages and beef burgers
- Luncheon meat
- Imitation crab meat
- Gravy powder and browning
- Self-basting turkeys
- Soups
- Brown rice syrup
- Soy sauce and other sauces
- Chutneys and pickles
- White pepper
- Supplements
- Some pharmaceutical products
- Oatmeal contaminated with gluten
- Communion wafers
- Instant coffee
- Potato crisps/chips
- Licorice
- Curry powder
- Some medicines containing starch or wheat derivatives
- Farina
- Matzo flour/meal
- Hydrolyzed vegetable protein
- Meat and fish pastes
- Salad dressings
- Hard candy
- Some toothpastes
- Play dough
- Some lipsticks
- Malt vinegar
- Some chocolates and drinking chocolate
- Mustards
- Blue cheese
- Shredded suet
- Baked beans
- Paté
- Seitan

most gluten proteins have been removed. Most patients with CD tolerate these products well, although a minority cannot.[20] These individuals should be advised to follow a strict GFD for which they ingest only commercial non–wheat starch–based gluten-free products. Symptomatic patients may be advised to avoid excessive milk ingestion in the first 6 months of following a GFD. Up to 70% of individuals with CD respond promptly to a GFD, showing improvement of symptoms within weeks or days.[21] In one study of 158 patients with CD evaluating the histologic recovery after initiation of a GFD showed an improvement in 65% of the patients within 2 years, 85.3% within 5 years, and 89.9% after 5 years of follow-up.[22]

Adhering to a strict GFD is particularly important, not only to improve symptoms and general well-being but also because of the significant effects on morbidity and mortality. With continued gluten ingestion, the resulting enteropathy may eventually lead to complications, such as osteoporosis, anemia, and vitamin D, copper, and zinc deficiency. These deficiencies can be partially reversed with a GFD.[23] Prompt and strict dietary treatment decreases all-cause mortality in patients with CD who adhere to a GFD.[24–27]

Some gluten-free products may contain trace amounts of gluten, and gluten contamination can also occur. This ingestion does not necessarily lead to treatment failure. The accepted daily intake of gluten in CD is 20 parts per million (ppm). One study involving 76 adults with CD evaluated the intake of 59 naturally gluten-free and 24 wheat starch–based gluten-free products. The gluten in these diets was quantified, and the intake of these products was compared with mucosal histology. Several naturally gluten-free (13 of 59) and wheat starch–based gluten-free (11 of 24) products were found to contain gluten from 20 to 200 ppm. The median daily flour consumption was 80 g (range: 10–300 g). Within these limits, the long-term mucosal recovery was good. Results of this study suggested that the safe level of gluten consumption is 100 ppm.[28] The exact daily gluten intake is difficult to quantify, because the actual gluten content of a typical GFD is unknown. Some medications may contain minimal gluten and must be avoided.

Total Versus Partial Gluten Exclusion

The risk of developing small intestinal lymphoma is increased in patients with CD who ingest a diet containing gluten.[29] Nutritional deficiencies are also more likely to occur. Therefore, recommending a strict GFD seems reasonable, even if patients are asymptomatic with a low gluten intake. Good dietary compliance should reduce the risk of osteoporosis in later life.

Need for Lifelong Treatment

Some adolescents might stop adhering to a GFD because they mistaken believe that they have "grown out of" their CD. If the diagnosis is doubted, a gluten challenge and repeat jejunal biopsy should be undertaken. If the diagnosis is established, lifelong treatment should be recommended.

Information and Support

Adherence to a GFD is not easy. Adolescence is often a particularly difficult time, when young patients may feel excluded from their peer group by their dietary restriction. Therefore, careful explanation and counseling is of great value, and the role of dietitians is vital to this process. Written advice should be provided whenever possible, and all patients should be encouraged to join celiac support groups.

CORRECTING NUTRITIONAL DEFICIENCIES
Vitamin D and Calcium Deficiency

Many individuals with CD have osteopenia (and less often osteoporosis). It can occur in patients without gastrointestinal symptoms.[23,30–32] Patients with advanced disease may have bone pain or deformity, but most patients are asymptomatic or have only hypocalcemia or raised serum levels of alkaline phosphatase.[33] Osteoporosis in CD is likely to be related to calcium malabsorption. Hypocalcemia can result in secondary hyperparathyroidism, which subsequently leads to increased bone turnover and cortical bone loss.[34] Vitamin D plays a less important role in osteopenia and osteoporosis in CD. However, individuals with CD may develop osteomalacia before they are diagnosed, which may affect the results of a dual-energy x-ray absorptiometry (DEXA) scan. In this case, vitamin D replacement is required.[35] The bone mineral density is positively related to calcium intake, body mass index, and menopausal age.[36] Significant improvement is seen 1 year after starting a GFD.[37] Loss of bone density in the peripheral skeleton may persist despite apparent normalization at axial skeletal sites.[38]

Considering a DEXA scan is usual practice for adults with newly diagnosed CD 1 year after initiation of a GFD, to allow for stabilization of bone density.[39] DEXA scans are not generally required in newly diagnosed pediatric patients with uncomplicated CD.[39] This evaluation may be repeated after 1 year in patients with osteopenia to monitor changes in the bone mineral density and response to treatment.[40] Vitamin D and calcium supplementation should be given to those deemed to be at high risk for osteoporosis or with proven osteoporosis. Younger men and premenopausal women require 1000 mg/d of elemental calcium, whereas men and women older than 50 years require up to 1500 mg/d. Vitamin D at a dosage of 400 to 800 IU/d is usually adequate in healthy individuals. Dosages of 1000 IU/d to 50,000 IU/wk may be required. Osteoporosis or worsening osteopenia may warrant treatment with bisphosphonates.

Other Nutritional Deficiencies

Many patients will be found to have dietary deficiencies at diagnosis, the most common being iron, zinc, folic acid, calcium, and vitamin B_{12}. Although these usually resolve spontaneously once the patient is following a GFD, it is reasonable to ensure rapid correction with appropriate supplements.

Iron, folic acid, calcium, vitamin D, and, rarely, thiamine, vitamin B_6, and B_{12} deficiency should be tested for and corrected. In more severe cases, mineral deficiencies (eg, copper, selenium, magnesium) can occur and should be replaced.

Patients with CD should be screened for nutritional deficiencies at the time of diagnosis (eg, parathyroid hormone; blood count; iron studies; vitamins A, E, and D; electrolytes; albumin; total protein; liver enzymes; clotting). They should have a follow-up appointment 3 to 6 months later to discuss any issues that may arise and ensure dietary compliance. This appointment is an opportunity to assess for any signs of complications and other autoimmune conditions. Patients should also be reviewed 1 year after starting a GFD and screened again for nutritional deficiency. If they are doing well, they could then be reviewed annually. If complications or poor compliance with diet are noted, they could be re-referred to the dietitian for counseling and education on maintaining a GFD.[41]

HYPOSPLENISM

Splenic dysfunction may occur secondary to a variety of reasons. In routine clinical practice, liver disease or CD are probably the 2 most common causes.[42] Patients with CD may have a degree of hyposplenism, which increases the risk of infections. Therefore, prophylactic pneumococcal vaccination should be offered.[43]

DERMATITIS HERPETIFORMIS

Dermatitis herpetiformis (DH) complicates 2% to 5% of cases of CD, and most cases of DH exhibit a degree of enteropathy. It is the most common skin disorder associated with CD.[44]

Improvement in DH after withdrawal of gluten may take between 6 and 12 months to occur compared with the response of the gastrointestinal clinical manifestations of the disease.[45] Dapsone is the preferred drug for achieving a rapid response, although it does have significant side effects. Patients should adhere strictly to the GFD, because this results in a significant improvement after 6 to 12 months and permits a reduction in the dose of, or elimination of the need for, dapsone. A few individuals are unable to tolerate dapsone because of side effects, which include a dose-dependent hemolytic anemia, methemoglobinemia, and headache. These patients can alternatively be treated with sulphapyridine.

MALIGNANCY
Lymphoma

The mechanism through which CD predisposes to intestinal lymphoma is unknown, although the association is not doubted. The commonest presentation involves the return of symptoms of diarrhea, associated with both weight loss and lassitude in patients with established CD. Standard investigations, including jejunal biopsy and small bowel barium studies, are likely to have a low yield, even when the lymphoma is suspected, because of the associated subtotal villous atrophy. The histologic appearance of peripheral lymph nodes, the liver, or bone marrow may be diagnostic, and ultrasound, CT, or nuclear MRI may be useful. Small bowel enteroscopy may be helpful through allowing direct visualization and biopsy of a greater proportion of the small intestine. Laparotomy or laparoscopy, with lymph node, liver, and full-thickness intestinal biopsies, is a useful diagnostic tool, and often the only way to achieve a definitive diagnosis. Treatment is difficult and usually involves surgery, radiotherapy, and chemotherapy. In addition to the rare enteropathy-associated T-cell lymphoma, patients with CD have an increased risk of non-Hodgkin's lymphoma.

Small Bowel Adenocarcinoma

Patients with CD have an increased risk of small bowel adenocarcinoma. It often presents with nonspecific symptoms, and diagnosis is often significantly delayed. As a result, patients often present with metastatic disease with poor prognosis. Surgery with consideration of chemotherapy is the mainstay of treatment. An increased prevalence of carcinoma of the esophagus is also seen.

ULCERATIVE JEJUNOILEITIS

Ulcerative jejunoileitis is an unusual complication in which unresponsive CD is associated with ulceration and structuring. The discrimination between this entity and lymphoma can normally only be made at surgery, and in some instances lymphoma seems to have developed on a background of jejunoileitis. Patients should be advised to continue with a GFD, but early surgery is indicated if symptoms do not resolve.

MICROSCOPIC COLITIS

Most patients experience concomitant colitis, which in some cases may be microscopic or lymphocytic. Appropriate therapy should be given, involving the use of mesalazine, bismuth, or, in resistant cases, low-dose systemic steroids.

AUTOIMMUNE DISEASES

Some studies found an association between duration of exposure to gluten in patients with CD and the development of other autoimmune disorders (such as type 1 diabetes mellitus, connective tissue diseases, Hashimoto thyroiditis, and Graves disease).[46,47] Other studies did not show a correlation between gluten exposure and development of autoimmune conditions.[48]

OTHER COMPLICATIONS
Lack of Dietary Fiber and Constipation

A GFD is low in fiber, and therefore symptoms of constipation or irritable bowel syndrome may be exacerbated. Adding roughage to the diet can avoid this problem, such as in the form of linseeds or psyllium seed husks.

Carbohydrate Intolerance

Carbohydrate intolerance may occur and individuals with ongoing symptoms despite gluten avoidance should be assessed for lactose, fructose or other intolorances.

Small Bowel Bacterial Overgrowth

In simple cases, small bowel bacterial overgrowth can be managed with probiotics. In more severe cases, antimicrobials that target intestinal microorganisms may need to be used.

Infertility

Infertility is common in undiagnosed and untreated patients. It can be avoided with patient education and a strict GFD.

Neurologic Complications

Neurologic complications may occur, although rarely. The risk is minimized through patient adherence to a GFD and replacement of nutritional deficiencies.

FOLLOW-UP

Patients diagnosed with CD should be offered a follow-up appointment to review their symptoms and answer any questions that may arise. Follow-up of patients with CD is vital to assess adherence to a GFD and prevent complications through early detection and management. Some experts suggest a repeat small bowel biopsy 4 to 6 months after commencing a strict GFD to assess adherence and response to treatment.[49] Other specialists in this field recommend performing a repeat small bowel biopsy in 1 to 2 years. Another approach is to follow-up with patients in 12 months and monitor response and adherence based on celiac serology.[41] No standard guidance or data exist to support any of these practiced methods, and many professionals follow the guidelines of their local institute or practice.

REFERENCES

1. Ludvigsson JF, Leffler DA, Bai JC, et al. The Oslo definitions for coeliac disease and related terms. Gut 2012. [Epub ahead of print].
2. Catassi C, Fasano A. New developments in childhood celiac disease. Curr Gastroenterol Rep 2002;4:238–43.
3. Talley NJ, Valdovinos M, Petterson TM, et al. Epidemiology of celiac sprue: a community-based study. Am J Gastroenterol 1994;89:843–6.
4. Rampertab SD, Pooran N, Brar P, et al. Trends in presentation of celiac disease. Am J Med 2006;119(4):355.e9–355.e14.
5. Rubio-Tapia A, Kyle RA, Kaplan EL, et al. Increased prevalence and mortality in undiagnosed celiac disease. Gastroenterology 2009;137(1):88–93.
6. Scanlon SA, Murray JA. Update on celiac disease—etiology, differential diagnosis, drug targets, and management advances. Clin Exp Gastroenterol 2011; 4:297–311.
7. Kemppainen TA, Heikkinen MT, Ristikankare MK, et al. Unkilned and large amounts of oats in the coeliac disease diet: a randomized, controlled study. Scand J Gastroenterol 2008;43:1094–101.
8. Lundin KE, Nilsen EM, Scott HG, et al. Oats induced villous atrophy in coeliac disease. Gut 2003;52:1649–52.
9. Selimoğlu MA, Karabiber H. Celiac disease: prevention and treatment. J Clin Gastroenterol 2010;44(1):4–8.
10. Catassi C, Fabiani E, Iacono G, et al. A prospective, double-blind, placebo-controlled trial to establish a safe gluten threshold for patients with celiac disease. Am J Clin Nutr 2007;85(1):160–6.
11. Koskinen O, Villanen M, Korponay-Szabo I, et al. Oats do not induce systemic or mucosal autoantibody response in children with coeliac disease. J Pediatr Gastroenterol Nutr 2009;48:559–65.
12. Holm K, Maki M, Vuolteenaho N, et al. Oats in the treatment of childhood coeliac disease: a 2-year controlled trial and a long-term clinical follow-up study. Aliment Pharmacol Ther 2006;23:1463–72.
13. Peraaho M, Kaukinen K, Mustalahti K, et al. Effect of an oats-containing gluten-free diet on symptoms and quality of life in coeliac disease. A randomized study. Scand J Gastroenterol 2004;39:27–31.
14. Garsed K, Scott BB. Can oats be taken in a gluten-free diet? A systematic review. Scand J Gastroenterol 2007;42:171–8.
15. Hall NJ, Rubin G, Charnock A. Systematic review: adherence to a gluten-free diet in adult patients with coeliac disease. Aliment Pharmacol Ther 2009;30: 315.
16. Abdulkarim AS, Burgart LJ, See J, et al. Etiology of nonresponsive celiac disease: results of a systematic approach. Am J Gastroenterol 2002;97:2016.
17. Leffler DA, Dennis M, Hyett B, et al. Etiologies and predictors of diagnosis in nonresponsive celiac disease. Clin Gastroenterol Hepatol 2007;5:445.
18. Cataldo F, Motalto G. CD in the developing countries: a new and challenging public health problem. World J Gastroenterol 2007;13(15):2153–9.
19. Ascher H, Krantz I, Kristiansson B. Increasing incidence of coeliac disease in Sweden. Arch Dis Child 1991;66(5):608–11.
20. Ciclitira PJ, Cerio R, Ellis HJ, et al. Evaluation of a gliadin-containing gluten-free product in coeliac patients. Hum Nutr Clin Nutr 1985;39(4):303–8.
21. Murray JA, Watson T, Clearman B, et al. Effect of a gluten-free diet on gastrointestinal symptoms in celiac disease. Am J Clin Nutr 2004;79:669–73.

22. Wahab PJ, Meijer JW, Mulder CJ. Histologic follow-up of people with celiac disease on a gluten-free diet: slow and incomplete recovery. Am J Clin Pathol 2002;118:459–63.
23. Shaker JL, Brickner RC, Findling JW, et al. Hypocalcemia and skeletal disease as presenting features of celiac disease. Arch Intern Med 1997;157:1013.
24. Holmes GK, Prior P, Lane MR, et al. Malignancy in coeliac disease–effect of a gluten free diet. Gut 1989;30:333.
25. Corrao G, Corazza GR, Bagnardi V, et al. Mortality in patients with coeliac disease and their relatives: a cohort study. Lancet 2001;358:356.
26. Askling J, Linet M, Gridley G, et al. Cancer incidence in a population-based cohort of individuals hospitalized with celiac disease or dermatitis herpetiformis. Gastroenterology 2002;123:1428.
27. Collin P, Reunala T, Pukkala E, et al. Coeliac disease–associated disorders and survival. Gut 1994;35:1215.
28. Collin P, Thorell L, Kaukinen K, et al. The safe threshold for gluten contamination in gluten-free products. Can trace amounts be accepted in the treatment of coeliac disease? Aliment Pharmacol Ther 2004;19:1277.
29. Kumar P. Coeliac disease and lymphoma. Eur J Gastroenterol Hepatol 2006;18: 131–2.
30. Walters JR, Banks LM, Butcher GP, et al. Detection of low bone mineral density by dual energy x ray absorptiometry in unsuspected suboptimally treated coeliac disease. Gut 1995;37:220.
31. Mustalahti K, Collin P, Sievänen H, et al. Osteopenia in patients with clinically silent coeliac disease warrants screening. Lancet 1999;354:744.
32. Meyer D, Stavropolous S, Diamond B, et al. Osteoporosis in a north American adult population with celiac disease. Am J Gastroenterol 2001;96:112.
33. Cooke WT, Holmes GK. Clinical presentation. In: Cooke WT, Holmes GK, editors. Coeliac disease. London: Churchill Livingston; 1984. p. 90.
34. Walters JR. Bone mineral density in coeliac disease. Gut 1994;35:150–1.
35. Scott EM, Gaywood I, Scott BB. Guidelines for osteoporosis in coeliac disease and inflammatory bowel disease. Gut 2000;46:i1–8.
36. McFarlane XA, Bhalla AK, Reeves DE, et al. Osteoporosis in treated adult coeliac disease. Gut 1995;36:710–4.
37. Valdimarsson T, Lofman O, Toss G, et al. Reversal of osteopenia with diet in adult coeliac disease. Gut 1996;38:322–7.
38. Selby PL, Davies M, Adams JE, et al. Bone loss in celiac disease is related to secondary hyperparathyroidism. J Bone Miner Res 1999;14:652.
39. American Gastroenterological Association medical position statement: guidelines on osteoporosis in gastrointestinal diseases. Gastroenterology 2003;124:791–4.
40. Scott EM, Gaywood I, Scott BB. Guidelines for osteoporosis in coeliac disease and inflammatory bowel disease. British Society of Gastroenterology. Gut 2000; 46(Suppl 1):i1–8.
41. Pietzak MM. Follow-up of patients with celiac disease: achieving compliance with treatment. Gastroenterology 2005;128:S135–41.
42. Brigden ML, Pattullo AL. Prevention and management of overwhelming postsplenectomy infection-An update. Crit Care Med 1999;27(4):836–42.
43. McKinley M, Leibowitz S, Bronzo R, et al. Appropriate response to pneumococcal vaccine in celiac sprue. J Clin Gastroenterol 1995;20(2):113–6.
44. Fry L. Dermatitis herpetiformis. Baillieres Clin Gastroenterol 1995;9:371.
45. Garioch JJ, Lewis HM, Sargent SA, et al. 25 years' experience of a gluten-free diet in the treatment of dermatitis herpetiformis. Br J Dermatol 1994;131:541.

46. Ventura A, Magazzù G, Greco L. Duration of exposure to gluten and risk for auto-immune disorders in patients with celiac disease. SIGEP Study Group for Autoimmune Disorders in Celiac Disease. Gastroenterology 1999;117:297.

47. Cosnes J, Cellier C, Viola S, et al. Incidence of autoimmune diseases in celiac disease: protective effect of the gluten-free diet. Clin Gastroenterol Hepatol 2008;6:753.

48. Sategna Guidetti C, Solerio E, Scaglione N, et al. Duration of gluten exposure in adult coeliac disease does not correlate with the risk for autoimmune disorders. Gut 2001;49:502.

49. Lee SK, Lo W, Memeo L, et al. Duodenal histology in patients with celiac disease after treatment with a gluten-free diet. Gastrointest Endosc 2003;57(2):187–91.

Mortality and Malignancy in Celiac Disease

Jonas F. Ludvigsson, MD, PhD[a,b,c,*]

KEYWORDS

- Autoimmunity • Cancer • Celiac • Death • Epidemiology • Gluten • Lymphoma
- Malignancy

KEY POINTS

- Patients with celiac disease (CD) are at a small increased risk of death.
- With the exception of an increased risk from lymphoproliferative malignancy, and potentially a small increased risk of gastrointestinal cancer, patients with CD do not seem to be at increased risk of malignancy.
- Undiagnosed CD is unlikely to confer a more than marginally increased risk of mortality or malignancy (if any), but follow-up in most earlier studies may have been insufficient to rule out excess mortality.
- The evidence that a GFD reduces the risk of mortality is weak, but there is some evidence suggesting that a GFD may reduce the risk of lymphoproliferative malignancy.

INTRODUCTION

Celiac disease (CD) is a chronic immune-mediated disease characterized by inflammation and villous atrophy (VA) in the small intestine.[1] It is found in people worldwide, occurring in about 1% to 2% of the Western population.[2,3]

Many patients with CD remain undiagnosed for several years before receiving a correct diagnosis and adequate treatment. Treatment consists of a lifelong

Disclosure/conflict of interest declaration: None.

Grant support (funding): JFL was supported by grants from the Swedish Society of Medicine, the Swedish Research Council – Medicine (522-2A09-195), the Swedish Celiac Society, and the Fulbright commission.

Independence (role of the sponsors): None of the funders had any role in the design and conduct of the study; collection, management, analysis, and interpretation of the data; and preparation, review, or approval of the article.

[a] Department of Pediatrics, Örebro University Hospital, Örebro 701 85, Sweden; [b] Clinical Epidemiology Unit, Department of Medicine, Karolinska Institutet, Stockholm 171 76, Sweden; [c] Division of Gastroenterology and Hepatology, Departments of Medicine and Immunology, Mayo Clinic College of Medicine, Rochester 55905, USA

* Department of Pediatrics, Örebro University Hospital, Örebro 701 85, Sweden.

E-mail address: jonasludvigsson@yahoo.com

gluten-free diet (GFD). Despite treatment with a GFD, most studies suggest that diagnosed CD is associated with increased mortality, as well as with certain types of cancer. Persistent inflammation with consequent malabsorption of micronutrients may be 1 explanation for this excess risk.

This article reviews a selection of studies on mortality and malignancy and describes how their results might influence the management of patients with CD.

MORTALITY
Diagnosed CD

Although several studies indicate that diagnosed CD is associated with increased mortality, data are contradictory with regards to the extent of such excess mortality. The first half of this article reviews the largest and most recent mortality studies, all of which included at least 1000 patients with CD.[4–8]

The first such study was an Italian multicenter study of 1072 individuals with CD.[8] In this study, adults with biopsy-proven CD from 11 gastroenterology units were identified (Table 1), and the investigators found a 2-fold increased risk of death in CD (standardized mortality ratio [SMR] 2.0; 95% confidence interval [CI] = 1.5–2.7).

The most important finding of that study was the association between severe clinical presentation and higher mortality (SMR = 2.5; 95% CI = 1.8–3.4). In contrast, no association was found in patients who had only mild CD (SMR = 1.1) or asymptomatic CD (SMR = 1.2).[8] The lack of excess mortality in these 2 groups indicates that patients with CD with mild symptoms have the same mortality risk as the general population.

A second finding of the Italian study was the relation between diagnostic delay and mortality.[8] Patients with more than 10 years of diagnostic delay were at a higher risk of death than those with less than 1 year of diagnostic delay. Although at first this finding seems reasonable, the increased risk of death in those with diagnostic delay is difficult to reconcile with the low SMR in those diagnosed in the oldest age group, in which diagnostic delay ought to have been longest.[8] One interpretation of the lower excess mortality in older patients with CD is that the relative importance of CD as a cause of death diminishes when more people (with or without CD) have other diseases.

In a second study, Peters and colleagues[7] investigated mortality in 10,032 Swedish patients with CD. The strength of this study is its statistical power, which allowed the investigators to calculate narrow CIs and to explore cause-specific death. Consistent with the Italian study,[8] the Swedish study found the lowest SMRs in the oldest age

Table 1					
Mortality ratios and rates in selected studies of patients with diagnosed CD					
Location	Study Period	Patients with CD	Risk Ratio[a]; 95% CI	Absolute Mortality/ 10,000 PYAR	Excess Mortality/ 10,000 PYAR
Italy[8]	1962–1998	1072	2.0; 1.5–2.7	82	41
Britain[4]	1987–2002	4732	1.31; 1.13–1.51	125	30
Britain[6]	1978–2006	1092	1.37; 1.16–1.62	141	38[b]
Sweden[7]	1964–1993	10,032	2.0; 1.8–2.1	102[c]	51[c]
Sweden[5]	1969–2008	29,096	1.39; 1.33–1.45	104	29

Abbreviation: PYAR, person-years at risk.
[a] Measures of association with the outcome are standardized mortality ratio (SMR)[6–8] and hazard ratio.[4,5]
[b] The absolute mortality risk in reference individuals was obtained by dividing 141 by the SMR (141/1.37 = 103). The excess mortality was the difference between 141 and 103.
[c] Estimated from data on number of deaths and person-years reported in the article.

group (SMR = 1.7), whereas adolescents with CD and young adults were at a more than 3-fold increased risk of death.[7] Two factors may have contributed to the high SMR for death in this study.[7] First, the study was based on inpatients with CD, although modern CD rarely requires hospital admission (although many patients with CD in Sweden in the 1960s to 1980s were admitted as part of the small intestinal biopsy procedure).[7] Inpatients may suffer from more advanced CD, with more symptoms, or more comorbid conditions. All these factors could have contributed to the 2-fold increased risk of death seen in the study by Peters and colleagues.[7] When Peters and colleagues restricted their dataset to patients who had only a diagnosis of CD and no other recorded comorbidity, the SMR decreased to 1.4. In all patients in this study, CD was diagnosed before 1994. The introduction of CD serology has since meant that CD is diagnosed in more patients with mild disease. Drawing from the evidence of Corrao and colleagues[8] that patients with asymptomatic CD had a lower mortality risk, it is reasonable to conclude that recently diagnosed patients have lower mortality risk (although contradicting data have also been reported).[6,7]

In contrast to the studies by Corrao and colleagues[8] and Peters and colleagues,[7] more recent studies[4–6] have found only modestly increased risks of death in CD. From 4732 patients with CD, West and colleagues[4] reported an overall mortality hazard ratio (HR) of 1.31, a figure that decreased to 1.17 after exclusion of the first year of follow-up. This study was able to adjust for smoking and body mass index (BMI, calculated as weight in kilograms divided by the square of height in meters) in a subset of patients (with no change of risk estimates) and estimate the absolute excess mortality (see **Table 1**). Taking advantage of long-term follow-up of a regional cohort, Grainge and colleagues[6] later examined the mortality in 1092 British patients from southern Derbyshire. That study found a 1.37-fold increased risk of death in CD. The study by Grainge and colleagues[6] focused on mortality change over time and confirmed Swedish data that mortality in CD has not changed substantially since the 1980s.[6]

The largest mortality study to date used histopathology data from Sweden's 28 pathology departments to identify more than 46,000 individuals with either CD (n = 29,096) or CD-related diseases (see later discussion).[5] The HR for death in biopsy-verified CD was 1.39 (95% CI = 1.33–1.45), decreasing to 1.26 when the first year of follow-up was excluded. After more than 5 years of follow-up, the HR remained slightly more than 1.[5] Several findings in this study are worth emphasizing. First, in contrast to a recent British study,[6] the Swedish study found similar HRs for death in men (1.28) and women (1.24).[5] Second, as in several other studies, excess mortality was lowest among those in whom CD was diagnosed at an older age.[5] If we accept the assumption that CD often begins at a younger age, the lack of excess mortality in those whose CD is diagnosed at an older age (supported by recent US findings[9]) could mean that long-standing untreated CD may have only a minimal effect on mortality.

Undiagnosed CD

Whereas 4 studies of undiagnosed CD have shown a similar mortality in patients and controls,[9–12] 2 studies have shown an increased risk of death in patients with undiagnosed CD.[13,14] There are 2 main reasons for a potentially increased risk of death in patients with undiagnosed CD: (1) CD may confer an inherent excess mortality independently of whether it is being diagnosed or not; and (2) undiagnosed CD, as opposed to diagnosed CD, remains untreated, with ongoing exposure to gluten.

In a German study, 15 of 63 individuals (24%) with positive antibodies to tissue transglutaminase (tTG) died during follow-up.[14] This finding corresponded to an HR of 2.53. Given that the investigators used only 1 serologic marker for their CD diagnosis (positive tTG), this HR is surprisingly high. Without confirming the tTG with either endomysial antibody (EMA) or small intestinal biopsy, a significant proportion of individuals should have false-positive results. The lack of confirmation of CD might then lead to dilution of data and a lower risk estimate for death. One potential reason for the high mortality HR in this study is that some patients with tTG positivity may not have had CD but rather had liver or heart disease, which could also cause tTG positivity and increase mortality.

The only other study showing substantial excess mortality in CD is an American study that used stored blood samples from young men at a US Air Force base (HR = 3.9).[13] Several facts are worth noting in this study by Rubio-Tapia and colleagues.[13] First, the follow-up period was longer than in any of the other studies. The excess mortality became apparent only after 15 to 20 years of follow-up. Potentially, the other studies with shorter follow-up may have failed to recognize an excess mortality that is evident only after a certain number of years with CD.[13] Second, the number of individuals with CD was small (n = 14) and the CI was wide (95% CI = 2.0–7.5). It cannot be ruled out that the high HR was a chance finding and that the true HR for death in this study was just more than 2 rather than about 4 (still within the 95% CI).[13] Third, because of the historical character of the study, the investigators were unable to verify the diagnosis of CD through biopsy, although all tTG-positive individuals required confirmation with EMA.[13] Fourth, among those who had positive CD serology, there may have been individuals with other (diagnosed or undiagnosed) diseases, such as certain liver and heart disease, which per se are associated with an increased risk of death. Because health care has vastly improved in the past 50 years, the HR for death of 3.9 in young men with undiagnosed CD in the 1940s and 1950s does not automatically mean that undiagnosed (and untreated) CD today is associated with a 4-fold increased risk of death. Nevertheless, the study by Rubio-Tapia and colleagues[13] constitutes one of the strongest arguments so far that undiagnosed CD may have severe adverse health effects.

The study by Godfrey and colleagues[9] found no increased risk of death in older patients (aged ≥50 years) with undiagnosed CD (HR = 0.80; 95% CI = 0.45–1.41). Of some 16,000 patients tested for CD, 0.8% had positive or borderline tTG and positive EMA.[9] However, this study had a significantly shorter follow-up than that of Rubio-Tapia and colleagues.[13] In addition, it is possible that the influence of CD (diagnosed or undiagnosed) diminishes at older ages, when the reference individuals acquire other diseases. In accordance with the lack of excess mortality, the investigators also found that seropositive and seronegative individuals had a similar BMI, and with the exception of slightly lower cholesterol and ferritin levels, they also had similar biochemical data (hemoglobin, vitamin B_{12}, folic acid, and albumin levels), suggesting that they did not have more than marginal malnutrition. The fact that CD was clinically detected in 15% of those with undiagnosed CD during follow-up (and presumably treated with a GFD) may also have affected the HR,[9] but cannot explain the lack of excess mortality, because studies of diagnosed CD show a positive association with death.

Finnish[11] and British[10] data indicate that patients with undiagnosed CD in these countries are not at increased risk of mortality. Both studies took advantage of centralized systems to identify recorded death dates, but the studies also adjusted for smoking.[10,11] The Finnish study used data from an earlier screening study (Mini-Finland) and identified 74 EMA-positive individuals and 204 Celikey tTG-positive individuals (Pharmacia Diagnostics, Uppsala)[15]; in addition, these individuals were all positive for a second type of tTG test.[11] The adjusted HR for death was 0.78 in

EMA-positive individuals and 1.19 in Celikey tTG-positive individuals. None of these risk estimates was statistically significant.

A British study examined 7527 individuals with blood samples from 2001.[10] Of these individuals, 87 were regarded as positive for CD (EMA-positive, but not confirmed through biopsy).[10] This study points to the necessity to adjust for risk factors when estimating risk of death. In the original unadjusted analyses, the HR for death was 0.73, but after adjustment for age, sex, socioeconomic group, and smoking status, this figure rose to 0.98 (95% CI = 0.57–1.69).[10] This finding is likely because of the low prevalence of smoking among British patients with CD[16]; however, this characteristic has not been confirmed in Swedish[17] or American data.[18]

Cause-Specific Mortality

The excess risk of death in patients with CD was long believed to be caused by malignancies.[11] This belief is only partly true. The commonest cause of death in patients with CD in our population-based Swedish cohort was cardiovascular death (1007 deaths during follow-up, compared with 773 deaths from malignancy).[5] That the relative risk of death from malignancy (HR = 1.55) is higher than that of cardiovascular disease (HR = 1.19) does not mean that malignancy causes more deaths than cardiovascular disease in patients with CD. Recent data indicate that patients with CD are at increased risk of ischemic heart disease,[5,7,19–21] stroke,[11,22,23] atrial fibrillation,[24,25] and potentially also autoimmune heart disease.[26,27] In the recent study by Canavan and colleagues[10] of undiagnosed CD (EMA-positivity), the adjusted risk of cardiovascular death (HR = 1.39, although nonsignificant: 95% CI = 0.66–2.92) was higher than that of death from malignancy (HR = 1.27; 95% CI = 0.57–2.85).

Several studies have reported an increased risk of respiratory death in CD[5,6] (with Lohi and colleagues[11] showing an increased risk of respiratory death in Celikey tTG-positive patients, whereas the risk was not statistically significantly increased in EMA-positive patients). This risk increase could be of multiple origins. Previous research has shown that patients with CD are at increased risk of pneumococcal infection,[28,29] which is expected given their predisposition to hyposplenism.[30] Other potential causes of respiratory death in patients with CD include pulmonary embolism,[31] tuberculosis,[32] and influenza.[33]

Although suicide is a rare condition, it constitutes an important cause of death in younger individuals in Western countries. It has also been suggested that some excess mortality noted in type 1 diabetes mellitus, another autoimmune disorder, is caused by suicide and external causes of death.[34] Psychiatric disease is more common in CD[35,36] (although probably not schizophrenia),[37] and psychiatric disease is a risk factor for suicide in patients with CD.[38] One smaller British study has also reported an increased risk of suicide in children with CD.[22] We therefore explored the risk of suicide in our cohort of biopsy-verified patients with CD and found a small but statistically significantly increased risk of suicide (HR = 1.55; 95% CI = 1.15–2.10; based on 54 completed suicides).[39]

Mortality in Children with CD

Few studies have investigated mortality in children with CD. Solaymani-Dodaran and colleagues[22] stratified their data set according to age at diagnosis and found a 2.6-fold increased risk of death in patients diagnosed with CD in childhood. What was especially concerning with this study was that deaths caused by accidents, suicide, and violence were increased (based on 7 deaths) and that excess mortality increased with longer follow-up (SMR was 3.32 after more than 5 years after diagnosis).[22]

Swedish data have since confirmed that childhood CD is associated with excess mortality (excluding the first year of follow-up: HR = 1.78) and remains increased after more than 5 years of follow-up (HR = 1.90).[5] Because of the concerns raised by Solaymani-Dodaran and colleagues[22] about deaths from external causes, we specifically looked at suicide rates in children and adolescents with CD in another population-based study.[39] In this study, we found no particular increase in suicide rates in patients diagnosed with CD before the age of 20 years (HR = 1.42). However because HRs were similar in all age strata in our cohorts,[39] we concluded that an early diagnosis of CD is unlikely to eliminate the increased suicide risk seen in CD.

Individuals Without VA

In our paper on biopsy-verified CD and future mortality, we also investigated mortality in patients undergoing small intestinal biopsy but who did not have CD.[40,41] A notable finding was that the mortality excess risk was higher in patients with inflammation (Marsh stage 1–2, intraepithelial lymphocytosis: HR = 1.72) than in those with VA (Marsh stage 3, CD: HR = 1.39).[5] There are several explanations for this finding. One is that patients without VA have traditionally not adopted a GFD. Hence, their inflammation is likely to remain active, whereas patients with VA (CD) would have received a GFD with a high chance of long-term mucosal healing (assuming that the GFD is protective against mortality). Another possible explanation is that not all duodenal inflammation is caused by CD. Whereas the heredity for CD was 12% in patients with VA in our study, it was lower in those with inflammation (5%), perhaps reflecting a more heterogeneous origin of this condition.[41] Mahadeva and colleagues[42] have reported that 40% of individuals with intraepithelial lymphocytosis develop CD (here defined as VA), but that most individuals do not. Still, when 2 researchers (independently) manually examined more than 1500 biopsy reports with VA or inflammation, few patients with inflammation had a non-CD diagnosis recorded in the biopsy register (inflammatory bowel disease was the most common other diagnosis and mentioned in 1.6% of the biopsy reports with Marsh 1–2).[41] It is therefore difficult to draw any conclusions regarding mortality in CD from our findings of an increased risk of death in patients with Marsh stage 1 to 2.

Underlying Mechanism for the Excess Mortality in CD

The dominant causes of death in patients with CD seem to be cardiovascular death and death from malignancy.[5–7,10,11] Because patients with CD often lack traditional cardiovascular risk factors (they have less hypertension[16] or no difference in blood pressure,[12] more beneficial lipid profile,[11,43] lower BMI,[44] [and most,[16,45–48] but not all,[17,18] studies suggest an inverse relation with smoking]), an explanation for the increased risk of cardiovascular death must be sought elsewhere. Some studies have found no or even a negative association between CD and cardiovascular disease, whereas the largest study so far (991 patients with CD developed ischemic heart disease during follow-up) found that patients with CD have about a 20% increased risk of cardiovascular disease.[21]

The most plausible link between CD and cardiovascular disease (as well as with death from malignancy) is the increase in inflammation, both before and after CD diagnosis.[49] Although Lewis and colleagues[43] did not compare C-reactive protein (CRP) values in patients with CD and controls, the average CRP level at diagnosis (based on 94 patients with CD) suggests that patients with CD have a normal CRP. However, other research has shown that patients with CD may have increased levels of other inflammatory markers (such as interleukin 4, 6, and 10, and tumor necrosis factor α) that could play a detrimental role for the risk of cardiovascular disease and malignancy.[50]

It is also probable that CD protects against certain types of disease because patients often have a slightly lower BMI[9] and smoke less often. Among diseases that may be less common in CD is breast cancer,[4,51] which is a common cause of death in women.

GFD and Mortality

A GFD is the only treatment of CD. Numerous reports confirm that treatment of CD results in better growth and overall health. The effect of GFD on mortality is less certain, and no prospective study on mortality has compared patients who adhere to a GFD with those who are nonadherent. Data on the role of GFD for mortality risk are therefore limited to retrospective data (often medical record reviews), which carry a strong risk of bias. In the study by Corrao and colleagues,[8] patients likely to have been on a GFD were at a nonsignificantly lower risk of death compared with the general population (SMR = 0.5; 95% CI = 0.2–1.1).[8] Those with uncertain dietary adherence had a 2-fold increased risk of dying, whereas those who were unlikely to have followed the diet were at a 6-fold increased risk of dying (95% CI = 4.0–8.8). However, a problem with these calculations is that most of the data in patients who died during the follow-up were obtained from relatives or friends, whereas individuals who were alive at the end of the follow-up were asked to grade their dietary adherence themselves. Thus, it cannot be ruled out that death per se influenced the relatives' responses and that patients who were alive overestimated their self-reported dietary adherence.

It could be argued that the higher mortality in patients diagnosed with CD in the 1970s and 1980s when strict adherence to GFD may not have been as widespread as it is currently is proof that a GFD is important to minimize excess mortality. Meanwhile, the lack of a major difference in mortality between individuals with VA (HR = 1.39) and those with normal mucosa but positive CD serology (HR = 1.35) suggests that a GFD may not have such a strong effect on mortality.[5] The main effect of a GFD is to heal the mucosa, but even individuals with normal mucosa seem to be at increased risk of death in this study.[5] However, a GFD may have other beneficial effects on the health of patients with CD. Some investigators have directly or indirectly[8,52] contended that a delay in the institution of a GFD increases the risk of other autoimmune comorbidities[52] (with detrimental effects on mortality) or affects the mortality risk per se.[8] One of our studies[5] showed increased risk of death in children with biopsy-verified CD, suggesting that short diagnostic delay in diagnosis may not prevent excess mortality.

Mortality: Implications for the Nondietary Management of CD

Given that cardiovascular disease is a common cause of death in patients with CD, general preventive measures are also relevant in patients with CD. Such measures include cessation of smoking, treatment of hypertension and hyperlipidemia, encouraging physical activity, and avoiding overweight. Although many of these risk factors are inversely related to CD, they are still highly prevalent in adults with CD.

A second theme of prevention deals with infectious and respiratory disease. Given the increased risk of both pneumococcal infections[28,29] and influenza,[33] immunization against these infections may be considered in patients with CD.

MALIGNANCY
Any Malignancy

Many studies on CD and malignancy typically identified patients with CD at 1 or a small number of referral centers, potentially leading to selection bias and overinflated risk estimates. Other studies have been limited by small number of cancers, leading to wide CIs and uncertainty regarding true risk estimates, whereas some older studies also included individuals with cancer diagnosed before or at the same time as CD or only examined death from cancer. Together, such limitations may lead to an over-estimation of cancer risk in CD.

Two large studies have examined the risk of any malignancy,[4,53] whereas the investigators of a third study chose to present data for lymphoproliferative malignancy (LPM) versus any solid malignancy separately.[54] Askling and colleagues[53] identified some 11,000 patients with an inpatient diagnosis of CD. Almost 3 of 4 patients were children at diagnosis, and patients were included until 1995[53] (in the 1970s–1990s, most patients were identified because of malabsorptive symptoms and diarrhea[55]). The over-all cancer risk was low in this Swedish study[53] (standardized incidence ratio [SIR] = 1.3; 95% CI = 1.2–1.5), but many of these patients (diagnosed in childhood) might not have been observed sufficiently long enough to reach an age when malignancy becomes more frequent. Insufficient follow-up might therefore explain the low relative risks. The SIRs for cancer decreased with follow-up. After more than 10 years of follow-up, patients with CD were no longer at a statistically increased risk of malignancy (SIR = 1.1; 95% CI = 0.9–1.4).[53] Another study characteristic that may have contributed to the low SIR in the study by Askling and colleagues[53] was the exclusion of the first year of follow-up after CD diagnosis. Many cancers are diagnosed just after CD diagnosis: the cancer may have caused the symptoms that led to the CD investigation, thereby creating falsely high risk estimates for cancer in CD; in addition, patients with CD are at increased risk of surveillance bias in the first year after diagnosis.

There have been at least 2 recent studies from Britain on malignancy in CD.[4,56] The larger, by West and colleagues,[4] found a statistically significantly increased risk of any malignancy with a relative risk (HR = 1.29; 95% CI = 1.06–1.55), which was almost identical to that of Askling and colleagues[53] The HR decreased to 1.10 (95% CI = 0.87–1.39) after exclusion of the first year of follow-up.[4] As noted earlier, West and colleagues[4] were able to adjust for smoking and BMI, although this had only marginal effects on the results. Although 12% of their study participants were children, the limited absolute number of children (n = 582) did not allow for any cancer estimates in this age group.[4] The second study (which had fewer participants, but longer follow-up for each participant than in the study by West and colleagues) found no overall increase in malignancy (SIR for all ages = 1.02).[56]

Although Elfström and colleagues[54] did not calculate the risk of any malignancy, our data suggest little or no increased risk of overall cancer. Beyond the first year of follow-up, the HR for any solid cancer was less than 1. Considering that the HR for LPM decreased to around 2 beyond the first year and that LPM made up only 15% of all cancers, the overall HR is likely to be less than 1.3, the SIR reported by an earlier Swedish study.[53] However, Swedish patients with biopsy-verified CD were at a 55% increased risk of dying from any cancer.[5]

All of these studies examined the risk of malignancy in patients with diagnosed CD.[4,54,56] Few data exist on malignancy in undiagnosed CD, and existing studies are limited by small sample sizes,[9,57] making it difficult to rule out an increased risk of malignancy. Godfrey and colleagues[9] reported that 24.4% of their patients with undiagnosed patients with CD versus 20.1% of controls had cancer during follow-up, corresponding to a nonsignificant odds ratio (OR) of 1.29 (95% CI = 0.77–2.15). Further, a Finnish study failed to show any association between undiagnosed CD and malignancy (relative risk in Celikey tTG-positive patients, 0.91, and in EMA-positive patients, 0.67).[57] A summary of selected studies calculating malignancy risk in CD is shown in **Table 2**.

Table 2
Malignancy ratios and rates in selected studies of patients with diagnosed CD

Location	Study Period	Patients with CD	Risk Ratio[a]; 95% CI	Absolute Risk/ 10,000 PYAR	Excess Risk/ 10,000 PYAR
Sweden[53]	1964–1994	11,019	1.3; 1.2–1.5	26[b]	6[b]
Britain[4]	1987–2002	4732	1.29; 1.06–1.55	72	16
Britain[56]	1978–2001	865	1.27[b]	76[b]	16[b]
Britain[86]	1970–2004	435	1.41; 1.09–1.78	63	18[b]

Abbreviation: PYAR, person-years at risk.
 [a] SIR,[53,56,86] HR.[4]
 [b] Calculated according to data on number of cancers and person-years supplied by the investigators. Excess risk was absolute risk – (absolute risk/relative risk). No CIs are given.

Lymphoproliferative Malignancy

Most modern studies have found a 2-fold to 6-fold increased risk of LPM in CD.[4,53,54,58–63] The largest study to date found an overall risk of LPM of 2.82 (95% CI = 2.36–3.37), decreasing to 2.25 during 1 to 5 years of follow-up after CD diagnosis and to 1.98 after more than 5 years of follow-up.[54]

Few studies have specifically addressed the risk of acute lymphocytic leukemia (ALL, which is an important cause of childhood malignancy), although the only study assessing this[63] failed to attain statistical significance between CD and later ALL (HR = 2.06; 95% CI = 0.84–5.04). Of the 4 largest studies examining Hodgkin lymphoma (HL), the 2 most recent ones found risk estimates between 2 and 3[54,61]; the other 2 studies reported a 4-fold to 5-fold increased risk of HL.[53,62]

Patients with CD are at increased risk of non-Hodgkin lymphoma (NHL). NHL has also been linked to several other autoimmune and inflammatory nonceliac conditions, including rheumatoid arthritis,[64] Sjögren syndrome,[65] systemic lupus erythematosus,[66] and Hashimoto thyroiditis.[67] Typically, the highest risks for NHL have been seen in the target organ of each disease (small intestine in CD, thyroid gland in Hashimoto disease, and parotid gland in Sjögren syndrome).

The highest NHL risk estimates in modern CD studies were reported by Lohi and colleagues[57] and found in patients with undiagnosed CD (defined as having EMA-positive, HR = 6.43). However, that risk estimate was based only on cases with both CD and NHL.[57] When the investigators defined undiagnosed CD as Celikey tTG-positive, the HR declined to 2.92, a nonsignificant result. The only other study of undiagnosed CD and LPM found only 2 patients with LPM (both in the small intestine) and was unable to calculate any risk estimates for LPM.[9]

The 2 largest studies of NHL in CD both found a 2-fold to 3-fold increased risk of NHL,[54,61] as did a European multicenter study (OR = 2.6).[60] The European multicenter study was able to distinguish between screen-detected CD and clinically detected CD; patients detected through screening were not at increased risk of NHL (OR = 1.3; 0.6–2.7).[60] Olén and colleagues,[68] exploring characteristics of patients with CD with LPM (57 of 58 lymphomas were NHL), reported that classic CD was a risk factor for the development of LPM. Both these studies[60,68] indicated that the risk of NHL is low in patients with mild or asymptomatic CD.

The lowest OR for NHL has been reported in a Swedish-Danish case-control study of 3055 patients with NHL cases and 3187 matched controls. In this study, all participants were interviewed about previous autoimmune and inflammatory conditions up to 1 year before the NHL diagnosis.[64] The risk of NHL was higher in patients with CD

(OR = 2.1; 95% CI = 1.0–4.8) than in patients with rheumatoid arthritis, a disease that is otherwise often seen as a benchmark for chronic inflammation.[64] A weakness of this study was that the diagnosis of CD was self-reported and false-positive CD may have driven the OR toward the null.[64]

The highest NHL relative risks in CD are those for T-cell NHL,[58,64,69,70] although recent data have provided evidence that B-cell NHL is also common in CD.[69] The risk estimates for T-cell NHL have varied markedly (17,[64] 19.2,[70] and 48,[54] although the CIs overlap). The lowest risk estimates for T-cell NHL were published by Anderson and colleagues[71] based on data from the SEER (Surveillance Epidemiology and End Results)-Medicare Database program of cancer registries. In that study, patients with CD were only at a 5.9-fold increased risk of T-cell NHL.[71] However, awareness of CD has long been low in the United States, and in the study by Anderson and colleagues, only 0.04% of the general population without NHL had a diagnosis of CD (eg, this was less than the number of patients with Addison disease), suggesting that their data may suffer from selection bias.

The most likely explanation for the high risk of LPM in CD is chronic inflammation. This explanation finds support in the study by Elfström and colleagues,[54] in which patients with VA (equal to CD in their study) had a statistically significantly higher risk of LPM than individuals with either Marsh 1 to 2 or Marsh 0 but positive CD serology (**Fig. 1**). That the degree of inflammation is crucial for LPM risk has also been noted for related diseases, especially in rheumatoid arthritis, in which researchers have shown that disease activity and not treatment (tumor necrosis factor α inhibitors) is the underlying cause of LPM development.[72] Long-standing inflammation in CD may lead to

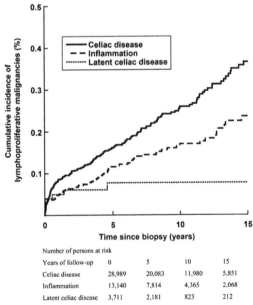

Fig. 1. Cumulative incidence of LPM according to underlying histopathology. Compared with individuals with CD, individuals with small intestinal inflammation (HR = 0.64; 95% CI = 0.50–0.83) or latent CD (HR = 0.38; 95% CI = 0.18–0.82) were at a statistically significantly lower risk of LPM. (*From* Elfstrom P, Granath F, Ekstrom Smedby K, et al. Risk of lymphoproliferative malignancy in relation to small intestinal histopathology among patients with celiac disease. J Natl Cancer Inst 2011;103:436–44; with permission.)

local LPM (thus the high risk of enteropathy-associated T-cell lymphoma) but also B-cell NHL. Even though CD does not show traditional signs of systemic inflammation (such as increased levels of CRP or erythrocyte sedimentation rate), cytokine levels are increased, signaling systemic inflammation.[50]

Refractory CD

Although most cases of nonresponsive CD are caused by gluten intake or the patient having a nonceliac diagnosis,[73] about 1% of adult patients with CD (and adherent to a GFD) develop refractory CD.[56,74] There are 2 types of refractory CD: type 1, in which the intraepithelial lymphocytes express a normal immunophenotype, and type 2, in which there is a clonal expansion of aberrant intraepithelial lymphocytes. Abnormal lymphocytes are characterized by the loss of normal surface markers. Patients with refractory CD are at high risk of T-cell lymphoma, although French reports of extremely high mortality[74] have not been replicated in British[56] or American[75] populations and risk estimates for malignancy in refractory CD are generally based on few cases with wide CIs.

Some researchers have argued that patients with type 2 refractory CD should undergo extensive regular radiological follow-up.[76] However, that decision must be weighed against the uncertainty of the malignancy risks of refractory CD, the potential risks of radiation exposure, costs, and the risk of overdiagnosing cancer.

Gastrointestinal Tract Malignancy

Most studies have reported an increased risk of gastrointestinal (GI) tract malignancy in CD. Some of these studies conclude that the relative risks are high,[59,77] whereas other studies suggest a risk ratio of approximately 2.[4] One of the largest studies to date is the Askling and colleagues[53] paper based on Swedish inpatient data on CD. That study found consistently increased relative risks of GI malignancies in patients with CD (oral cavity: 2.3; esophagus: 4.2; small intestine: 10; large intestine 1.9; liver: 2.7; and pancreas: 1.9).[53] However, the SIRs of the study may constitute an overestimate of the true relative risk of GI malignancy because hospital admission was required for a diagnosis of CD in that study.[53] In contrast, using primary care data, West and colleagues[4] found a 1.85-fold increased risk of GI cancer. That figure included the first year of follow-up, when surveillance bias may have contributed to the high HR. Excluding the first year, the HR in this British study decreased to 1.65 (borderline statistical significance; 95% CI = 0.99–2.76).[4] In their Derbyshire study, with a long follow-up, the same researchers reported that GI malignancy occurred in 9 patients with CD (expected = 5.7), corresponding to an overall SIR of 1.58.[56]

Elfström and colleagues[63] also found high relative risks of GI malignancy in the first year after CD diagnosis. What was particularly notable with this study was that the risk of GI cancer was increased in all patients undergoing small intestinal biopsy, independently of the underlying histopathology (with an increased risk in patients with CD but also in patients with normal mucosa).[63] The high initial risk was followed by normal HRs for GI cancer beyond the first year, strongly suggesting that the increased risk of GI cancer is caused by surveillance bias, or more likely, that patients with diffuse GI cancer symptoms undergo CD investigations, and in some patients, the CD diagnosis is confirmed before the cancer is diagnosed. The only subtypes of GI cancers with an increased risk beyond the first year of follow-up in our recent cohort study were small intestinal cancer (HR = 2.22; 95% CI = 1.19–4.14) and liver cancer (HR = 1.78; 95% CI = 1.22–2.60).[63] A null relation between CD and colorectal neoplasia or cancer has also been confirmed in American data.[78,79]

Breast Cancer

It has long been noted that CD protects against breast cancer. One of the first research teams to note this was Swinson and colleagues[80] in 1983. However, the low relative risk of breast cancer in that study may partly be caused by the large number of LPMs and GI cancers. Thus, a deficit of another cancer was natural given the researchers' study design.[80] However, later studies have shown a decrease in breast cancer rates, including the studies of Askling and colleagues[53] and West and colleagues.[4] Both of these studies[4,53] found a relative risk of approximately 0.3. Regional[56] or single-center[81] data have since found slightly higher or even null associations with breast cancer. The largest study to date, including more breast cancer cases than all previous studies combined, found a negative association with breast cancer but only of borderline significance (HR = 0.85; 95% CI = 0.72–1.01).[51] The same study reported reduced risks of endometrial and ovarian cancer in women with CD.[51] Overall, data clearly point toward an inverse relation with breast cancer in CD but the differences in the results among different studies are intriguing. Potential explanations include varying severity of CD, different smoking patterns, and socioeconomic status of patients with CD. Both inflammation and malnutrition typically seen in patients with severe CD[82] may in some circumstances protect against breast cancer.

Malignancy in Childhood CD

Beyond case reports, there are sparse data on malignancy in children with CD. Although Solaymani-Dodaran and colleagues[22] used death as their outcome, the increased SMR for any malignancy in patients with a childhood diagnosis of CD (5 deaths vs 1.39 expected) indicates that an early diagnosis of CD does not preclude future excess malignancy. In contrast, Askling and colleagues[53] did not find any malignancy increase in patients with CD diagnosed before 10 years of age (2 observed cases vs 1.4–1.5 expected; SIR = 1.4). In a recent study of childhood CD based on histopathology reports, Elfström and colleagues[54] found no increased risk of LPM (HR = 0.75; 6 observed cases vs 8 expected). However, only Solaymani-Dodaran and colleagues[22] had a long follow-up (median follow-up in children was 34 years). Thus, it is possible that their study[22] was the only one that could detect an increase in LPM in children.

The Role of the GFD

It is widely assumed that a GFD protects against malignancy, especially LPM, in patients with CD. Given the abundance of literature supporting an association between inflammatory diseases and LPM, it is reasonable to assume that a GFD can protect against this type of cancer, but firm evidence is still lacking and individual studies have noted substantial risk increases for NHL in patients adhering to a GFD.[59,83] Most of the studies that have evaluated the role of GFD have been limited by small numbers (number of patients with CD developing LPM or NHL: n = 9,[84] 9,[83] and 9[59]), with only 1 study exceeding 50 cases with both CD and LPM.[68] Of the first 3 studies, 2 suggest that GFD is protective against LPM,[83,84] whereas the third concluded that the risk of NHL persists despite a GFD (although this is not equal to ruling out a protective effect from GFD).[59] However, none of these studies compared patients with CD on a GFD with nonadhering patients with CD.

Through a nested case-control approach, Olén and colleagues[68] used blinded patient medical record data to compare poor compliance with good compliance. The degree of compliance was independently graded by 2 reviewers.[68] Although

Olén and colleagues found an increased risk of LPM in the CD group with low adherence (OR = 1.83), their data were not statistically significant (95% CI = 0.78–4.31). Furthermore, Olén and colleagues[68] found no evidence that diet adherence would protect against T-cell lymphoma (OR in poor compliance = 1.01; 95% CI = 0.32–3.15). In contrast, there was a strong suggestion that adherence protected against B-cell lymphoma (OR in poor compliance = 4.74; 95% CI = 0.89–25.3). The Swedish study also evaluated several potential risk factors for future LPM in patients with CD and found no influence of duration of symptoms, degree of VA at CD diagnosis, number of additional autoimmune diagnoses, or duration of symptoms on LPM risk.[68] The only laboratory parameter that was positively associated with future LPM was vitamin B_{12} deficiency (for LPM occurring more than 3 years after CD diagnosis).[68]

IMPLICATIONS FOR SCREENING

Several studies noted in this paper on mortality and malignancy in CD shed light on the debate over screening for CD in the general population, and specifically argue against screening. Corrao and colleagues[8] reported that mortality was increased only in symptomatic individuals, the consequence being that asymptomatic patients with undiagnosed CD are unlikely to benefit from a CD diagnosis in relation to mortality risk. Recent data suggest that individuals with dermatitis herpetiformis, which is regarded as a milder form of CD by some, are at no increased risk of mortality or malignancy.[85] Further, in our study of patients undergoing biopsy, we saw no increased risk of death after 5 years of follow-up in patients with positive CD serology (tTG, EMA, or antigliadin antibodies) but normal mucosa.[5]

Neither Godfrey and colleagues[9] nor Lohi and colleagues[57] found any evidence of excess malignancy in patients with undiagnosed CD. Hence, screening of the general population for CD does not seem to be of benefit in relation to risk of malignancy.

SUMMARY

It seems that patients with diagnosed CD are at a small increased risk of mortality. With the exception of an increased risk of LPM and a modest, short-term excess risk of GI malignancy, patients with CD do not seem to be at increased risk of malignancy. Future research should focus on the importance of dietary adherence to reduce existing risks, identify other risk factors for mortality and LPM in patients with CD, and evaluate the risk for mortality and malignancy in individuals with undiagnosed CD followed up for more than 20 to 30 years. Currently, general population-based screening for CD is unlikely to reduce mortality or malignancy.

REFERENCES

1. Green PH, Cellier C. Celiac disease. N Engl J Med 2007;357:1731–43.
2. Dube C, Rostom A, Sy R, et al. The prevalence of celiac disease in average-risk and at-risk Western European populations: a systematic review. Gastroenterology 2005;128:S57–67.
3. Walker MM, Murray JA, Ronkainen J, et al. Detection of celiac disease and lymphocytic enteropathy by parallel serology and histopathology in a population-based study. Gastroenterology 2010;139:112–9.
4. West J, Logan RF, Smith CJ, et al. Malignancy and mortality in people with coeliac disease: population based cohort study. BMJ 2004;329:716–9.
5. Ludvigsson JF, Montgomery SM, Ekbom A, et al. Small-intestinal histopathology and mortality risk in celiac disease. JAMA 2009;302:1171–8.

6. Grainge MJ, West J, Card TR, et al. Causes of death in people with celiac disease spanning the pre- and post-serology era: a population-based cohort study from Derby, UK. Am J Gastroenterol 2011;106(5):933–9.
7. Peters U, Askling J, Gridley G, et al. Causes of death in patients with celiac disease in a population-based Swedish cohort. Arch Intern Med 2003;163: 1566–72.
8. Corrao G, Corazza GR, Bagnardi V, et al. Mortality in patients with coeliac disease and their relatives: a cohort study. Lancet 2001;358:356–61.
9. Godfrey JD, Brantner TL, Brinjikji W, et al. Morbidity and mortality among older individuals with undiagnosed celiac disease. Gastroenterology 2010;139:763–9.
10. Canavan C, Logan RF, Khaw KT, et al. No difference in mortality in undetected coeliac disease compared with the general population: a UK cohort study. Aliment Pharmacol Ther 2011;34:1012–9.
11. Lohi S, Maki M, Rissanen H, et al. Prognosis of unrecognized coeliac disease as regards mortality: a population-based cohort study. Ann Med 2009;41:508–15.
12. Johnston SD, Watson RG, McMillan SA, et al. Coeliac disease detected by screening is not silent–simply unrecognized. QJM 1998;91:853–60.
13. Rubio-Tapia A, Kyle RA, Kaplan EL, et al. Increased prevalence and mortality in undiagnosed celiac disease. Gastroenterology 2009;137:88–93.
14. Metzger MH, Heier M, Maki M, et al. Mortality excess in individuals with elevated IgA anti-transglutaminase antibodies: the KORA/MONICA Augsburg cohort study 1989-1998. Eur J Epidemiol 2006;21:359–65.
15. Maki M, Mustalahti K, Kokkonen J, et al. Prevalence of celiac disease among children in Finland. N Engl J Med 2003;348:2517–24.
16. West J, Logan RF, Hill PG, et al. Seroprevalence, correlates, and characteristics of undetected coeliac disease in England. Gut 2003;52:960–5.
17. Ludvigsson JF, Montgomery SM, Ekbom A. Smoking and celiac disease: a population-based cohort study. Clin Gastroenterol Hepatol 2005;3:869–74.
18. Patel AH, Loftus EV Jr, Murray JA, et al. Cigarette smoking and celiac sprue: a case-control study. Am J Gastroenterol 2001;96:2388–91.
19. Ludvigsson JF, de Faire U, Ekbom A, et al. Vascular disease in a population-based cohort of individuals hospitalised with coeliac disease. Heart 2007;93: 1111–5.
20. Wei L, Spiers E, Reynolds N, et al. Association between coeliac disease and cardiovascular disease. Aliment Pharmacol Ther 2007;27:514–9.
21. Ludvigsson JF, James S, Askling J, et al. Nationwide cohort study of risk of ischemic heart disease in patients with celiac disease. Circulation 2011;123: 483–90.
22. Solaymani-Dodaran M, West J, Logan RF. Long-term mortality in people with celiac disease diagnosed in childhood compared with adulthood: a population-based cohort study. Am J Gastroenterol 2007;102:864–70.
23. Ludvigsson JF, West J, Card T, et al. Risk of stroke in 28,000 patients with celiac disease: a Nationwide Cohort Study in Sweden. J Stroke Cerebrovasc Dis 2011. [Epub ahead of print].
24. Emilsson L, Smith JG, West J, et al. Increased risk of atrial fibrillation in patients with coeliac disease: a nationwide cohort study. Eur Heart J 2011;32(19):2430–7.
25. West J, Logan RF, Card TR, et al. Risk of vascular disease in adults with diagnosed coeliac disease: a population-based study. Aliment Pharmacol Ther 2004;20:73–9.
26. Fonager K, Sorensen HT, Norgard B, et al. Cardiomyopathy in Danish patients with coeliac disease. Lancet 1999;354:1561.

27. Elfstrom P, Hamsten A, Montgomery SM, et al. Cardiomyopathy, pericarditis and myocarditis in a population-based cohort of inpatients with coeliac disease. J Intern Med 2007;262:545–54.
28. Ludvigsson JF, Olen O, Bell M, et al. Coeliac disease and risk of sepsis. Gut 2008;57:1074–80.
29. Thomas HJ, Wotton CJ, Yeates D, et al. Pneumococcal infection in patients with coeliac disease. Eur J Gastroenterol Hepatol 2008;20:624–8.
30. Di Sabatino A, Rosado MM, Cazzola P, et al. Splenic hypofunction and the spectrum of autoimmune and malignant complications in celiac disease. Clin Gastroenterol Hepatol 2006;4:179–86.
31. Ludvigsson JF, Welander A, Lassila R, et al. Risk of thromboembolism in 14,000 individuals with coeliac disease. Br J Haematol 2007;139:121–7.
32. Ludvigsson JF, Sanders DS, Maeurer M, et al. Risk of tuberculosis in a large sample of patients with coeliac disease–a nationwide cohort study. Aliment Pharmacol Ther 2011;33:689–96.
33. Marild K, Fredlund H, Ludvigsson JF. Increased risk of hospital admission for influenza in patients with celiac disease: a nationwide cohort study in Sweden. Am J Gastroenterol 2010;105:2465–73.
34. Wibell L, Nystrom L, Ostman J, et al. Increased mortality in diabetes during the first 10 years of the disease. A population-based study (DISS) in Swedish adults 15-34 years old at diagnosis. J Intern Med 2001;249:263–70.
35. Fera T, Cascio B, Angelini G, et al. Affective disorders and quality of life in adult coeliac disease patients on a gluten-free diet. Eur J Gastroenterol Hepatol 2003; 15:1287–92.
36. Ludvigsson JF, Reutfors J, Osby U, et al. Coeliac disease and risk of mood disorders–a general population-based cohort study. J Affect Disord 2007;99: 117–26.
37. West J, Logan RF, Hubbard RB, et al. Risk of schizophrenia in people with coeliac disease, ulcerative colitis and Crohn's disease: a general population-based study. Aliment Pharmacol Ther 2006;23:71–4.
38. Tidemalm D, Langstrom N, Lichtenstein P, et al. Risk of suicide after suicide attempt according to coexisting psychiatric disorder: Swedish cohort study with long term follow-up. BMJ 2008;337:a2205.
39. Ludvigsson JF, Sellgren C, Runeson B, et al. Increased suicide risk in coeliac disease–a Swedish nationwide cohort study. Dig Liver Dis 2011;43: 616–22.
40. Ludvigsson JF, Brandt L, Montgomery SM. Symptoms and signs in individuals with serology positive for celiac disease but normal mucosa. BMC Gastroenterol 2009;9:57.
41. Ludvigsson JF, Brandt L, Montgomery SM, et al. Validation study of villous atrophy and small intestinal inflammation in Swedish biopsy registers. BMC Gastroenterol 2009;9:19.
42. Mahadeva S, Wyatt JI, Howdle PD. Is a raised intraepithelial lymphocyte count with normal duodenal villous architecture clinically relevant? J Clin Pathol 2002; 55:424–8.
43. Lewis NR, Sanders DS, Logan RF, et al. Cholesterol profile in people with newly diagnosed coeliac disease: a comparison with the general population and changes following treatment. Br J Nutr 2009;102:509–13.
44. Olen O, Montgomery SM, Marcus C, et al. Coeliac disease and body mass index: a study of two Swedish general population-based registers. Scand J Gastroenterol 2009;44:1198–206.

45. Snook JA, Dwyer L, Lee-Elliott C, et al. Adult coeliac disease and cigarette smoking [see comments]. Gut 1996;39:60–2.
46. Vazquez H, Smecuol E, Flores D, et al. Relation between cigarette smoking and celiac disease: evidence from a case-control study. Am J Gastroenterol 2001;96: 798–802.
47. Austin AS, Logan RF, Thomason K, et al. Cigarette smoking and adult coeliac disease. Scand J Gastroenterol 2002;37:978–82.
48. Suman S, Williams EJ, Thomas PW, et al. Is the risk of adult coeliac disease causally related to cigarette exposure? Eur J Gastroenterol Hepatol 2003;15: 995–1000.
49. Lee SK, Lo W, Memeo L, et al. Duodenal histology in patients with celiac disease after treatment with a gluten-free diet. Gastrointest Endosc 2003;57: 187–91.
50. Manavalan JS, Hernandez L, Shah JG, et al. Serum cytokine elevations in celiac disease: association with disease presentation. Hum Immunol 2009;71:50–7.
51. Ludvigsson JF, West J, Ekbom A, et al. Reduced risk of breast, endometrial, and ovarian cancer in women with celiac disease. Int J Cancer 2012;131(3): E244–50.
52. Ventura A, Magazzu G, Greco L. Duration of exposure to gluten and risk for auto-immune disorders in patients with celiac disease. SIGEP Study Group for Autoimmune Disorders in Celiac Disease. Gastroenterology 1999;117:297–303.
53. Askling J, Linet M, Gridley G, et al. Cancer incidence in a population-based cohort of individuals hospitalized with celiac disease or dermatitis herpetiformis. Gastroenterology 2002;123:1428–35.
54. Elfstrom P, Granath F, Ekstrom Smedby K, et al. Risk of lymphoproliferative malignancy in relation to small intestinal histopathology among patients with celiac disease. J Natl Cancer Inst 2011;103:436–44.
55. Rampertab SD, Pooran N, Brar P, et al. Trends in the presentation of celiac disease. Am J Med 2006;119(355):e9–14.
56. Card TR, West J, Holmes GK. Risk of malignancy in diagnosed coeliac disease: a 24-year prospective, population-based, cohort study. Aliment Pharmacol Ther 2004;20:769–75.
57. Lohi S, Maki M, Montonen J, et al. Malignancies in cases with screening-identified evidence of coeliac disease: a long-term population-based cohort study. Gut 2009;58:643–7.
58. Catassi C, Bearzi I, Holmes GK. Association of celiac disease and intestinal lymphomas and other cancers. Gastroenterology 2005;128:S79–86.
59. Green PH, Fleischauer AT, Bhagat G, et al. Risk of malignancy in patients with celiac disease. Am J Med 2003;115:191–5.
60. Mearin ML, Catassi C, Brousse N, et al. European multi-centre study on coeliac disease and non-Hodgkin lymphoma. Eur J Gastroenterol Hepatol 2006;18: 187–94.
61. Gao Y, Kristinsson SY, Goldin LR, et al. Increased risk for non-Hodgkin lymphoma in individuals with celiac disease and a potential familial association. Gastroenterology 2009;136:91–8.
62. Goldacre MJ, Wotton CJ, Yeates D, et al. Cancer in patients with ulcerative colitis, Crohn's disease and coeliac disease: record linkage study. Eur J Gastroenterol Hepatol 2008;20:297–304.
63. Elfstrom P, Granath F, Ye W, et al. Low risk of gastrointestinal cancer among patients with celiac disease, inflammation, or latent celiac disease. Clin Gastroenterol Hepatol 2012;10(1):30–6.

64. Smedby KE, Hjalgrim H, Askling J, et al. Autoimmune and chronic inflammatory disorders and risk of non-Hodgkin lymphoma by subtype. J Natl Cancer Inst 2006;98:51–60.
65. Theander E, Henriksson G, Ljungberg O, et al. Lymphoma and other malignancies in primary Sjogren's syndrome: a cohort study on cancer incidence and lymphoma predictors. Ann Rheum Dis 2006;65:796–803.
66. Bjornadal L, Lofstrom B, Yin L, et al. Increased cancer incidence in a Swedish cohort of patients with systemic lupus erythematosus. Scand J Rheumatol 2002;31:66–71.
67. Mellemkjaer L, Pfeiffer RM, Engels EA, et al. Autoimmune disease in individuals and close family members and susceptibility to non-Hodgkin's lymphoma. Arthritis Rheum 2008;58:657–66.
68. Olen O, Askling J, Ludvigsson JF, et al. Coeliac disease characteristics, compliance to a gluten free diet and risk of lymphoma by subtype. Dig Liver Dis 2011; 43(11):862–8.
69. Smedby KE, Akerman M, Hildebrand H, et al. Malignant lymphomas in coeliac disease: evidence of increased risks for lymphoma types other than enteropathy-type T cell lymphoma. Gut 2005;54:54–9.
70. Catassi C, Fabiani E, Corrao G, et al. Risk of non-Hodgkin lymphoma in celiac disease. JAMA 2002;287:1413–9.
71. Anderson LA, Gadalla S, Morton LM, et al. Population-based study of autoimmune conditions and the risk of specific lymphoid malignancies. Int J Cancer 2009;125:398–405.
72. Baecklund E, Iliadou A, Askling J, et al. Association of chronic inflammation, not its treatment, with increased lymphoma risk in rheumatoid arthritis. Arthritis Rheum 2006;54:692–701.
73. Leffler DA, Dennis M, Hyett B, et al. Etiologies and predictors of diagnosis in nonresponsive celiac disease. Clin Gastroenterol Hepatol 2007;5:445–50.
74. Cellier C, Delabesse E, Helmer C, et al. Refractory sprue, coeliac disease, and enteropathy-associated T-cell lymphoma. French Coeliac Disease Study Group. Lancet 2000;356:203–8.
75. Roshan B, Leffler DA, Jamma S, et al. The incidence and clinical spectrum of refractory celiac disease in a North American referral center. Am J Gastroenterol 2011;106:923–8.
76. Malamut G, Afchain P, Verkarre V, et al. Presentation and long-term follow-up of refractory celiac disease: comparison of type I with type II. Gastroenterology 2009;136:81–90.
77. Harris OD, Cooke WT, Thompson H, et al. Malignancy in adult coeliac disease and idiopathic steatorrhoea. Am J Med 1967;42:899–912.
78. Lebwohl B, Stavsky E, Neugut AI, et al. Risk of colorectal adenomas in patients with coeliac disease. Aliment Pharmacol Ther 2010;32:1037–43.
79. Landgren AM, Landgren O, Gridley G, et al. Autoimmune disease and subsequent risk of developing alimentary tract cancers among 4.5 million US male veterans. Cancer 2011;117:1163–71.
80. Swinson CM, Slavin G, Coles EC, et al. Coeliac disease and malignancy. Lancet 1983;1:111–5.
81. Viljamaa M, Kaukinen K, Pukkala E, et al. Malignancies and mortality in patients with coeliac disease and dermatitis herpetiformis: 30-year population-based study. Dig Liver Dis 2006;38:374–80.
82. Michels KB, Ekbom A. Caloric restriction and incidence of breast cancer. JAMA 2004;291:1226–30.

83. Holmes GK, Prior P, Lane MR, et al. Malignancy in coeliac disease–effect of a gluten free diet. Gut 1989;30:333–8.
84. Silano M, Volta U, Vincenzi AD, et al. Effect of a gluten-free diet on the risk of enteropathy-associated T-cell lymphoma in celiac disease. Dig Dis Sci 2008; 53(4):972–6.
85. Lewis NR, Logan RF, Hubbard RB, et al. No increase in risk of fracture, malignancy or mortality in dermatitis herpetiformis: a cohort study. Aliment Pharmacol Ther 2008;27:1140–7.
86. Grainge MJ, West J, Solaymani-Dodaran M, et al. The long-term risk of malignancy following a diagnosis of coeliac disease or dermatitis herpetiformis: a cohort study. Aliment Pharmacol Ther 2012;35:730–9.

Non-celiac Gluten Sensitivity

Knut E.A. Lundin, MD, PhD[a],*, Armin Alaedini, PhD[b],*

KEYWORDS

- Gluten sensitivity • Celiac disease • Antibody • Food challenge
- Irritable bowel syndrome

KEY POINTS

- Nonceliac gluten sensitivity (NCGS) has emerged as a frequently encountered entity in the clinical setting. Individuals with self-reported NCGS appear to far outnumber those with celiac disease, and may be increasing.
- A better understanding of NCGS is hampered by the lack of objective clinical diagnostic criteria and absence of specific biomarkers.
- The financial burden on patients is considerable.
- In countries where reimbursement or prescription for gluten-free diet exists, the clinician must be aware of the condition and carefully consider the health economic aspects.

INTRODUCTION

Celiac disease (CD) is an autoimmune enteropathy triggered by ingestion of wheat gluten and related cereal proteins in genetically predisposed individuals.[1] The ensuing inflammatory response in the small intestine leads to villous atrophy, crypt hyperplasia, and lymphocytic infiltration. Elimination of the gluten proteins from diet generally leads to clinical and histologic improvement.[2] CD is a multigenic disorder, with genes for specific class II human leukocyte antigens (HLA) conferring about 40% of the genetic susceptibility. The primary HLA association is with DQ2 (DQA1 *05/ DQB1 02) and DQ8 (DQA1 *0301/DQB1 *0302).[3] The HLA-DQ2 and HLA-DQ8 molecules confer susceptibility for CD by having the important role of presenting specific immunogenic gluten peptides to gluten-specific T cells in the small intestine. The major antibody responses in CD are targeted at (1) gluten proteins, (2) deamidated gluten sequences, and (3) the transglutaminase 2 (TG2) enzyme autoantigen.[4] Among these antibodies, the immunoglobulin A (IgA) anti-TG2 antibody is currently

Disclosures: Dr Lundin has received speaker fees from MSD, Abbott, Ferring. He has received meeting honorarium from Glaxo and ImmunsanT.
a Department of Gastroenterology, Oslo University Hospital Rikshospitalet, Center for Immune Regulation, University of Oslo, Sognsvannsveien 20, Oslo N-0372 Norway; b Department of Medicine, Celiac Disease Center, and Institute of Human Nutrition, Columbia University Medical Center, 1130 Saint Nicholas Avenue, Room 937, New York, NY 10032, USA
* Corresponding authors.
E-mail addresses: k.e.a.lundin@medisin.uio.no; knut.lundin@ous-hf.no; aa819@columbia.edu

considered the most sensitive and specific serologic marker of CD.[5,6] Immunoglobulin G (IgG) and IgA antibodies to deamidated gliadin have also been shown to have high sensitivity and specificity for CD. Antibodies to native gliadin proteins have low specificity for CD, and have been reported to be elevated in several other conditions. The presence of these antibodies has been suggested in some studies to be a marker of immune sensitivity to gluten, even in the absence of CD. CD is now understood to have a wide range of clinical manifestations, both intestinal and extraintestinal.[4]

Some of the CD-associated symptoms experienced in response to ingestion of wheat are also reported by individuals who do not have the typical serologic, histologic, or genetic markers of CD, and who also do not experience the immunoglobulin E (IgE) serologic response associated with wheat allergy. The term nonceliac gluten sensitivity (NCGS) has been proposed to refer to the spectrum of conditions reported by these patients.[1] The term nonceliac gluten intolerance has also been used in the past, but is not recommended.[1]

DEFINITION OF NCGS

A precise and widely agreed definition of NCGS does not yet exist. NCGS is currently understood as a condition associated with the experiencing of various symptoms in response to ingestion of foods containing wheat, rye, and barley, and the resolution of symptoms on removal of those foods from diet in individuals in whom CD and wheat allergy have been ruled out. The symptoms may be accompanied with an increase in levels of antibody to gluten. The majority of symptoms associated with NCGS are subjective, including abdominal pain, headache, "brain fog," tingling and/or numbness in hands and feet, fatigue, and musculoskeletal pain. However, other symptoms such as rash and diarrhea, as well as more severe neurologic and psychiatric conditions including schizophrenia and cerebellar ataxia, have also been reported to be associated with NCGS. **Table 1** lists the most commonly reported symptoms associated with NCGS in comparison with those of CD and wheat allergy.

Table 1
Some of the symptoms reported to be associated with CD, wheat allergy, and NCGS

	CD	Wheat Allergy	NCGS
Gastrointestinal	Abdominal pain Diarrhea Constipation	Abdominal pain Vomiting Diarrhea	Abdominal pain Diarrhea Constipation Nausea Vomiting
Neurologic/ psychiatric	Headache Musculoskeletal pain Brain fog Tingling and/or numbness in hands and feet Fatigue Ataxia	Dizziness Headache	Headache Musculoskeletal pain Brain fog Tingling and/or numbness in hands and feet Fatigue Other neurologic and psychiatric conditions
Other	Dermatitis herpetiformis Weight loss	Eczema Asthma Rhinitis Nausea Itchiness	Rash Nausea Weight loss

PAST STUDIES OF NCGS

Although NCGS has garnered increased attention during the last few years, there have been earlier reports suggesting that the condition is a distinct clinical entity. A study in 1980 described 8 female subjects with abdominal pain and chronic diarrhea who had dramatic relief on a gluten-free diet and a return of symptoms on gluten challenge.[7] CD was ruled out by lack of villous atrophy on a gluten-containing diet, but it was noted that the gluten challenge induced a jejunal cellular infiltrate. The clinical description of these patients is similar to that for patients who are now frequently found in clinical practice and are thought to have NCGS.

In a study using rectal challenge of gluten for investigation of CD, it was shown that about half of nonceliac siblings of CD patients respond to gluten, with epithelial changes and an increase in intraepithelial lymphocyte numbers.[8] It is interesting that this rectal response was not dependent on the presence of HLA-DQ2. The observation suggests that an immune response to gluten can happen in the absence of the HLA-DQ2–restricted, gluten-specific T cells that are central to the development of CD.[9]

Kaukinen and colleagues[10] observed further that intolerance to cereals is not specific for overt or latent CD. Ninety-three adults reporting symptoms in response to ingestion of gluten were recruited. Only 8 patients were found to have CD, 7 could be said to have latent CD, and 19 were positive for allergy tests. Similar data were reported from Campanella and colleagues.[11] One hundred eighty patients on a gluten-free diet because of a diagnosis of CD not based on proper diagnostic criteria were reanalyzed in a tertiary referral setting. In 112 patients gluten was reintroduced to their diet. A definite diagnosis of CD was made in 51 of these patients. Gluten exposure induced clinical symptoms in 71% of the CD patients and in 54% of the nonceliac subjects. The investigators concluded that a clinical response to either withdrawal or reintroduction has no role in the diagnosis of CD. These data correlate well with a recent publication from the Oslo group.[12] Thirty-five patients on a strict, self-introduced, gluten-free diet were recruited after newspaper advertisement and from gastroenterological outpatient clinics. These patients were selected from more than 100 responders based on positivity for HLA-DQ2. Subjects were challenged with gluten-containing sandwich bread for 3 days, and examined with gastroscopy and a newly developed HLA-DQ2–deamidated gliadin peptide tetramer test on the sixth day of challenge.[13] Only 3 of the 35 HLA-DQ2[+] patients were diagnosed with CD. The nonceliac patients reported more symptoms than the CD patients.[14]

GLUTEN SENSITIVITY AND NEUROPSYCHIATRIC DISEASE

A connection between CD and certain specific neurologic and psychiatric disorders has been proposed in the last few decades, based primarily only on findings of elevated antibodies to gliadin in affected patients.[15,16] Some of the most discussed and debated among these include schizophrenia, peripheral neuropathy, cerebellar ataxia, and autism. Recently published reports by two independent groups in the United States[17,18] using large patient cohorts demonstrate increased circulating levels of antibody to gluten in about a quarter of individuals with schizophrenia. However, new data indicate that the antigluten immune response in these patients differs significantly from that in CD, displaying a unique antigenic specificity that is apparently independent of the action of transglutaminase enzyme and presentation by HLA-DQ2 and HLA-DQ8 molecules.[18] As such, the majority of such patients may belong to the NCGS category rather than the CD category. Case reports and small studies indicate improvement in response to gluten-free diet in some patients with schizophrenia, although double-blinded and placebo-controlled trials are still lacking.[19]

Similarly, elevated antibody reactivity to gluten has been reported in up to 40% of patients with idiopathic sporadic ataxia.[20,21] Other investigators have shown similarly higher prevalence of increased antibody reactivity to gliadin in both sporadic and hereditary ataxias.[22,23] Most of these patients do not appear to have the specific serologic markers of CD and may again fit more appropriately within the NCGS spectrum.[23] A study with a cohort of patients with ataxia and elevated antigliadin antibodies has shown a positive response to gluten-free diet in some individuals.[24] However, the pathogenic relevance of the increased antibody response to gliadin in the different forms of ataxia and the potential effect of gluten-free diet on disease remain subjects of debate.[25,26]

A possible association between autism and CD was first discussed by Dohan more than 40 years ago.[27] In both the scientific and lay literature, dietary gluten proteins have been suggested to be associated with or to play a role in the etiopathogenesis of autism, either directly as circulating partially digested peptides with opioid-like properties, or through the body's immune response to them.[28–31] Whereas some studies have pointed to an increase in the prevalence of CD, family history of CD, or antibodies to gluten among autistic children,[32,33] others have ruled out an association.[34–36] The inconsistency in results has been attributed to methodological differences in assaying, variation in patient diagnostic instruments, and the lack or incompleteness of controls. In addition, the effect of gluten-free diet on autism-spectrum disorders has received considerable attention. Diets that exclude gluten are becoming increasingly popular in the autism community, although their effectiveness has not been shown in controlled studies.[37] A Cochrane database systematic review in 2008 reported that the evidence for a gluten- and casein-free diet in autism was weak,[38] calling for large-scale, good-quality randomized controlled trials.

It is becoming increasingly clear that at least some of the neurologic and psychiatric deficits previously thought to be associated with CD may be more aptly attributed to NCGS. Substantial additional work is needed to understand whether and how gluten may contribute to the pathogenesis of certain neuropsychiatric conditions.

EPIDEMIOLOGY AND GENETICS

Reliable epidemiologic studies of NCGS have not been published. According to an article in *The Wall Street Journal*, some experts think as many as 1 in 20 Americans may have some form of NCGS.[39] The data behind such an estimate remain elusive. It is also estimated that the market for gluten-free food, as of 2010, was $2.6 billion. This figure would suggest that a considerable proportion of the United States population is consuming gluten-free foods. Data from both scientific and lay literature suggest that there is greater public recognition of gluten sensitivity than of CD.[40] Whereas the "low-carb diet" was widely adopted in the years after 2000, this diet has shown a steady decline since 2005. On the other hand, the popularity of the gluten-free diet has shown a steady increase since 2008 and is expected to increase further. Although the prevalence of CD in the United States is around 1%,[41] most of these patients are undiagnosed and the known celiacs make up a relatively small fraction of the consumers of gluten-free products. High-quality genetic studies on the NCGS population have not been performed as yet. There are no data suggesting that the condition follows the same HLA-DQ2/-DQ8 association as CD.

DIAGNOSIS OF NCGS

In clinical practice, it is typical to meet patients who have commenced a gluten-free diet without formal evaluation for food sensitivity. There are many reasons as to why they have started the diet. Some receive suggestions from family members and relatives who may have CD. Others have received advice from dieticians or "alternatively orientated doctors." In many cases, their diet has resolved their symptoms. In other cases, the patients continue their diet although the symptoms remain uncontrolled. In the authors' experience, NCGS patients usually maintain a strict gluten-free diet, even though they might not have received professional advice. In addition, there is a high rate of misdiagnosis among patients with a formal diagnosis of CD, shown to be as much as 20% in one study.[42]

The clinical workup for diagnosis of NCGS usually focuses initially on the exclusion of CD and wheat allergy. Serologic testing is particularly useful in this regard, including testing for IgA antibodies to TG2, as well as IgG and IgA antibodies to deamidated gliadin for CD, and IgE antibodies to wheat proteins for wheat allergy. HLA typing may also be particularly useful, as negativity for HLA-DQ2 and HLA-DQ8 has an excellent negative predictive value for CD.[43] Skin-prick testing is an additional tool for ruling out wheat allergy. The task of exclusion is difficult in the case of a patient already on a strict gluten-free diet. If the patient in fact has CD, the mucosa may have recovered and the serology could also be negative. However, in many cases the mucosal damage persists for a definite diagnosis, so a small intestinal biopsy can be taken and serologic tests performed, even if the patient is on a gluten-free diet already.[12] In other cases, a short gluten challenge may be necessary.

The definitive diagnosis of NCGS can so far only be made through gluten challenge. It is reasonable to demand that the patients' symptoms be under good control before initiation of a gluten challenge. The clinical response after gluten challenge might be variable but usually overlaps with symptoms of CD to a large degree. The need for performing a double-blinded, placebo-controlled food challenge (DBPCFC) is a controversial issue. A single-day DBPCFC with capsules containing wheat flour has been used and is recommended, but has been disappointing in the authors' hands (Rudihaugen J, unpublished results, 2006). The American Gastroenterological Association technical review from 2001 recommended a DBPCFC,[44] and this was also recommended in a recent review[45] and a workgroup report.[45] Others have emphasized the limitations and impracticality of the DBPCFC and consider the procedure not suitable in a normal clinical setting.[46] Virtually none of these publications have addressed the investigation of NCGS as the clinical entity encountered today.

The authors generally perform an open challenge with 4 slices of white sandwich bread (approximately 4 g gluten per slice). As this challenge is not blinded, one could expect a substantial placebo effect. However, the clinical responses picked up by this method seem to overlap with those seen after blinded challenge.[47] There is no clear agreement on how to perform symptom evaluation after challenge. The authors have used symptom scoring with the following questionnaires: Short Form (36) Health Survey (SF-36), Scoring System for Subjective Health Complaints (SHC), and Gastrointestinal Symptom Rating Scale for IBS (GSRS-IBS).[48] None of the validated CD-specific symptom questionnaires have been applied to NCGS investigation. A consensus among clinicians on how to diagnose NCGS is urgently needed. **Fig. 1** shows a proposed algorithm for the diagnosis of NCGS.

SEROLOGY

At present, there are no known specific serologic markers for NCGS. Wahnschaffe and colleagues[49] reported that a high proportion of NCGS patients have increased levels of IgG antibodies to gliadin. More recently, Volta and colleagues[50] studied 78 patients with NCGS and 80 patients with untreated CD in a tertiary referral setting.

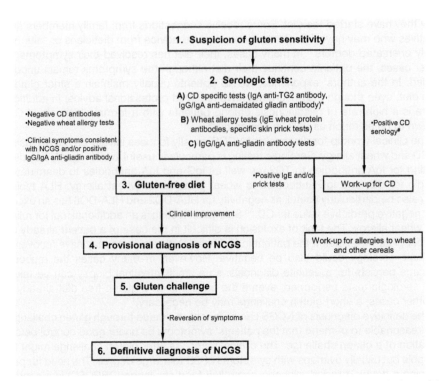

Fig. 1. Proposed diagnostic algorithm for NCGS. * HLA typing may also be particularly useful here, as the absence of HLA-DQ2 and -DQ8 has an excellent negative predictive value for CD. # The clinician may proceed with the work-up for CD in the less common cases of negative serology but high clinical suspicion.

Their criteria for NCGS were (1) exclusion of CD by determination of normal histology and negative CD-specific serology, (2) exclusion of wheat allergy by normal specific IgE and negative skin-prick test, (3) a 6- to 12-month trial of gluten-free diet with disappearance of symptoms, and (4) relapse of symptoms by open gluten challenge for 1 month. IgG antigliadin antibodies were found to be positive in 56.4% of NCGS patients and 81.2% of CD patients. A control group was not included, but the investigators refer to 2% to 8% positivity in the general population and healthy blood donors. Another recently published study by Ruuskanen and colleagues[51] showed that patients with antibodies to gliadin and celiac-specific HLA markers (DQ2 and/or DQ8) have more gastrointestinal symptoms than do antibody-negative individuals. The gastrointestinal symptoms in these individuals were mild to severe, ranging from flatulence to diarrhea, constipation, and abdominal pain.

The antigenic specificity of the antibody response to gluten has not been studied well in NCGS in comparison with CD. In patients with schizophrenia, a substantially different pattern of antibody response to gluten has been observed in comparison with CD, further underlining the fact that the mechanisms of the immune response to gluten in the 2 conditions are probably very different.[52] As such, detailed molecular characterization of the antigenic specificity of antigluten antibody response in NCGS may reveal novel biomarkers for the identification of specific subsets of patients.

EXPERIMENTAL MODELS

It has now been established that the pathogenesis of CD involves both the adaptive and the innate immune responses. Uptake and presentation of gluten peptides through the HLA-DQ2/-DQ8 molecules of antigen-presenting cells to gluten-specific T cells is an essential process in the mechanism of CD. In contrast to CD, however, there are no data showing T-cell reactivity against gluten peptides in NCGS. Taken together with the lack of an HLA-DQ2/-DQ8 association in NCGS, this suggests that the adaptive immune responses in these 2 conditions are fundamentally different.

There is a large body of literature indicating that gluten can affect cell function in cell-culture systems, apparently in the absence of involvement by the immune system. Gluten has been shown to induce agglutination of K562(S) myelogenous leukemia cells, cause actin rearrangement, and trigger apoptosis in Caco-2 cells.[53–55] Gluten has also been found to lower the threshold for immune activation through maturation of antigen-presenting cells, without production of classic pro- or anti-inflammatory mediators,[56] and to induce an increase in intestinal permeability by binding to the chemokine receptor CXCR3.[57] The molecular mechanisms behind these effects remain largely unknown, and it is not known if they have any role in the pathogenesis of NCGS.

In addition to gluten's direct effect on cells, the antibody response to gluten may exert a pathogenic effect through cross-reactivity toward autoantigens. Antibodies to gliadin have been found to bind Purkinje cells of the cerebellum[58] and to cross-react with synapsin I,[59] a neuronal phosphoprotein involved in the regulation of neurotransmitter release. As synapsin I is a protein that is relatively specific to the nervous system, the possibility that it might be associated with neurologic deficits is intriguing, although a pathogenic effect for this cross-reactivity remains to be demonstrated.

The effect of gluten has also been studied in several animal models.[60] Those that have been designed to specifically explore CD are not discussed here. Several studies have shown that gluten can have a potent diabetogenic effect in BB-dp rats and NOD mice.[61,62] The presence, amount, and timing of the introduction of gluten appears to influence this effect. However, recent work indicates that gluten enrichment may also prevent diabetes in NOD mice.[63] The relevance of these findings to NCGS is not yet clear. At present, the closest and best characterized animal model of gluten sensitivity is perhaps one that has been generated in rhesus macaques.[64] When fed with a diet rich in gluten, those animals identified as being gluten-sensitive show signs and symptoms of chronic diarrhea, malabsorptive steatorrhea, intestinal lesions, and elevated antigliadin antibodies. A gluten-free diet appears to reverse these effects. Despite the high antigliadin antibody reactivity and clinical symptoms after ingestion of gluten, these macaques do not generate a robust anti-TG2 antibody response. The immune response to gluten in the macaques is therefore likely to be significantly different from CD, perhaps more closely resembling NCGS. It may therefore serve as a useful model for the study of gluten sensitivity in the absence of CD.

PATHOPHYSIOLOGY

Although many questions about the mechanism of CD remain unresolved, the disease is one of the best understood autoimmune disorders. By contrast, little is known about the pathophysiology of NCGS. Sapone and colleagues[65] studied 42 patients with CD and 26 with NCGS. The diagnosis of NCGS was based on positive response to gluten challenge after 4 months under clinical supervision. At the end of challenge, examinations including CD serology and endoscopy with duodenal biopsies were done. The CD patients were untreated patients with supportive serology and demonstration of villous atrophy. Unlike the individuals with CD, NCGS patients did not exhibit increased intestinal permeability as measured by a lactulose and mannitol probe. Gene-expression analyses showed the NCGS patients to have increased expression of Toll-like receptor 2 and reduced expression of the T-regulatory cell marker FOXP3. The NCGS patients had increased density of intraepithelial lymphocytes (IELs), although not to the same level as untreated CD patients. The IELs expressed the T-cell receptor α/β, but not the γ/δ subtype. The investigators concluded that the NCGS patients showed signs of increased innate, rather than adaptive, immune activation.

A more recent study by Brottveit et al., (Unpublished data, 2012) further supports the presence of mucosal immune activation in NCGS, but one that may also involve the adaptive response. Thirty HLA-DQ2$^+$ NCGS patients were challenged with 4 slices of gluten-containing bread daily for 3 days, according to the protocol first described by Anderson and colleagues.[66,67] NCGS patients displayed an increased density of intraepithelial CD3$^+$ T cells before initiation of challenge. Following gluten challenge there was a significantly increased expression of interferon-γ mRNA in NCGS duodenal biopsies. It can be concluded that although the pathophysiology of NCGS is currently far from clear, the available data suggest immune activation to be a common denominator in both CD and NCGS.

Despite the selected terminology for NCGS, there is no clear evidence indicating that gluten proteins are in fact the sole or main trigger molecules for the condition. It is in fact possible that nongluten proteins of wheat are partially, or wholly, responsible for the associated symptoms in at least a subset of patients with NCGS. Better characterization of the trigger molecules in NCGS will be a major step toward gaining a better understanding of the pathogenic mechanism of the condition, identifying specific biomarkers, and devising more effective treatment strategies.

OVERLAP WITH IRRITABLE BOWEL SYNDROME

Irritable bowel syndrome (IBS) is considered by many to be a functional gastrointestinal disorder, in the sense that the patients' complaints cannot be explained by laboratory or biopsy testing. However, the Rome criteria emphasize pain as a dominant and necessary feature of IBS.[68] The authors' experience with NCGS, however, shows that while some of these patients may have pain, much more prominent are bloating, flatulence, and diarrhea. Thus it is difficult to give such patients a diagnosis of IBS. In addition, the diagnosis of IBS in patients who experience full recovery after withdrawal of gluten from their diet raises a semantic question: do they suffer from food intolerance with IBS-like symptoms or do they suffer from food-induced IBS? It is likely that careful investigations of NCGS patients would reveal subgroups both with and without IBS. In a previous investigation of NCGS, all participants also fulfilled the criteria for IBS.[47] There may be several reasons why a gluten-free diet would have a positive effect in IBS. It may be partially because a gluten-free diet is deficient in dietary fiber, making it more easily digestible, even in patients without any gluten sensitivity.[69] In addition, subsets of NCGS and IBS patients could have somatization disorders as a common denominator. It has been found that the IBS population suffers from substantial psychiatric comorbidity.[70] In a study of CD and HLA-DQ2$^+$ NCGS patients, however, the authors found that the NCGS patients did not exhibit a tendency for general somatization.[14] In addition, the psychometric profiles of the 2 cohorts were completely overlapping, as was their quality of life as measured by SF-36.

SUMMARY

NCGS has emerged as a frequently encountered entity in the clinical setting. The number of individuals with self-reported NCGS appears to far outnumber those with

CD and may be increasing. Better understanding of NCGS is hampered by the lack of objective clinical diagnostic criteria and the absence of specific biomarkers. The financial burden on patients is considerable. In countries where reimbursement or prescription for gluten-free diet exists, clinicians must be aware of the condition and carefully consider the health economic aspects.

REFERENCES

1. Ludvigsson J, Leffler DA, Bai J, et al. The Oslo definitions for coeliac disease and related terms. Gut 2012. [Epub ahead of print].
2. Alaedini A, Green PH. Narrative review: celiac disease: understanding a complex autoimmune disorder. Ann Intern Med 2005;142:289–98.
3. Louka AS, Sollid LM. HLA in coeliac disease: unravelling the complex genetics of a complex disorder. Tissue Antigens 2003;61:105–17.
4. Briani C, Samaroo D, Alaedini A. Celiac disease: from gluten to autoimmunity. Autoimmun Rev 2008;7:644–50.
5. Rostami K, Kerckhaert J, Tiemessen R, et al. Sensitivity of antiendomysium and antigliadin antibodies in untreated celiac disease: disappointing in clinical practice. Am J Gastroenterol 1999;94:888–94.
6. Alaedini A, Green PH. Autoantibodies in celiac disease. Autoimmunity 2008;41:19–26.
7. Cooper BT, Holmes GK, Ferguson R, et al. Gluten-sensitive diarrhea without evidence of celiac disease. Gastroenterology 1980;79:801–6.
8. Troncone R, Greco L, Mayer M, et al. In siblings of celiac children, rectal gluten challenge reveals gluten sensitization not restricted to celiac HLA. Gastroenterology 1996;111:318–24.
9. Sollid LM, Lundin KE. Diagnosis and treatment of celiac disease. Mucosal Immunol 2009;2:3–7.
10. Kaukinen K, Turjanmaa K, Maki M, et al. Intolerance to cereals is not specific for coeliac disease. Scand J Gastroenterol 2000;35:942–6.
11. Campanella J, Biagi F, Bianchi PI, et al. Clinical response to gluten withdrawal is not an indicator of coeliac disease. Scand J Gastroenterol 2008; 43:1311–4.
12. Brottveit M, Raki M, Bergseng E, et al. Assessing possible celiac disease by an HLA-DQ2-gliadin tetramer test. Am J Gastroenterol 2011;106:1318–24.
13. Raki M, Fallang LE, Brottveit M, et al. Tetramer visualization of gut-homing gluten-specific T cells in the peripheral blood of celiac disease patients. Proc Natl Acad Sci U S A 2007;104:2831–6.
14. Brottveit M, Vandvik PO, Wojniusz S, et al. Absence of somatization in non-coeliac gluten sensitivity. Scand J Gastroenterol 2012;47:770–7.
15. Green PH, Alaedini A, Sander HW, et al. Mechanisms underlying celiac disease and its neurologic manifestations. Cell Mol Life Sci 2005;62:791–9.
16. Bushara KO. Neurologic presentation of celiac disease. Gastroenterology 2005; 128:S92–7.
17. Cascella NG, Kryszak D, Bhatti B, et al. Prevalence of celiac disease and gluten sensitivity in the United States clinical antipsychotic trials of intervention effectiveness study population. Schizophr Bull 2009;37:94–100.
18. Dickerson F, Stallings C, Origoni A, et al. Markers of gluten sensitivity and celiac disease in recent-onset psychosis and multi-episode schizophrenia. Biol Psychiatry 2010;68:100–4.
19. Kalaydjian AE, Eaton W, Cascella N, et al. The gluten connection: the association between schizophrenia and celiac disease. Acta Psychiatr Scand 2006;113:82–90.

20. Burk K, Bosch S, Muller CA, et al. Sporadic cerebellar ataxia associated with gluten sensitivity. Brain 2001;124:1013–9.
21. Hadjivassiliou M, Grunewald RA, Chattopadhyay AK, et al. Clinical, radiological, neurophysiological, and neuropathological characteristics of gluten ataxia. Lancet 1998;352:1582–5.
22. Abele M, Schols L, Schwartz S, et al. Prevalence of antigliadin antibodies in ataxia patients. Neurology 2003;60:1674–5.
23. Bushara KO, Goebel SU, Shill H, et al. Gluten sensitivity in sporadic and hereditary cerebellar ataxia. Ann Neurol 2001;49:540–3.
24. Hadjivassiliou M, Davies-Jones GA, Sanders DS, et al. Dietary treatment of gluten ataxia. J Neurol Neurosurg Psychiatr 2003;74:1221–4.
25. Wills AJ, Unsworth DJ. Gluten ataxia 'in perspective'. Brain 2003;126:E4.
26. Hadjivassiliou M, Grunewald R. Reply to: gluten ataxia 'in perspective'. Brain 2003;126:E5.
27. Dohan FC. Coeliac disease and schizophrenia. Lancet 1970;1:897–8.
28. Knivsberg AM, Reichelt KL, Hoien T, et al. A randomised, controlled study of dietary intervention in autistic syndromes. Nutr Neurosci 2002;5:251–61.
29. Cade RJ, Privette RM, Fregly M, et al. Autism and schizophrenia: intestinal disorders. Nutr Neurosci 2000;3:57–72.
30. Vojdani A, O'Bryan T, Green JA, et al. Immune response to dietary proteins, gliadin and cerebellar peptides in children with autism. Nutr Neurosci 2004;7: 151–61.
31. Jyonouchi H, Sun S, Itokazu N. Innate immunity associated with inflammatory responses and cytokine production against common dietary proteins in patients with autism spectrum disorder. Neuropsychobiology 2002;46:76–84.
32. Barcia G, Posar A, Santucci M, et al. Autism and coeliac disease. J Autism Dev Disord 2008;38:407–8.
33. Valicenti-McDermott MD, McVicar K, Cohen HJ, et al. Gastrointestinal symptoms in children with an autism spectrum disorder and language regression. Pediatr Neurol 2008;39:392–8.
34. Pavone L, Fiumara A, Bottaro G, et al. Autism and celiac disease: failure to validate the hypothesis that a link might exist. Biol Psychiatry 1997;42:72–5.
35. McCarthy DM, Coleman M. Response of intestinal mucosa to gluten challenge in autistic subjects. Lancet 1979;2:877–8.
36. Batista IC, Gandolfi L, Nobrega YK, et al. Autism spectrum disorder and celiac disease: no evidence for a link. Arq Neuropsiquiatr 2012;70:28–33.
37. Elder JH. The gluten-free, casein-free diet in autism: an overview with clinical implications. Nutr Clin Pract 2008;23:583–8.
38. Millward C, Ferriter M, Calver S, et al. Gluten- and casein-free diets for autistic spectrum disorder. Cochrane Database Syst Rev 2008;(2):CD003498.
39. Beck M. Clues to gluten sensitivity. The Wall Street Journal; Available at: http://online.wsj.com/article/SB10001424052748704893604576200393522456636.html. Accessed August 8, 2012.
40. Simpson S, Lebwohl B, Sanders DS, et al. Awareness of gluten-related disorders: a survey of the general public, chefs and patients. E Spen Eur E J Clin Nutr Metab, 2011;6:e227–e231.
41. Fasano A, Berti I, Gerarduzzi T, et al. Prevalence of celiac disease in at-risk and not-at-risk groups in the United States: a large multicenter study. Arch Intern Med 2003;163:286–92.
42. Biagi F, Bianchi PI, Campanella J, et al. The impact of misdiagnosing celiac disease at a referral centre. Can J Gastroenterol 2009;23:543–5.

43. Sollid LM, Lie BA. Celiac disease genetics: current concepts and practical applications. Clin Gastroenterol Hepatol 2005;3:843–51.
44. Sampson HA, Sicherer SH, Birnbaum AH. AGA technical review on the evaluation of food allergy in gastrointestinal disorders. American Gastroenterological Association. Gastroenterology 2001;120:1026–40.
45. Lieberman JA, Sicherer SH. Diagnosis of food allergy: epicutaneous skin tests, in vitro tests, and oral food challenge. Curr Allergy Asthma Rep 2011;11: 58–64.
46. Asero R, Fernandez-Rivas M, Knulst AC, et al. Double-blind, placebo-controlled food challenge in adults in everyday clinical practice: a reappraisal of their limitations and real indications. Curr Opin Allergy Clin Immunol 2009;9:379–85.
47. Biesiekierski JR, Newnham ED, Irving PM, et al. Gluten causes gastrointestinal symptoms in subjects without celiac disease: a double-blind randomized placebo-controlled trial. Am J Gastroenterol 2011;106:508–14 [quiz: 515].
48. Wiklund IK, Fullerton S, Hawkey CJ, et al. An irritable bowel syndrome-specific symptom questionnaire: development and validation. Scand J Gastroenterol 2003;38:947–54.
49. Wahnschaffe U, Schulzke JD, Zeitz M, et al. Predictors of clinical response to gluten-free diet in patients diagnosed with diarrhea-predominant irritable bowel syndrome. Clin Gastroenterol Hepatol 2007;5:844–50 [quiz: 769].
50. Volta U, Tovoli F, Cicola R, et al. Serological tests in gluten sensitivity (nonceliac gluten intolerance). J Clin Gastroenterol 2011. [Epub ahead of print].
51. Ruuskanen A, Luostarinen L, Collin P, et al. Persistently positive gliadin antibodies without transglutaminase antibodies in the elderly: gluten intolerance beyond coeliac disease. Dig Liver Dis 2011;43:772–8.
52. Samaroo D, Dickerson F, Kasarda DD, et al. Novel immune response to gluten in individuals with schizophrenia. Schizophr Res 2010;118:248–55.
53. Auricchio S, De Ritis G, De Vincenzi M, et al. Agglutinating activity of gliadin-derived peptides from bread wheat: implications for coeliac disease pathogenesis. Biochem Biophys Res Commun 1984;121:428–33.
54. Silano M, Vincentini O, Luciani A, et al. Early tissue transglutaminase-mediated response underlies K562(S)-cell gliadin-dependent agglutination. Pediatr Res 2012;71:532–8.
55. Giovannini C, Sanchez M, Straface E, et al. Induction of apoptosis in caco-2 cells by wheat gliadin peptides. Toxicology 2000;145:63–71.
56. Naiyer AJ, Hernandez L, Ciaccio EJ, et al. Comparison of commercially available serologic kits for the detection of celiac disease. J Clin Gastroenterol 2008;43(3): 225–32.
57. Lammers KM, Lu R, Brownley J, et al. Gliadin induces an increase in intestinal permeability and zonulin release by binding to the chemokine receptor CXCR3. Gastroenterology 2008;135:194–204.e3.
58. Hadjivassiliou M, Boscolo S, Davies-Jones GA, et al. The humoral response in the pathogenesis of gluten ataxia. Neurology 2002;58:1221–6.
59. Alaedini A, Okamoto H, Briani C, et al. Immune cross-reactivity in celiac disease: anti-gliadin antibodies bind to neuronal synapsin I. J Immunol 2007;178:6590–5.
60. Marietta EV, David CS, Murray JA. Important lessons derived from animal models of celiac disease. Int Rev Immunol 2011;30:197–206.
61. Scott FW. Food-induced type 1 diabetes in the BB rat. Diabetes Metab Rev 1996; 12:341–59.
62. Funda DP, Kaas A, Bock T, et al. Gluten-free diet prevents diabetes in NOD mice. Diabetes Metab Res Rev 1999;15:323–7.

63. Funda DP, Kaas A, Tlaskalova-Hogenova H, et al. Gluten-free but also gluten-enriched (gluten+) diet prevent diabetes in NOD mice; the gluten enigma in type 1 diabetes. Diabetes Metab Res Rev 2008;24:59–63.

64. Bethune MT, Borda JT, Ribka E, et al. A non-human primate model for gluten sensitivity. PLoS One 2008;3:e1614.

65. Sapone A, Lammers KM, Casolaro V, et al. Divergence of gut permeability and mucosal immune gene expression in two gluten-associated conditions: celiac disease and gluten sensitivity. BMC Med 2011;9:23.

66. Anderson IH, Levine AS, Levitt MD. Incomplete absorption of the carbohydrate in all-purpose wheat flour. N Engl J Med 1981;304:891–2.

67. Anderson RP, Degano P, Godkin AJ, et al. In vivo antigen challenge in celiac disease identifies a single transglutaminase-modified peptide as the dominant A-gliadin T-cell epitope. Nat Med 2000;6:337–42.

68. Thompson WG, Longstreth GF, Drossman DA, et al. Functional bowel disorders and functional abdominal pain. Gut 1999;45(Suppl 2):II43–7.

69. Clemente G, Giacco R, Lasorella G, et al. Homemade gluten-free pasta is as well or better digested than gluten-containing pasta. J Pediatr Gastroenterol Nutr 2001;32:110–3.

70. Ladabaum U, Boyd E, Zhao WK, et al. Diagnosis, comorbidities, and management of irritable bowel syndrome in patients in a large health maintenance organization. Clin Gastroenterol Hepatol 2012;10:37–45.

Small Bowel Imaging in Celiac Disease

Christina A. Tennyson, MD[a], Carol E. Semrad, MD[b],*

KEYWORDS

• Enteroscopy • Small intestine • Enterography • Imaging • Celiac disease

KEY POINTS

- Recent advances in small bowel imaging technologies have improved the care of patients with small bowel diseases. Small bowel endoscopic and radiologic technologies are complementary and are often used in conjunction.
- In patients with celiac disease and gastrointestinal symptoms, radiologic imaging may be diagnostic of celiac disease.
- It is critical that radiologists and gastroenterologists are familiar with findings suggestive of celiac disease with new imaging modalities.
- Video capsule endoscopy, enterography, and device-assisted enteroscopy are usually reserved for those with alarm symptoms, refractory celiac disease, or suspicion of small bowel lymphoma/adenocarcioma.

INTRODUCTION

The small intestine is the longest organ of the gastrointestinal tract, which is fanned on the mesenteric stalk in the abdominal cavity. The multiple folds of small bowel loops in the abdominal cavity and peristalsis make it difficult to examine using standard endoscopic and radiologic imaging techniques. As a result, the small intestine has long been considered the black hole of the gastrointestinal tract. Upper endoscopy, push enteroscopy, and colonoscopy allow examination of only a small portion of the jejunum and distal ileum. Radiologic imaging by small bowel barium study and traditional abdominal computed tomography (CT) show luminal findings suggestive of celiac disease but provide poor examination of the small bowel wall. In addition, small bowel series is a time-consuming, operator-dependent study that has fallen out of favor for CT imaging. Recent advances in endoscopic imaging technologies (capsule and device-assisted eneroscopy) have enabled detailed visualization of the

[a] Department of Medicine, Columbia University College of Physicians and Surgeons, 180 Fort Washington Avenue, Room 936, New York, NY 10032, USA; [b] Department of Medicine, The University of Chicago Medicine, 5841 South Maryland Avenue, MC 4080, Chicago, IL 60637, USA
* Corresponding author.
E-mail address: csemrad@medicine.bsd.uchicago.edu

Gastrointest Endoscopy Clin N Am 22 (2012) 735–746
http://dx.doi.org/10.1016/j.giec.2012.07.013
1052-5157/12/$ – see front matter © 2012 Elsevier Inc. All rights reserved.

entire small bowel mucosa. Radiologic advances (CT enterography [CTE] and magnetic resonance enterography [MRE]) have markedly improved examination of the small bowel wall and surrounding structures. Intraoperative enteroscopy, considered the gold standard of complete enteroscopy, has largely been replaced. New imaging technologies provide less-invasive methods, with excellent reader agreement, for examining the small bowel. These technologies have improved the diagnosis and management of patients with small bowel diseases, such as small bowel bleeding, Crohn, disease, and celiac disease.

Celiac disease is a common inflammatory disease of the small bowel that affects 1% of the white population.[1] It is triggered, in genetically predisposed individuals, by the ingestion of gluten, a protein component of wheat, rye, and barley.[2] Most individuals are diagnosed with celiac disease in adult life. Celiac disease may present with classic (diarrhea-predominant) symptoms or atypical symptoms or may be asymptomatic and detected via screening.[3] Atypical presentations of celiac disease include nonspecific abdominal pain/dyspepsia, constipation, bloating, reflux, infertility, anemia, osteoporosis, dental enamel defects, short stature, vitamin deficiencies, fatigue, or neurologic problems, such as neuropathy or ataxia.[4] The rash of dermatitis herpetiformis is virtually always associated with celiac disease whereas intestinal biopsy may be normal with gluten ataxia. Serology for the antibodies directed against tissue transglutaminase (tTG IgA) is the best screening test for celiac disease.[5] The gold standard for diagnosis is upper endoscopy with small bowel biopsy. Patients with positive serology should have an upper endoscopy performed with 4 to 6 biopsies of the small intestine with samples from both the bulb and the second portion of the duodenum to maximize yield.[6,7] If the suspicion for celiac disease is high, endoscopy with biopsy should be performed despite negative serology results. Endoscopic findings of celiac disease include loss of folds and scalloping, a mosaic pattern, and fissuring of mucosa (**Fig. 1**).[8,9] Endoscopic abnormalities are not present in all cases and biopsies should be obtained even if the duodenum appears normal. Marsh[10] and Oberhuber and colleagues[11] described the histologic changes of celiac disease as increased intraepithelial lymphocytes, crypt hyperplasia, and villous atrophy. These findings largely account for abnormalities detected on radiologic imaging studies. Endoscopic biopsies of the duodenum may be normal if the disease is patchy. Jejunal biopsies may improve diagnostic yield in such patients.

The only current available treatment of celiac disease is a gluten-free diet. Up to 30% of celiac patients experience continued symptoms on a gluten-free diet or incomplete histologic recovery and are considered nonresponsive.[12,13] Other causes of ongoing symptoms include continued gluten exposure, microscopic colitis, small intestinal bacterial overgrowth, lactose or fructose intolerance, pancreatic exocrine insufficiency, and refractory celiac disease (RCD).[14] RCD is defined as persistent diarrhea with villous atrophy, crypt hyperplasia, and inflammation, despite adherence to a strict gluten-free diet for 6 to 12 months.[15,16] Its prevalence is unknown. RCD is classified into type 1 and type 2 depending on intraepithelial lymphocyte expression.[17] In RCD type 1, intraepithelial lymphocytes have normal surface expression of both CD3 and CD8 with a polyclonal T-cell receptor. In RCD type 2, however, an abnormal lymphocyte population is present with a loss of surface CD3 and CD8 expression, retention of intracellular CD3, and a monoclonal T-cell receptor rearrangement. In a study of 57 patients with RCD, the 5-year survival rate was 93% in patients with RCD type 1 and 44% with RCD type 2.[18] Enteropathy-associated T-cell lymphoma (EATL) occurs in more than 50% of patients with RCD type 2 and is a significant cause of mortality.[17–20] Evaluation of poorly responsive and refractory celiac patients includes consultation with a skilled dietician, endoscopy with biopsy, stool studies,

A Normal

B Scalloping

C Fissuring

D Mosaic pattern

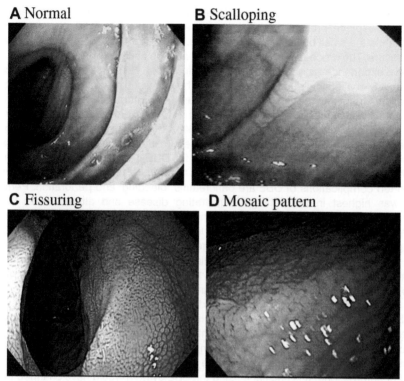

Fig. 1. Endoscopic findings in the duodenum in celiac disease. (*A*) Normal. (*B*) Scalloping. (*C*) Fissuring. (*D*) Mosaic pattern.

hydrogen breath testing, and, in cases of alarm symptoms and refractory disease, video capsule endoscopy, enterography, and deep enteroscopy if a suspicious lesion is identified. This review focuses on the role of standard radiologic imaging, enterography, and device-assisted enteroscopy in celiac disease.

DEVICE-ASSISTED ENTEROSCOPY

Device-assisted enteroscopy allows for diagnosis, tissue sampling, and therapy. The procedure can be performed using balloons or a spiral element attached to the endoscope. Therapeutic options can be performed during enteroscopy, such as hemostasis, lesion marking, and stricture dilation/stenting. The majority of published literature has involved double-balloon enteroscopy (DBE) because it has been available for the longest period of time.

Balloon-Assisted Enteroscopy

DBE, or push-and-pull enteroscopy, was introduced in 2003 and allows complete examination of the small bowel via the oral (antegrade) or rectal (retrograde) approach or both approaches.[21,22] The DBE system (Fujinon, Wayne, New Jersey) consists of a 140-cm polyurethane overtube back-loaded on a 200-cm enteroscope with 2 latex balloons attached at the tips of the overtube and enteroscope. Single-balloon enteroscopy (SBE) (Olympus Optical, Tokyo, Japan) uses a stiffer enteroscope and single, latex-free, balloon on the end of the overtube. A series of push-and-pull maneuvers are performed with serial inflation and deflation of the balloons. These maneuvers hold the bowel in place, prevent looping, and allow advancement deep into the small bowel by pleating the small bowel onto the overtube. The exact depth of insertion is difficult to measure. The procedure is time consuming and the average procedure time of DBE in initial experience ranged from 70 to 110 minutes.[23–26] The retrograde approach is particularly challenging due to retroflexion of the thin flexible endoscope in the cecum on advancement into the ileocecal valve with unstable intubation of the terminal ileum. In several initial studies, the overall diagnostic yield of DBE ranged from 43% to 80% and total enteroscopy varied from 5% to 86%.[23–26] Success of total enterosocpy is influenced by endoscopist experience, procedure time, patient body habitus, and prior abdominal surgery. Complication rates for DBE in an international multicenter study were 0.8% and 4.3% for diagnostic and therapeutic procedures, respectively.[27] Reported complications of DBE are pancreatitis, bleeding, and perforation. Perforation was highest in the setting of ulcerating disease and altered small bowel anatomy.[27,28] The absolute contraindications to balloon-assisted enteroscopy is small bowel obstruction, and in the case of DBE, latex allergy with relative contraindications being coagulopathy, pancreatitis, and large esophageal varices.[29] When compared with push enteroscopy, DBE had higher diagnostic yield (63% vs 44%) and greater depth of insertion (230 cm vs 80 cm).[30] In 1 study, carbon dioxide insufflation rather than air, increased the depth of insertion and reduced patient discomfort.[31]

In small studies comparing the DBE and SBE techniques, diagnostic yields were similar, but total enteroscopy rate was higher with DBE.[32,33] In a prospective, multicenter trial, the DBE system had a significantly higher diagnostic yield and total enteroscopy rate when 2 balloons were used compared with a single balloon used at the tip of the overtube.[34] This study did not use the actual SBE system, which contains a stiffer enteroscope. It is unclear if using the SBE system would have changed these results.

The literature on the use of enteroscopy in celiac disease is limited. A small series using DBE for the evaluation of malabsorption suggests DBE was useful in excluding complications of celiac disease (**Figs. 2** and **3**).[35] Because balloon-assisted enteroscopy is time consuming and invasive, it best complements video capsule endoscopy and enterography when suspicious lesions are identified. In a series of 21 patients with RCD, DBE was useful in detecting or excluding complications, such as EATL or ulcerative jejunitis.[36] In this study, low-risk lesions were defined as a reduction

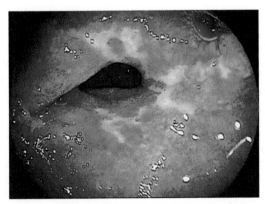

Fig. 2. Endoscopic findings in RCD using device-assisted enteroscopy. Ulcerative jejunitis with stensosis. (*Courtesy of* Suzanne Lewis, Columbia University, New York.)

A White nodules

B Ulcerated lesion

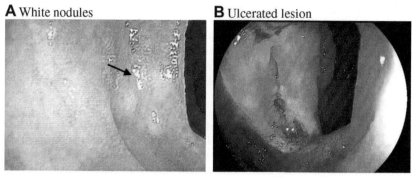

Fig. 3. Endoscopic findings of small bowel lymphoma using device-assisted enteroscopy. (*A*) White nodules. (*B*) Ulcerated lesion.

(<3 per endoscopic field of view) or loss of folds, scalloping, nodularity, and presence of visible vessels after air insufflations. High-risk lesions were defined as stenosis and ulcerations more than 5 mm in diameter. Hadithi and colleagues[36] detected EATL in 5 of 21 patients (24%) that appeared as circumferential, discrete, or confluent ulcerations whereas 2 of 21 patients (9%) were diagnosed with ulcerative jejunitis in the absence of EATL. DBE helped to exclude EATL in 4 patients with CT findings suggestive of malignancy due to small bowel wall thickening. A recent small case series examined the role of DBE using virtual chromoendoscopy (Fujinon intelligent color enhancement [FICE]). There was no improvement in the detection of features of celiac disease using FICE.[37]

Spiral Enteroscopy

Spiral enteroscopy (SE) is a method of device-assisted enteroscopy that uses rotational energy to pleat the small bowel. The Endo-Ease Discovery SB (Olympus Optical), a 118-cm polyvinyl chloride overtube with a 21-cm spiral element at the tip, can be back-loaded and locked onto an enteroscope. Using clockwise rotation, the device pleats the small bowel on to the overtube until the device can no longer be advanced. The enteroscope is subsequently unlocked and advanced through the overtube with a subsequent series of hook-and-suction maneuvers to further pleat small bowel. Advantages of SE include reduced procedure times and stability for therapeutics deep in the small intestine, because the enteroscope can be removed and reinserted through the overtube. In the initial experience, mean procedure time was 36.5 minutes and diagnostic yield 33%.[38] In a subsequent prospective multicenter study of SE, the diagnostic yield was 65% and average procedure time 45 minutes.[39] In a small, prospective, crossover, single-center study comparing SE and DBE, SE had a reduced examination time (43 minutes vs 65 minutes) but decreased insertion depth compared with DBE (250 cm vs 310 cm).[40] Although there are no published studies of SE in celiac disease, the device has been used in celiac patients without complications (personal experience).

RADIOLOGIC SMALL BOWEL IMAGING

Abnormal findings on radiologic imaging have been described in celiac disease since 1934.[41,42] These findings are not specific for celiac disease but reflect changes that occur with small bowel inflammation, fluid secretion, and altered motility. Radiologic examinations of the small bowel are frequently obtained in individuals with abdominal pain and diarrhea and, therefore, it is important to be familiar with radiologic findings that are suggestive of celiac disease. Although video capsule endoscopy provides a noninvasive means to visualize the small bowel mucosa, the miss rate for isolated mass lesions is up to 20%.[43] Ongoing advancement of enterography technology makes detection of ever-smaller bowel wall lesions possible. CTE and MRE are both useful in the examination of the bowel wall and extraluminal structures.

Small Bowel Barium Study

Several radiologic findings have been described in celiac disease using barium.[44] Jejunal dilation, fold thickening, hypomotility, and intussusceptions are nonspecific findings that can be found with other diseases, such as tropical sprue, scleroderma, and hypoalbuminemia. Small bowel intussusceptions are usually transient and may be multiple without a lead point (**Fig. 4**).[45,46] They may be related to laxity of the bowel wall. Specific barium findings for celiac disease include decreased jejunal fold pattern and increased ileal fold pattern (jejunization of ileum), so-called reversal of fold pattern (see **Fig. 4**). In a small study of celiac patients with active disease, 3 or fewer folds per inch of proximal jejunum were found in 73% of patients[47] and not in other inflammatory conditions or control subjects (greater than 5 folds per inch). The cause of decreased or absent jejunal fold pattern is unclear but may be associated with bowel dilation and barium retention in the segment. An increase of ileal fold thickness greater than 1 mm was found in 78% of patients with celiac disease. It likely reflects the high capacity for ileal adaptation in the setting of decreased jejunal nutrient absorption[48] and is usually found with long-standing disease. Celiac individuals with milder inflammation may not show these findings. Reversal of fold pattern can be found on cross-sectional abdominal imaging as well.

The use of small bowel barium studies remains relevant as in 1 study of 280 adults diagnosed with celiac disease[49]; 49 patients had barium studies before their diagnosis of celiac disease due to diarrhea, weight loss, or abdominal pain. Almost all studies showed findings suggestive of celiac disease that aided in the diagnosis. Severe celiac disease with bowel wall edema may mimic small bowel ischemia on barium study (see **Fig. 4**).

Abdominal CT Scan

With advancement in imaging technology, abdominal CT scan has surpassed barium study in the evaluation of abdominal symptoms and has the advantage of luminal and extraluminal examination. In a recent large study of CT findings in adults with celiac disease, a pattern of findings was identified suggestive of celiac disease.[50] Most of these findings stem from bowel inflammation and fluid secretion in the intestinal lumen. The pattern of CT findings suggestive of celiac disease included (1) dilated, fluid-filled loops of small bowel, (2) flocculation (flecks of precipitated barium in dilated loops), (3) telescoping/intussusception of bowel loops, (4) prominence of upper mesenteric lymph nodes, (5) large colon volume with gas and cecal plume of fluid, (6) small bowel wall thickening, (7) duodenal and jejunal wall fat, (8) hypervascular mesentery, (9) hyposplenism, and (10) mesenteric cavitary lymph node. The reversal of fold pattern is difficult to define on cross-sectional CT imaging due to poor localization of jejunal and ileal folds. This problem has been overcome by the use of CT enterography (CTE), a powerful tool in the evaluation of small bowel disease. Reversal of jejunoileal fold pattern in celiac disease has been identified using negative contrast and coronal reformatted images that demonstrated loss of valvulae conniventes in jejunum and thickened folds in ileum.[51] CT enteroclysis in adults with active celiac disease also identified reversal of jejunoileal fold pattern.[52]

Small bowel intussusception
A (coiled-spring appearance)

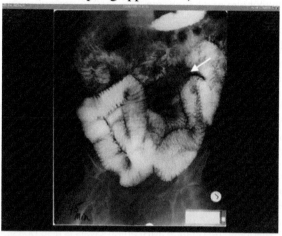

Reversal of jejunal and
B ileal fold patterns   **C** Severe small bowel wall edema

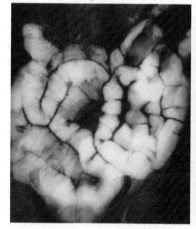
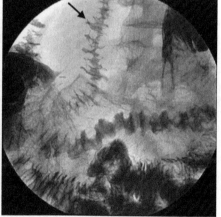

Fig. 4. Small bowel barium findings in celiac disease. (*A*) Small bowel intussusception (coiled-spring appearance). (*B*) Reversal of jejunal and ileal fold patterns. (*C*) Severe small bowel wall edema. (*Courtesy of* Arunas Gasparaitis, The University of Chicago, Illinois.)

CT enterography

Improvements in technology have allowed multidetector row CT scans to rapidly acquire high-resolution images and create multiplanar reconstructions. In CTE, a large volume (1350–2000 mL) of neutral or negative oral contrast is rapidly ingested to distend the entire small intestinal lumen and intravenous dye is administered while thin-slice (1–3 mm) images are acquired using a helical CT scanner.[53] Enteroclysis refers to contrast administration via a nasojejunal catheter. Although this achieves uniform filling of the bowel lumen, it is uncomfortable and invasive. CT enteroclysis and CTE have similar diagnostic accuracies of 88% and 80%.[54] CTE provides detailed visualization of the small bowel wall as well as the mesentery, lymph nodes, and external structures in a short time. Contraindications to CTE include pregnancy, renal insufficiency, or contrast allergy.

CTE is useful to examine celiac patients for signs of severe disease, such as dilated small bowel, hyposplenism, and mesenteric (sometimes cavitary) adenopathy, as well as ulceration with stricture and lymphoma (**Fig. 5**). CTE performs well in the detection of small bowel tumors. In a study comparing endoscopy, enteroscopy, video capsule endoscopy, CT enteroclysis, and clinical follow-up, enteroclysis detected tumors as small as 5 mm with a reported sensitivity and specificity of 95% and 100%.[55] Mucosal enhancement, mural thickening, fatty proliferation, and dilated vasa recta are imaging parameters of active inflammation, although these have been studied primarily in patients with Crohn disease, not celiac disease.[53] CT enteroclysis findings of reversed jejunoileal fold pattern, ileal fold thickening, vascular engorgement, and splenic atrophy strongly correlated with active celiac disease.[52] Other CT findings in celiac disease include small bowel intussusception, dilation, increased splanchnic circulation, and mesenteric and retroperitoneal lymphadenopathy.[56,57]

Magnetic resonance enterography

MRI has the advantage of high-quality imaging without radiation exposure and provides more detailed imaging of soft tissue structures when compared with CT. Disadvantages of MRE include higher cost, motion artifact, and increased length of the examination. Magnetic resonance (MR) enteroclysis is also possible using a nasojejunal catheter. The technique for MRE requires an overnight fast, the rapid ingestion of a large volume of contrast (1350–2000 mL), and use of an antispasmodic agent in some protocols to decrease bowel peristalsis.[58,59] MRI has the benefit of safety in pregnancy and renal disease[58] when contrast agent is contraindicated. There is a limited literature comparing CTE and MRE; sensitivities are comparable (95.2% and 90.5%, respectively) for detecting small bowel inflammation.[60] In this study, CTE had higher-quality images when compared with MRE, possibly from more rapid image acquisition.

MRE and MR enteroclysis have been used to examine for features of the celiac disease and complications, including malignancy. MRI is often more commonly performed in European centers. An MR enteroclysis score has been validated to help differentiate RCD type 2 patients using parameters of mesenteric fat infiltration, bowel wall thickening, and loss of jejunal folds.[61] A positive score was defined as 2 or more of the following features associated with RCD type 2: fewer than 10 folds per 5 cm jejunum, mesenteric fat infiltration, and bowel wall thickening. The score was positive in 13 of 15 patients with RCD type 2 (sensitivity 0.87) and negative in 24 of 25 patients without RCD type 2 (specificity 0.96). In those patients with a positive score, the 5-year survival rate was 56% versus 95% in patients with a negative score ($P<.0001$). MR

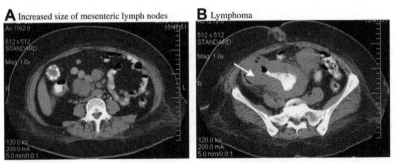

Fig. 5. Abdominal CT findings in celiac disease. (*A*) Increased size of mesenteric lymph nodes. (*B*) Lymphoma. (*Courtesy of* Aytekin Oto, The University of Chicago, Illinois.)

enteroclysis also helped identify 7 of 8 malignancies. MRE has also been used to evaluate morphologic traits in a small series of 10 patients with non-Hodgkin lymphoma. Lymphoma can be seen as a smooth, single, long (>10 cm) continuous bowel segment with aneurysmal dilation in the absence of a distinct mesenteric or antimesenteric distribution.[62] Luminal stricturing was present in cases of low-grade lymphoma whereas mesenteric fat infiltration was found in high-grade lymphoma. A recent small study performed by 2 radiologists blinded to clinical history reported an association of intestinal fold pattern on MRE with clinical presentation in celiac patients.[63] Patients with a normal intestinal fold pattern were more likely to have silent celiac disease whereas those with reversal of jejunoileal fold pattern had typical celiac disease.

Ultrasound

Although abdominal ultrasound is a noninvasive, safe, inexpensive, and portable modality that can provide high-quality images, it is rarely used in the United States to visualize the small intestine.[64] During abdominal ultrasound, the small intestine is examined for wall thickening, stenosis, dilatation, and motility as well as duplex imaging of the celiac and superior mesenteric arteries. Limitations include impaired depth of penetration in obese patients and limited view when luminal gas is present. Ultrasound in celiac disease is not well studied, but features include fluid-filled distended intestinal loops, increased peristalsis, and enlarged mesenteric lymph nodes.[65]

SUMMARY

Recent advances in small bowel imaging technologies have improved the care of patients with small bowel diseases. Small bowel endoscopic and radiologic technologies are complementary and are often used in conjunction. In patients with celiac disease and gastrointestinal symptoms, radiologic imaging may be diagnostic of celiac disease. It is critical that radiologists and gastroenterologists are familiar with findings suggestive of celiac disease with new imaging modalities. Video capsule endoscopy, enterography, and device-assisted enteroscopy are usually reserved for those with alarm symptoms, refractory celiac disease, or suspicion of small bowel lymphoma/adenocarcioma.

REFERENCES

1. Fasano A, Berti I, Gerarduzzi T, et al. Prevalence of celiac disease in at-risk and not-at-risk groups in the United States: a large multicenter study. Arch Intern Med 2003;163:286–92.
2. Green PH, Cellier C. Celiac disease. N Engl J Med 2007;357:1731–43.
3. Lo W, Sano K, Lebwohl B, et al. Changing presentation of adult celiac disease. Dig Dis Sci 2003;48:395–8.
4. Green PH. The many faces of celiac disease: clinical presentation of celiac disease in the adult population. Gastroenterology 2005;128(Suppl 1):S74–8.
5. Rostom A, Dubé C, Cranney A, et al. The diagnostic accuracy of serologic tests for celiac disease: a systematic review. Gastroenterology 2005;128:S38–46.
6. Rostom A, Murray JA, Kagnoff MF. American Gastroenterological Association (AGA) Institute technical review on the diagnosis and management of celiac disease. Gastroenterology 2006;131:1981–2002.
7. Gonzalez S, Gupta A, Cheng J, et al. Prospective study of the role of duodenal bulb biopsies in the diagnosis of celiac disease. Dig Dis Sci 2011;56:805–11.

8. Magazzu G, Bottari M, Tuccari G, et al. Upper gastrointestinal endoscopy can be a reliable screening tool for celiac sprue in adults. J Clin Gastroenterol 1994;19: 255–7.

9. Maurino E, Capizzano H, Niveloni S, et al. Value of endoscopic markers in celiac disease. Dig Dis Sci 1993;38:2028–33.

10. Marsh MN. Gluten, major histocompatibility complex, and the small intestine. A molecular and immunobiologic approach to the spectrum of gluten sensitivity (celiac sprue). Gastroenterology 1992;102:330–54.

11. Oberhuber G, Granditsch G, Vogelsang H. The histopathology of coeliac disease: a time for a standardized report scheme for pathologists. Eur J Gastroenterol Hepatol 1999;11:1185–94.

12. O'Mahony S, Howdle PD, Losowsky MS, et al. Review article: management of patients with non-responsive coeliac disease. Aliment Pharmacol Ther 1996;10:671–80.

13. Abdulkarim AS, Burgart LJ, See J, et al. Etiology of nonesponsive celiac disease: results of a systemic approach. Am J Gastroenterol 2002;97:2016–21.

14. Rubio-Tapia A, Murray JA. Classification and management of refractory coeliac disease. Gut 2010;59:547–57.

15. Biagi F, Corazza GR. Defining gluten refractory enteropathy. Eur J Gastroenterol Hepatol 2001;13:561–5.

16. Al-toma A, Verbeek WH, Mulder CJ. The management of complicated celiac disease. Dig Dis 2007;25:230–6.

17. Cellier C, Delabesse E, Helmer C, et al. Refractory sprue, coeliac disease, and enteropathy-associated T-cell lymphoma. French Coeliac Disease Study Group. Lancet 2000;356:203–8.

18. Malamut G, Afchain P, Verkarre V, et al. Presentation and long-term follow-up of refractory celiac disease: comparison of type I with type II. Gastroenterology 2009;136:81–90.

19. Rubio-Tapia A, Kelly DG, Lahr BD, et al. Clinical staging and survival in refractory celiac disease: a single center experience. Gastroenterology 2009;136:99–107.

20. Al-Toma A, Verbeek WH, Hadithi M, et al. Survival in refractory coeliac disease and enteropathy-associated T-cell lymphoma: retrospective evaluation of single-centre experience. Gut 2007;56:1373–8.

21. Yamamoto H, Sekine Y, Sato Y, et al. Total enteroscopy with a nonsurgical steerable double-balloon method. Gastrointest Endosc 2001;53:216–20.

22. Yamamoto H, Yano T, Kita H, et al. New system of double balloon enteroscopy for diagnosis and treatment of small intestinal disorders. Gastroenterology 2003;125: 1556.

23. May A, Nachbar L, Ell C. Double-balloon enteroscopy (push-and-pull enteroscopy) of the small bowel: feasibility and diagnostic and therapeutic yield in patients with suspected small bowel disease. Gastrointest Endosc 2005;62:62–70.

24. Mehdizadeh S, Ross A, Gerson L, et al. What is the learning curve associated with double balloon enteroscopy? Technical details and early experience in 6 U.S. Tertiary Care Centers. Gastrointest Endosc 2006;64:740–50.

25. Di Caro S, May A, Heine DG, et al. The European experience with double-balloon enteroscopy: indications, methodology, safety, and clinical impact. Gastrointest Endosc 2005;62:545–50.

26. Yamamoto H, Kita H, Sunada K, et al. Clinical outcomes of double-balloon endoscopy for the diagnosis and treatment of small intestinal diseases. Clin Gastroenterol Hepatol 2004;2:1010–6.

27. Mensink P, Haringsma J, Kucharzik TF, et al. Complications of double balloon enteroscopy (DBE): a multicenter study. Endoscopy 2007;39:613–5.

28. Gerson LB, Tokar J, Chiorean M, et al. Complications associated with double balloon enteroscopy at nine US centers. Clin Gastroenterol Hepatol 2009;7: 1177–82.
29. Gerson L, Flodin J, Miyabayashi K. Balloon-assisted enteroscopy: technology and troubleshooting. Gastrointest Endosc 2008;68:1158–67.
30. May A, Nachbar L, Schneider M, et al. Prospective comparison of push entero-scopy and push-and-pull enteroscopy in patients with suspected small-bowel bleeding. Am J Gastroenterol 2006;101:2016–24.
31. Domagk D, Bretthauer M, Lenz P, et al. Carbon dioxide insufflation improves intu-bation depth in double-balloon enteroscopy: a randomized, controlled, double-blind trial. Endoscopy 2007;39:1064–7.
32. Domagk D, Mensink P, Aktas H, et al. Single- vs. double balloon enteroscopy in small bowel diagnostics: a randomized multicenter trial. Endoscopy 2011;43:472–6.
33. Takano N, Yamada A, Watabe H, et al. Single-balloon versus double-balloon endoscopy for achieving total enteroscopy: a randomized, controlled trial. Gas-trointest Endosc 2011;73:734–9.
34. May A, Färber M, Aschmoneit I, et al. Prospective multicenter trial comparing push-and-pull enteroscopy with the single- and double-balloon techniques in patients with small-bowel disorders. Am J Gastroenterol 2010;105:575–81.
35. Fry L, Bellutti M, Neumann H, et al. Utility of double ballon enteroscopy for the evaluation of malabsorption. Dig Dis 2008;26:134–9.
36. Hadithi M, Al-toma A, Oudejans J, et al. The value of double-balloon enteroscopy in patients with refractory celiac disease. Am J Gastroenterol 2007;102:987–96.
37. Neumann H, Fry LC, Bellutti M, et al. Double-balloon enteroscopy-assisted virtual chromoendoscopy for small-bowel disorders: a case series. Endoscopy 2009;41: 468–71.
38. Akerman PA, Agrawal D, Chen W, et al. Spiral enteroscopy: a novel method of enteroscopy by using the Endo-Ease Discovery SB overtube and a pediatric co-lonoscope. Gastrointest Endosc 2009;69:327–32.
39. Morgan D, Upchurch B, Draganov P, et al. Spiral enteroscopy: prospective U.S. multicenter study in patients with small bowel disorders. Gastrointest Endosc 2010;72:992–8.
40. May A, Manner H, Aschmoneit I, et al. Prospective, cross-over, single-center trial comparing oral double-balloon enteroscopy and oral spiral enteroscopy in patients with suspected small-bowel vascular malformations. Endoscopy 2011; 43:477–83.
41. Kanto JL. The roentgen diagnosis of idiopathic steatorrhea and allied conditions: practical value of the "moulage sign". Am J Roentgenol 1939;41:758–78.
42. Marshak RH, Wolf BS, Adlersberg D. Roentgen studies of the small intestine in sprue. Am J Roentgenol Radium Ther Nucl Med 1954;72:380–400.
43. Lewis BS, Eisen GM, Friedman S. A pooled analysis to evaluate results of capsule endoscopy trials [Erratum appears in Endoscopy 2007;39:303]. Endoscopy 2005;37:960–5.
44. Kumar P, Bartram CI. Relevance of the barium follow-through examination in the diagnosis of adult celiac disease. Gastrointest Radiol 1979;14:285–9.
45. Ruoff M, Lindner AE, Marshak RH. Intussusception in sprue. Am J Roentgenol Radium Ther Nucl Med 1968;104:525–8.
46. Cohen MD, Lintott DJ. Transient small bowel intussusception in adult coeliac disease. Clin Radiol 1978;29:529–34.
47. Herlinger H, Maglinte DD. Jejunal fold separation in adult celiac disease: rele-vance of enteroclysis. Radiology 1986;158:605–11.

48. Bova JG, Friedman AC, Weser E, et al. Adaptation of the ileum in nontropical sprue: reversal of the jejuno-ileal pattern. AJR Am J Roentgenol 1985;144: 299–302.
49. La Seta F, Cuccellato A, Albanese M, et al. Radiology and adult celiac disease. Current indication of small bowel barium examinations. Radiol Med 2004;108: 515–21.
50. Scholz FJ, Afnan J, Behr SC. CT findings in adult celiac disease. Radiographics 2011;31:977–92.
51. Paulsen SR, Huprich JE, Fletcher JG, et al. CT enterography as a diagnostic tool in evaluating small bowel disorders: review of clinical experience with over 700 cases. Radiographics 2006;26:641–62.
52. Soyer P, Boudiaf M, Dray X, et al. CT enteroclysis features of uncomplicated celiac disease: retrospective analysis of 44 patients. Radiology 2009;253: 416–24.
53. Bruining DH. CT enterography: is it the current state-of-the-art for small bowel diagnostics? Dig Dis 2010;28:429–32.
54. Wold PB, Fletcher JG, Johnson CD, et al. Assessment of small bowel Crohn disease: noninvasive peroral CT enterography compared with other imaging methods and endoscopy—feasibility study. Radiology 2003;229:275–81.
55. Boudiaf M, Jaff A, Soyer P, et al. Small-bowel diseases: prospective evaluation of multi-detector row helical CT enteroclysis in 107 consecutive patients. Radiology 2004;233:338–44.
56. Gonda TA, Khan SU, Cheng J, et al. Association of intussusception and celiac disease in adults. Dig Dis Sci 2010;55:2899–903.
57. Elsayes KM, Al-Hawary MM, Jagdish J, et al. CT enterography: principles, trends, and interpretation of findings. Radiographics 2010;30:1955–70.
58. Fidler JL, Guimaraes L, Einstein DM. MR imaging of the small bowel. Radiographics 2009;29:1811–25.
59. Feuerbach S. MRI enterography: the future of small bowel diagnostics? Dig Dis 2010;28:433–8.
60. Siddiki HA, Fidler JL, Fletcher JG, et al. Prospective comparison of state-of-the-art MR enterography and CT enterography in small-bowel Crohn's disease. Am J Roentgenol 2009;193:113–21.
61. Van Weyenberg SJ, Meijeerink MR, Jacobs M, et al. MR enteroclysis in refractory celiac disease: proposal and validation of a severity scoring system. Radiology 2011;259:151–61.
62. Lohan DG, Alhajeri AN, Cronin CG, et al. MR enterography of small-bowel lymphoma: potential for suggestion of histologic subtype and the presence of underlying celiac disease. Am J Roentgenol 2008;190:287–93.
63. Tomei E, Diacinti D, Stagnitti A, et al. MR enterography: relationship between intestinal fold pattern and the clinical presentation of adult celiac disease. J Magn Reson Imaging 2012;36:183–7.
64. Nylund K, Ødegaard S, Hausken T, et al. Sonography of the small intestine. World J Gastroenterol 2009;15:1319–30.
65. Fraquelli M, Colli A, Colucci A, et al. Accuracy of ultrasonography in predicting celiac disease. Arch Intern Med 2004;164:169–74.

Video Capsule Endoscopy in Celiac Disease

Christina A. Tennyson, MD*, Edward J. Ciaccio, PhD,
Suzanne K. Lewis, MD

KEYWORDS

- Celiac disease • Capsule endoscopy • Video

KEY POINTS

- Capsule endoscopy is a safe, noninvasive way to visualize the small intestine.
- Capsule endoscopy is helpful in patients with suspected celiac disease who are unable or unwilling to undergo capsule endoscopy, those with positive celiac serology and normal duodenal biopsies, and in patients with established celiac disease with alarm symptoms.
- The limitations of capsule endoscopy include the inability to obtain biopsies, erratic motion of the capsule, incomplete examinations, and subjective interpretation.
- Computer applications may assist in standardizing the assessment of villous atrophy in capsule endoscopy studies of patients with celiac disease.

INTRODUCTION

Celiac disease is a common multisystem autoimmune disorder affecting approximately 1% of the population, which is triggered by the ingestion of gluten (a protein component of wheat, rye, and barley) in genetically susceptible individuals.[1] Screening for celiac disease is available via serologic testing, with excellent reported sensitivity and specificity.[2] Antibodies available for celiac disease screening include anti-tissue transglutaminase (TTG) immunoglobulin A (IgA) antibody, anti-endomysial (EMA) IgA antibody, and the more recently developed anti–deamidated gliadin peptide IgA/IgG antibodies. The gold standard for the diagnosis of celiac disease still remains small intestinal biopsy performed during upper endoscopy. Features of celiac disease appreciated on conventional upper endoscopy include a mosaic mucosal pattern, scalloping, villous atrophy, and flattening of folds.[3,4] In patients with partial villous atrophy, however, the small intestine may seem endoscopically normal and biopsies should be obtained regardless of the appearance if celiac disease is suspected. Histologic features suggestive of celiac disease include increased intraepithelial lymphocytes, crypt hyperplasia, and villous atrophy.[5,6] Marsh[5] developed an initial grading system to classify the histologic

Celiac Disease Center at Columbia University, Division of Digestive Diseases, Columbia University, 180 Fort Washington Avenue, Room 936, New York, NY 10032, USA
* Corresponding author.
E-mail address: ct2398@columbia.edu

Gastrointest Endoscopy Clin N Am 22 (2012) 747–758
http://dx.doi.org/10.1016/j.giec.2012.07.011
1052-5157/12/$ – see front matter © 2012 Published by Elsevier Inc.

changes associated with celiac disease and this was later refined by Oberhuber.[5,6] These histologic features are not unique to celiac disease and can be found in other conditions, such as tropical sprue and autoimmune enteropathy.[1]

Small bowel biopsy during upper endoscopy has several limitations. Upper endoscopy is an invasive procedure and sedation is routinely administered. Patients often require an escort home and miss work. During routine upper endoscopy, a very small portion of the small bowel is examined. Celiac disease may be patchy, and biopsies may fail to sample areas demonstrating disease. Some physicians may not obtain the suggested 4 to 6 biopsies during upper endoscopy when evaluating patients for suspected celiac disease.[7] Interpretation of histology may also be problematic because pathologists in some settings, particularly in commercial laboratories or community hospitals, may fail to recognize the features of celiac disease.[8] Histologic samples may also be poorly oriented, and the interpretation may be hindered.

VIDEO CAPSULE ENDOSCOPY: TECHNOLOGY AND ADMINISTRATION

Video capsule endoscopy (VCE) provides an alternative means to conventional upper endoscopy to visualize the small intestine. VCE was first introduced in 2001, and there are several systems currently available worldwide: PillCam SB2, Given Imaging, Yoqneam, Israel; Endo Capsule, Olympus America Inc, Center Valley, Pennsylvania; OMOM, Jinshan Science and Technology, Chongqing, China; and MiroCam, IntroMedic, Seoul, South Korea.[9,10] Currently, the PillCam SB2 and Endo Capsule endoscopes are available in the United States. The capsule endoscopes typically measure 11 × 26 mm and contain a battery, lens, light-emitting diodes (LEDs), and transmitter. The camera lens is surrounded by 6 LEDs that illuminate the mucosal surface of the gastrointestinal tract during the capsule passage. The capsules typically obtain 2 pictures every second and transmit images to a recording device worn by patients. The study is typically 8 hours, but an extended 12-hour capsule has recently been introduced. When the battery on the capsule endoscope is discharged, the study is complete. Images are subsequently downloaded to a workstation and reviewed. A real-time viewer is also available to assess the capsule location while the study is being conducted.

Before VCE, bowel purgatives or other preparations are not routinely recommended. Patients are often instructed to ingest a clear-liquid diet for 1 day and fast after midnight the night before the examination. A prospective randomized trial of 150 patients demonstrated similar VCE completion rates, yield, and image quality with and without the use of purgatives and prokinetics.[11] Conversely, a recent meta-analysis suggested that purgatives before VCE resulted in enhanced mucosal visualization and slightly increased the yield when compared with clear-liquid preparations.[12] In VCE studies of patients with celiac disease, the use of purgatives may be helpful to improve the visualization of the mucosa. Simethicone reduces intestinal bubbles and enhances mucosal visualization during VCE.[13] In patients with celiac disease whereby mucosal visualization is paramount, the authors' center has been using a 2 L PEG–based bowel purgative preparation the night before the examination and a 60-mg simethicone dose administered with the capsule endoscope.

INDICATIONS FOR VCE IN CELIAC DISEASE

According to an international consensus conference, VCE can be considered as an imaging modality in cases of known or suspected celiac disease in select situations (**Box 1**).[14] VCE can be performed when a person is unable or unwilling to have a conventional upper endoscopy. Examples include patients with cardiopulmonary instability or history of bleeding disorders. VCE may also be performed in cases of

---

Box 1
Indications for VCE in patients with celiac disease

1. Initial evaluation in patients unable or unwilling to have conventional upper endoscopy with suspected celiac disease

2. Positive celiac serology (TTG or EMA) and normal duodenal histology

3. History of celiac disease with warning signs, particularly refractory celiac disease type II

---

positive serology (TTG or EMA) and normal duodenal histology to visualize more distal portions of the small intestine for features of celiac disease. In patients with known celiac disease who develop warning signs, such as weight loss, bleeding, and/or abdominal pain, VCE can be used to evaluate the intestine. These concerning symptoms may occur on the initial presentation of celiac disease or after an extended period on a gluten-free diet. If there is concern for refractory celiac disease or malignancy, VCE is usually performed in combination with conventional upper endoscopy, colonoscopy, and often radiographic enterography.[1] These studies assist in excluding malignancy, particularly adenocarcinoma and lymphoma. In patients with refractory celiac disease type II whereby a clonal population of cells is present, particular concern exists for enteropathy-associated T-cell lymphoma (EATL).[15] If an abnormal area is detected on VCE, enteroscopy using a device-assisted approach can be performed to sample tissue.[16]

ROLE OF VCE IN CELIAC DISEASE

The use of VCE in celiac disease is an area of active research. It is an appealing imaging modality for patients with celiac disease because it is a relatively noninvasive and safe procedure. Because capsule endoscopes are unable to obtain biopsies, and small bowel histology remains the gold standard for the diagnosis of celiac disease, VCE serves a complementary role to conventional endoscopy. Features of celiac disease visualized during VCE are similar to those seen during conventional upper endoscopy: scalloping of folds, mosaic appearance, fissures, flat mucosa, and stacking of folds (**Fig. 1**).[17,18]

VCE examines the whole intestine and can be used to determine the extent of enteropathy. Interestingly, in a study of 38 patients with untreated biopsy-proven celiac disease, VCE detected villous atrophy in 92% of patients, but the extent of enteropathy did not correlate with clinical symptoms.[19] In this study by Murray and colleagues,[19] 59% of patients with untreated celiac disease had extensive enteropathy, 32% had duodenal enteropathy, and less than 1% had jejunal enteropathy alone.

The sensitivity and specificity for detecting features of celiac disease has varied in several clinical studies when compared with the gold standard of duodenal histology. In an initial multicenter trial by Rondonotti and colleagues[17] of 43 patients with suspected celiac disease who underwent both upper endoscopy and VCE, VCE had a sensitivity of 87.5%, specificity of 90.9%, positive predictive value of 96.5%, and negative predictive value of 71.4% for the detection of villous atrophy as compared with duodenal histology. In a study of 21 patients with suspected celiac disease (positive EMA) and 23 control patients having both upper endoscopy and VCE, 17 out of 20 patients with suspected celiac disease with villous atrophy on biopsy had abnormal VCE studies.[20] In this study by Hopper,[20] the sensitivity, specificity, positive predictive value, and negative predictive value of VCE as compared with duodenal histology was 85.0%, 100%, 100%, and 88.9%, respectively. When the small bowel mucosa was evaluated in VCE studies of patients with celiac disease, Crohn disease, and irritable

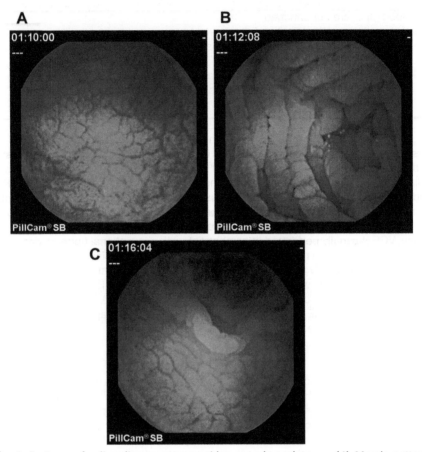

Fig. 1. Features of celiac disease seen on video capsule endoscopy. (*A*) Mosaic pattern, mucosal fissures; (*B*) scalloping; (*C*) villous atrophy.

bowel syndrome by 3 blind observers, the sensitivity ranged from 90% to 95%, whereas the specificity was only 63.6%.[21] In this study, VCE had only moderate agreement with histologic pattern with a Kappa statistic for observer 1, 2, and 3 of 0.45, 0.49, and 0.51, respectively. In a recent meta-analysis including 166 individuals using VCE in the diagnosis of celiac disease, the overall pooled VCE sensitivity was 89% (95% confidence interval 89%–98%) and the specificity was 95% (95% confidence interval 82%–94%).[22] If suspicion for celiac disease remains following a normal VCE study, upper endoscopy with biopsy should be performed.

The role of VCE in monitoring patients with celiac disease is less clear. Up to 30% of patients with celiac disease may fail to improve on a gluten-free diet alone.[23] In these patients, a systematic approach is used to exclude causes, such as gluten contamination; bacterial overgrowth; fructose/lactose intolerance; microscopic colitis; pancreatic exocrine function; refractory celiac disease; and associated malignancy, such as EATL.[24] VCE has been suggested in the evaluation of these patients combined with dietary counseling, breath testing, upper endoscopy, colonoscopy, radiologic imaging, and enteroscopy when indicated.[1] There is still limited evidence, however, to support the use of VCE in patients with nonresponsive celiac disease.

VCE was not included in a recent proposed algorithm for patients with celiac disease with persistent symptoms on a gluten-free diet, but the investigators currently use VCE in their evaluation of patients with suspected refractory celiac disease.[25] In a blinded pilot comparison study of 19 patients with unresponsive celiac disease, 53% had normal VCE studies, 47% demonstrated features of celiac disease, 11% (2 patients) had ulcers, but no small bowel tumors were found.[26] In a study performed at the authors' center, 47 patients were examined with features of complicated celiac disease: abdominal pain, weight loss, diarrhea, iron deficiency anemia, occult blood positive stool, long-standing untreated celiac disease, or a history of small bowel cancer /adenoma.[18] In this study, VCE detected lesions suspicious for lymphoma in 2 patients with refractory celiac disease type II, a case of carcinoma, a submucosal mass, a stricture, and a case of intussusception. In this study, ulcerations were found in 45% of subjects and villous atrophy was detected in 68% of subjects.

The sensitivity for detecting villous atrophy may vary in patients with treated celiac disease. In an analysis of VCE studies of patients with nonresponsive celiac disease reviewed by a single reader with expertise in celiac disease, 31% of patients had villous atrophy on VCE, but the sensitivity of VCE for detecting villous atrophy was only 56%, whereas specificity was 85%.[27] Nonresponsive celiac disease was defined as persistent or recurrent symptoms, including diarrhea, weight loss, and abdominal pain, after at least 6 months on a gluten-free diet. In this study by Atlas,[27] the presence of ulcerations was associated with the use of nonsteroidal medications; but, importantly, a case of ulcerative jejunitis or lymphoma was detected in a patient with refractory celiac disease type II and adenocarcinomas were reported. There was also weak agreement of capsule endoscopy and histology in the patients with nonresponsive celiac disease ($\kappa = 0.44$).

The literature concerning VCE in patients with refractory celiac disease is particularly limited. Daum and colleagues[28] examined 14 patients with refractory celiac disease (7 type I, 7 type II) who had VCE and abdominal imaging performed via computed tomography or magnetic resonance tomography. No abnormalities were detected in the patients with refractory celiac disease type 1 via any method, but VCE and radiologic imaging each detected signs of ulcerative jejunitis or lymphoma in separate patients with refractory celiac disease type II. Not all erosions or ulcerations represent significant abnormalities because these can be found in healthy patients, patients with treated celiac disease, and patients with nonresponsive celiac disease.[27] Although there is limited evidence to support its use, VCE should be considered in patients with refractory celiac disease type II, but it is likely of limited yield in patients with refractory celiac disease type I.

Finally, an international consensus conference recommended VCE as an imaging modality to examine the distal small intestine for features of celiac disease in cases of positive TTG antibodies and normal duodenal histology, but there is little data to support its use. Capsule endoscopy has not been shown to have any added benefit for detecting villous atrophy in patients with positive celiac serology and normal duodenal histology.[29] In this small prospective single-center study by Lidums and colleagues,[29] 8 patients with positive TTG or EMA and normal duodenal histology had normal VCE studies. In addition, only 9 out of 14 patients (64%) had a complete evaluation of the small intestine, whereas the remainder of the patients had incomplete examinations.

LIMITATIONS

VCE has several important limitations (**Box 2**). The capsule endoscopes obtain images deep in the small bowel but are presently unable to obtain biopsies or perform therapy.

Box 2
Limitations of VCE in patients with celiac disease

1. Unable to obtain biopsies or perform therapy
2. Possibility of incomplete studies and missed lesions
3. Subjective, labor-intensive analysis without a standardized scoring system for celiac disease
4. May fail to detect partial villous atrophy

Using available technology, it may be possible to develop lighter video capsules equipped with small motors that can perform biopsies.[30]

VCE studies of the small intestine may be incomplete, fail to visualize an area of interest, or the reader may miss the area of abnormality. In approximately 15% to 20% of capsule endoscopy studies, the cecum is not entered during the study.[31] Lesions may also be missed during capsule endoscopy because of the tumbling and erratic motion of the capsule.[32] In a pooled analysis of 530 VCE examinations, the overall miss rate for VCE was 10.8%, with mass lesions missed in 19% of cases when compared with other modalities, such as push enteroscopy, small bowel series, and colonoscopy with ileoscopy.[33] Importantly, for cases of celiac disease, the proximal duodenum is often poorly visualized in VCE studies, which is likely because of the speed at which the capsule passes through this fixed portion.[34]

Analysis of VCE images is subjective and labor intensive with a large number of images to view for each patient. Over an 8-hour study period, at a frame rate of 2/s, more than 50 000 frames are generated; subtle details may be overlooked during analysis. Bulges and red spots may be prone to misinterpretation.[35] VCE interpretation of features of celiac disease may be particularly difficult, and VCE may fail to detect partial villous atrophy. There is no standardized VCE scoring system applied to celiac disease. The Lewis score is an instrument to assess inflammatory change in the small intestine based on villous appearance, ulcerations, and stenosis but has not been applied regularly to celiac disease.[36] Other limitations in the literature include the frequent use of older-generation capsule technology. Newer VCEs have improved optics and field of view, but it is not certain that this would increase the sensitivity and specificity of detecting celiac disease.

The interobserver agreement for VCE in celiac disease has been moderate in some clinical studies. In the multicenter study by Rondonotti,[17] the interobserver agreement ranged between 79.2% and 94.4%, with kappa values ranging between 0.56 and 0.87.[17] However, in another study of 38 patients with untreated celiac disease, there was excellent overall interobserver agreement of 86.5% for 2 experienced VCE readers.[19]

The main risk of capsule endoscopy is capsule retention, which is defined as the retention of the capsule in the gastrointestinal tract for more than 2 weeks.[37] Capsule retention occurs less than 1% of the time in patients having a capsule endoscopy for obscure gastrointestinal bleeding, but the risk varies by indication.[38] There are no data on the incidence of capsule retention in celiac disease, but one would expect it to be low except in cases of lymphoma, adenocarcinoma, or ulcerative jejunitis with stricturing disease. If symptoms of obstruction are present, it is advisable to perform radiologic imaging of the small bowel before VCE. A dissolving patency capsule may also be used to screen for possible retention. The patency capsule consists of a dissolving lactose shell, and imaging is performed 30 hours following ingestion to ensure passage of the capsule. Rare case reports of aspiration of the capsule endoscope have also been reported.[39]

FUTURE DIRECTION: QUANTIFICATION OF VCE IMAGES IN CELIAC DISEASE

Because VCE is limited by its subjective and labor-intensive nature, performing an analysis with the assistance of a computerized method would be helpful. There is no computer system to definitively diagnose celiac disease or villous atrophy, but recent research has focused on computer analysis of VCE imaging to detect areas of abnormality.

As the capsule endoscope tumbles during small intestinal passage, the camera angle, with respect to the mucosal surface, varies greatly and continuously. Because only 2 frames are obtained per second, it is not possible to develop a contiguous map of the small intestine based on the succession of image frames. Rather, each frame is a discreet sample of the luminal surface. The quantification of VCE images has used the PillCam SB2 system, and images acquired are 576 × 576 pixels in dimension. The spatial resolution depends on the camera angle and the distance to the luminal surface, with a maximal resolution of 0.1 mm. The camera field of view is fixed for the previously mentioned system at 156°. The resolution per pixel can be estimated using a formula incorporating the field of view and average distance from the mucosal surface. As the camera angle becomes more oblique with respect to the luminal surface, the resolution is reduced. For analysis in several initial pilot studies, the authors have used an approach that assumes a mean distance and mean viewing angle of the capsule with respect to the luminal surface are constant over time. Using this approximation, any variations in distance and camera angle are treated as random phase noise. Performing an analysis of 2-dimensional image sequences, the authors have estimated the 3-dimensional mucosal structure, luminal motility, and the textural properties of the image itself.

An approximation of the 3-dimensional mucosal structure, using shape-from-shading principles, can be useful to detect and possibly quantify villous atrophy.[40] The method supposes that the camera-to-lumen distance is directly proportional to the image gray-scale level, with darker pixels indicating greater distance and lighter pixels indicating lesser distance. Using this approximation, a 3-dimensional representation is obtained. In **Fig. 2**A, an example is shown of a video-capsule image acquired

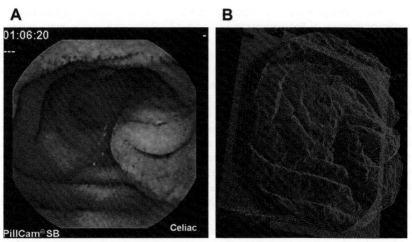

Fig. 2. (*A*) An example of a video capsule image acquired from a patient with celiac disease with villous atrophy. The original color image converted to a gray-scale image. The 3-dimensional representation of this image is shown in (*B*).

from a patient with celiac disease with villous atrophy, with the original color image converted to a gray-scale image for simplicity. The 3-dimensional representation of this image is shown in **Fig. 2**B. Small protrusions, valleys, and folds appear as distinct structures in the 3-dimensional structure. The 3-dimensional structure can then be used for measurement using a process called *syntactic analysis* in which the structures to be examined are stated in computer syntax. The authors have hypothesized that the most important structures that would differ in patients with celiac disease with villous atrophy as compared with control-patient images are mucosal protrusions. These mucosal protrusions are detected in each image by computer analysis; and the height, width, and number per image can be tabulated.[40] As compared with VCE images from control patients, patients with celiac disease with villous atrophy had more blunted protrusions (less height and greater diameter).

Image analysis has also been used to quantify texture, which is the variance in pixel gray-scale level over a predefined surface area.[40–42] Texture can be measured as the variance in gray-scale level over an image, but this would not capture localized spatial variations. In the authors' analysis, selected 10 × 10 pixel areas, termed *subimages*, were used. The authors hypothesized that the statistical variance measured in each of these subimages would be representative of regional textural differences in VCE images. A total of 56 × 56 subimages were analyzed in each of the celiac and control images, exclusive of edge pixels. In VCE images of patients with celiac disease, there is significantly greater texture, as measured by a higher degree of variance, when compared with control-patient images.[40–42] The images of patients with celiac disease were darker overall, likely because of abnormalities on both a microscopic level (where actual villous atrophy is more apparent) and at the macroscopic level (fissures, scalloping of luminal folds, mosaic pattern). Because these features in the VCE images of patients with celiac disease increase the heterogeneity of pixel gray-scale values, and also the darkness of the average pixel level, there is a correlation between microscopic and macroscopic properties in the small intestinal mucosa. An example is shown in **Fig. 3**. **Fig. 3**A, B shows control images that have the appearance of smoothness and uniformity. **Fig. 3**C, D shows images of a patient with celiac disease at areas with villous atrophy, which have the appearance of substantial structural variation manifested as fissuring, mosaic pattern, and scalloping of folds.

Quantitative image analysis can also be useful to estimate motility by evaluating the dynamic properties of the sequence of images.[43] Reference points were noted on each image in the sequence, and the variation of these reference points was used as a measure of motility. For simplicity, the authors selected the 10,000 darkest pixels in each image as reference points from 331, 776 (576 × 576) pixels in each frame, representing 3% of the total pixel content. Generally, the darkest pixels are concentrated in the direction along the luminal axis. Both the centroid (the average change in centroid location in the x and y directions) and the maximal width of the darkest region were used to estimate motility. An example is shown in **Fig. 4**, with the original image in **Fig. 4**A after conversion to gray scale, and the darkest pixels with the maximum contiguous width being given in **Fig. 4**B as a whitened area with a gray line. The standard deviations in these parameters are used as estimates of motility and found to be different in patients with celiac disease at areas of evident villous atrophy as compared with control patients.[43] Mechanical function as well as absorption may be altered in areas of villous atrophy in celiac disease.

The authors have also developed another method to estimate motility, which is based on the frequency spectrum that can be generated from a series of VCE images.[44,45] The spectral peak with the greatest magnitude indicates the main cycle length, or repetition rate, for that image series. The inverse of the frequency of this

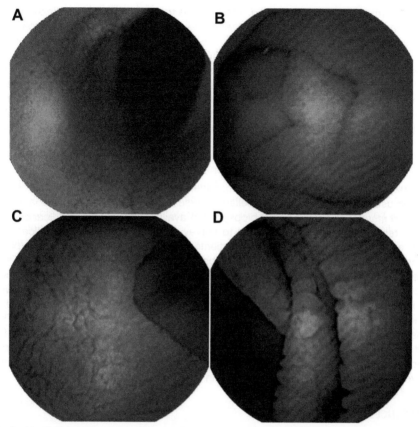

Fig. 3. (*A, B*) Control images that have the appearance of smoothness and uniformity. (*C, D*) Images of patient with celiac disease at areas with villous atrophy, which have the appearance of substantial structural variation (manifested as fissuring), mosaic pattern, and scalloping of folds.

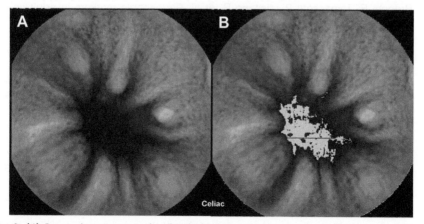

Fig. 4. (*A*) Conversion to gray scale. The darkest pixels with maximum contiguous width are shown in (*B*) as a whitened area with gray line.

peak is termed the *dominant period*. There seems to be a decreased dominant period (ie, slower periodicity) in patients with celiac disease with villous atrophy as compared with controls.[44,45]

The previously mentioned methods of quantifying video-capsule images have the potential to be used in monitoring patients with newly diagnosed celiac disease as well as those with established celiac disease. Pilot studies have been performed in small numbers of patients with celiac disease with villous atrophy but show promising results. Prospective analysis in a larger study population would assist in validating the utility of these methods for the quantitative characterization of celiac disease.

SUMMARY

The role of capsule endoscopy in the management of celiac disease is still evolving. VCE is useful in the diagnosis of celiac disease in special circumstances in which the gold standard of small bowel biopsy is not available because of medical or individual reasons. It is also being used to survey the small bowel for complications, such as malignancies, particularly in patients with refractory celiac disease type II. Capsule endoscopy examines the small bowel and can be helpful to detect distal disease and to direct more invasive endoscopic or surgical procedures. Limitations occur because of the nature of the capsule's passage, where areas may not be well visualized, as well as with interobserver differences in interpretation. Classic villous changes, however, are well defined and easily identified on capsule endoscopy. The most challenging situations include patients with mild mucosal changes that are difficult to identify, such as in individuals with positive celiac serology but normal duodenal biopsies. The role of computerized analysis of villous changes and motility by quantitative image analysis may be most useful in these more ambiguous cases.

REFERENCES

1. Green PH, Cellier C. Celiac disease. N Engl J Med 2007;357:1731–43.
2. Leffler DA, Schuppan D. Update on serologic testing in celiac disease. Am J Gastroenterol 2010;105:2520–4.
3. Brocchi E, Corazza GR, Caletti G, et al. Endoscopic demonstration of loss of duodenal folds in the diagnosis of celiac disease. N Engl J Med 1988;319:741–4.
4. Brocchi E, Tomassetti P, Misitano B, et al. Endoscopic markers in adult celiac disease. Dig Liver Dis 2002;34:177–82.
5. Marsh MN. Gluten, major histocompatibility complex, and the small intestine. A molecular and immunobiologic approach to the spectrum of gluten sensitivity (celiac sprue). Gastroenterology 1992;102:330–54.
6. Oberhuber G, Granditsch G, Vogelsang H. The histopathology of coeliac disease: a time for standardized report scheme for pathologists. Eur J Gastroenterol Hepatol 1999;11:1185–94.
7. Lebwohl B, Kapel RC, Neugut AI, et al. Adherence to biopsy guidelines increases celiac disease diagnosis. Gastrointest Endosc 2011;74:103–9.
8. Arguelles-Grande C, Tennyson CA, Lewis SK, et al. Variability in small bowel histopathology reporting between different pathology practice settings: impact on the diagnosis of coeliac disease. J Clin Pathol 2012;63:242–7.
9. Iddan G, Meron G, Glukhovsky A, et al. Wireless capsule endoscopy. Nature 2000;405:417.
10. Leighton JA. The role of endoscopic imaging of the small bowel in clinical practice. Am J Gastroenterol 2011;106:27–36.

11. Postgate A, Tekkis P, Patterson N, et al. Are bowel purgatives and prokinetics useful for small-bowel capsule endoscopy? A prospective randomized controlled study. Gastrointest Endosc 2009;69:1120–8.

12. Rokkas T, Papaxoinis K, Triantafyllou K, et al. Does purgative preparation influence the diagnostic yield of small bowel video capsule endoscopy? A meta-analysis. Am J Gastroenterol 2009;104:219–27.

13. Wu L, Cao Y, Liao C, et al. Systematic review and meta-analysis of randomized controlled trials of simethicone for gastrointestinal endoscopic visibility. Scand J Gastroenterol 2011;46:227–35.

14. Cellier C, Green PH, Collin P, et al. ICCE consensus for celiac disease. Endoscopy 2005;37:1055–9.

15. Cellier C, Delabesse E, Helmer C, et al. Refractory sprue, coeliac disease, and enteropathy–associated T-cell lymphoma. French Coeliac Disease Study Group. Lancet 2000;356:203–8.

16. Hadithi M, Al-toma A, Oudejans J, et al. The value of double-balloon enteroscopy in patients with refractory celiac disease. Am J Gastroenterol 2007;102:987–96.

17. Rondonotti E, Spada C, Cave D, et al. Video capsule enteroscopy in the diagnosis of celiac disease: a multicenter study. Am J Gastroenterol 2007;102:1624–31.

18. Culliford A, Daly J, Diamond B, et al. The value of wireless capsule endoscopy in patients with complicated celiac disease. Gastrointest Endosc 2005;62:55–61.

19. Murray JA, Rubio-Tapia A, Van Dyke CT. Mucosal atrophy in celiac disease: extent of involvement, correlation with clinical presentation, and response to treatment. Clin Gastroenterol Hepatol 2008;6:186–93.

20. Hopper AD, Sidhu R, Hurlstone DP, et al. Capsule endoscopy: an alternative to duodenal biopsy for the recognition of villous atrophy in coeliac disease? Dig Liver Dis 2007;39:140–5.

21. Biagi F, Rondonotti E, Campanella J, et al. Video capsule endoscopy and histology for small bowel mucosa evaluation: a comparison performed by blinded observers. Clin Gastroenterol Hepatol 2006;4:998–1003.

22. Rokkas T, Niv Y. The role of video capsule endoscopy in the diagnosis of celiac disease: a meta-analysis. Eur J Gastroenterol Hepatol 2012;24:303–8.

23. O'Mahony S, Howdle PD, Losowsky MS, et al. Review article: management of patients with non-responsive coeliac disease. Aliment Pharmacol Ther 1996;10:671–80.

24. Abdulkarim AS, Burgart LJ, See J, et al. Etiology of nonresponsive celiac disease: results of a systematic approach. Am J Gastroenterol 2002;97:2016–21.

25. Dewar DH, Donnelly SC, McLaughlin SD, et al. Celiac disease: management of persistent symptoms in patients on a gluten-free diet. World J Gastroenterol 2012;18:1348–56.

26. Maiden L, Elliot T, McLaughlin SD, et al. A blinded pilot comparison of capsule endoscopy and small bowel histology in unresponsive celiac disease. Dig Dis Sci 2009;54:1280–3.

27. Atlas DS, Rubio-Tapia A, Van Dyke CT, et al. Capsule endoscopy in nonresponsive celiac disease. Gastrointest Endosc 2011;74:1315–22.

28. Daum S, Wahnschaffe U, Glasenapp R, et al. Capsule endoscopy in refractory celiac disease. Endoscopy 2007;39:455–8.

29. Lidums I, Cummins AG, Teo E. The role of capsule endoscopy in suspected celiac disease patients with a positive serology. Dig Dis Sci 2011;56:499–505.

30. Swain P. The future of wireless capsule endoscopy. World J Gastroenterol 2008;14:4142–5.

31. Rondonotti E, Villa F, Mulder CJ, et al. Small bowel capsule endoscopy in 2007: indications, risks and limitations. World J Gastroenterol 2007;13:6140–9.

32. Cave DR, Fleischer DE, Leighton JA, et al. A multicenter randomized comparison of the Endocapsule and the Pillcam SB. Gastrointest Endosc 2008;68: 487–94.

33. Lewis BS, Eisen GM, Friedman S. A pooled analysis to evaluate results of capsule endoscopy trials [erratum in: Endoscopy 2007;39:303]. Endoscopy 2005;37: 960–5.

34. Selby WS, Prakoso E. The inability to visualize the ampulla of Vater is an inherent limitation of capsule endoscopy. Eur J Gastroenterol Hepatol 2011;23:101–3.

35. Gerson L. Capsule endoscopy and deep enteroscopy: indications for the practicing clinician. Gastroenterology 2009;137:1197–201.

36. Gralnek IM, Defranchis R, Seidman E, et al. Development of a capsule endoscopy scoring index for small bowel mucosal inflammatory change. Aliment Pharmacol Ther 2008;27:146–54.

37. Cave D, Legnani P, de Franchis R, et al. 2005 reference for capsule retention. Endoscopy 2005;37:1065–7.

38. Li F, Gurudu SR, De Petris G, et al. Retention of the capsule endoscope: a single center experience of 1000 capsule endoscopy procedures. Gastrointest Endosc 2008;68:174–80.

39. Koulaouzidis A, Pendlebury J, Douglas S, et al. Aspiration of video capsule: rare but potentially life-threatening complication to include in your consent form. Am J Gastroenterol 2009;104:1602–3.

40. Ciaccio EJ, Tennyson CA, Lewis SK, et al. Distinguishing patients with celiac disease by quantitative analysis of video capsule endoscopy images. Comput Methods Programs Biomed 2010;100:39–48.

41. Ciaccio EJ, Tennyson CA, Bhagat G, et al. Classification of video capsule endoscopy image patterns: comparative analysis between patients with celiac disease and normal individuals. Biomed Eng Online 2010;9:44.

42. Ciaccio EJ, Bhagat G, Tennyson CA, et al. Quantitative assessment of endoscopic images for degree of villous atrophy in celiac disease. Dig Dis Sci 2011;56:805–11.

43. Ciaccio EJ, Tennyson CA, Bhagat G, et al. Quantitative estimates of motility from video capsule endoscopy images are useful to distinguish celiac patients from controls. Dig Dis Sci 2012. [Epub ahead of print].

44. Ciaccio EJ, Tennyson CA, Bhagat G, et al. Robust spectral analysis of video capsule images acquired from celiac disease patients. Biomed Eng Online 2011;10:78.

45. Ciaccio EJ, Tennyson CA, Bhagat G, et al. Transformation of video capsule images to detect small bowel mucosal differences in celiac versus control patients. Comput Methods Programs Biomed 2012;108(1):28–37.

Refractory Celiac Disease

Georgia Malamut, MD, PhD[a,b,c], Joseph A. Murray, MD, PhD[d,*],
Christophe Cellier, MD, PhD[a,b,c]

KEYWORDS

- Refractory celiac disease • Aberrant intraepithelial lymphocytes
- Immunosuppressive treatments

KEY POINTS

- Novel concepts of refractory celiac disease have recently emerged and refer to 2 distinct entities sustained by 2 different pathogenic mechanisms.
- Type I refractory celiac disease (RCDI) is indistinguishable from uncomplicated active celiac disease except in its autonomy toward gluten exposure.
- RCDII resembles a low-grade lymphoma characterized by clonal expansion of small aberrant intraepithelial lymphocytes (IELs).
- Diagnosis is based on specialized small bowel investigations (enteroscopy, videocapsule endoscopy) and techniques of IEL analyses (immunohistochemistry, molecular biology, flow cytometry).
- Survival of patients with RCDI has been described as being inferior to that of those with celiac disease, and is associated with passage of RCDI to RCDII and onset of overt lymphoma.
- Prognosis of RCDII is poor because of severe malnutrition and very high risk of overt lymphoma.
- Recent advances in understanding of the pathogenesis of both forms of refractory celiac disease (RCD) offer new targeted strategies to cure RCD and prevent overt lymphoma.

Novel concepts of refractory celiac disease (RCD) have recently emerged and refer to 2 distinct entities sustained by 2 different pathogenic mechanisms. Type I RCD (RCDI) is indistinguishable from uncomplicated active celiac disease except in its autonomy toward gluten exposure. Pathogenesis probably involves self-perpetuated inflammation caused by autoimmunity. Type II RCD (RCDII) resembles a low-grade lymphoma characterized by clonal expansion of small aberrant intraepithelial lymphocytes (IELs). Diagnosis is based on specialized small bowel investigations (enteroscopy, videocapsule

[a] Université Paris Descartes, 15 rue de l'école de Médecine, 75006 Paris, France; [b] Gastroenterology Department, Hôpital Européen Georges Pompidou APHP, 20 rue Leblanc, 75015 Paris, France; [c] Insem U989, 154 rue de Vaugirard, 75015 Paris, France; [d] Division of Gastroenterology and Hepatology, Mayo Clinic, 200 First Street SW, Rochester, MN 55905, USA
* Corresponding author.
E-mail address: murray.joseph@mayo.edu

Gastrointest Endoscopy Clin N Am 22 (2012) 759–772
http://dx.doi.org/10.1016/j.giec.2012.07.007
1052-5157/12/$ – see front matter © 2012 Elsevier Inc. All rights reserved.

endoscopy) and techniques of IEL analyses (immunohistochemistry, molecular biology, flow cytometry). Survival of patients with RCDI has been described as being inferior to that of those with celiac disease, and is associated with passage of RCDI to RCDII and onset of overt lymphoma.[1,2] Prognosis of RCDII is poor because of severe malnutrition and very high risk of overt lymphoma. Altogether, these rare but resistant and severe forms of celiac disease require efficient treatments. Recent advances in the understanding of the pathogenesis of both forms of RCD offer new targeted strategies to cure RCD and prevent overt lymphoma.

BACKGROUND

Celiac disease is an enteropathy related to autoimmune diseases induced by gluten in genetically predisposed individuals with HLA-DQ2 and HLA-DQ8 genotypes. The rate of diagnosis has been rising dramatically, although, with a prevalence of 1% of Caucasians in Europe and the Americas, most cases remain undetected.[3–5] Its clinical presentation is extremely variable, and diagnosis relies on the detection of specific serum antibodies and the demonstration of intestinal villous atrophy.[6] Treatment relies on strict adherence to a lifelong gluten-free diet (GFD), which generally prevents bone, autoimmune, and malignant complications. An initial nonresponse to a GFD is mainly from accidental or deliberate gluten contamination of the diet. Once gluten contamination and other causes of symptoms and villous atrophy have been ruled out, a small subgroup of patients with celiac disease remain who may have a primarily or secondary resistance to a GFD because of an authentic RCD. This article describes the diagnosis and treatment of the different types of RCD to provide guidance for the care of this rare but serious condition.

DIAGNOSIS OF RCD
Definition

RCD can be defined as persistent or recurrent severe enteropathy and symptomatic malabsorption in patients with previously confirmed celiac disease who have been on a GFD for at least 12 months (see exception mentioned later) and whose enteropathy or symptoms are not otherwise explained by other conditions or gluten conatamination.[1,2] A very small subgroup of patients with celiac disease develop primary or secondary resistance to a GFD. Incomplete exclusion of dietary gluten must first be eliminated, because as many as 50% of patients are less than optimally compliant.[7] Persistent or recurrent symptoms of malabsorption with intestinal villous atrophy for at least 12 months of a strict GFD characterize RCD. Diagnosis of this condition is made after other small bowel diseases are excluded, such as autoimmune enteropathy,[8] tropical sprue,[9] or common variable immunodeficiency,[10] and the other conditions that are highly likely to explain the symptoms (**Fig. 1**). RCD has been subdivided into 2 subgroups: type I (RCDI), defined by persisting villous atrophy despite a strict GFD associated with an increased number of IELs bearing a normal phenotype with surface CD3 and CD8 expression, and type II (RCDII) characterized by clonal expansion of abnormal IELs lacking surface markers CD3, CD8, and T-cell receptors, and preserved expression of intracellular CD3.[11,12]

Epidemiology

Frequency of RCDI and RCDII remain unknown. In the Derby cohort, West and Holmes[13] report that 0.7% of 713 patients with celiac disease had RCDII. In this latest study, diagnosis of patients with RCDII was based only on aspects of ulcerative jejunitis,[13] which could have either caused an underestimation of RCDII from lack of application of molecular techniques or overestimation from confounding with RCDI.

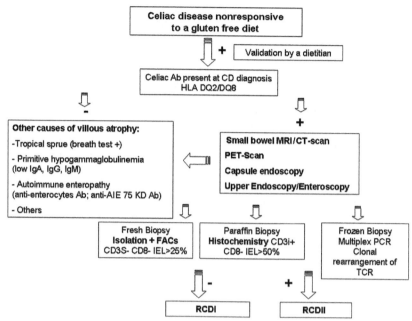

Fig. 1. Diagnostic approach in celiac disease refractory to a GFD.

Incidence of T-cell lymphoma associated with celiac disease has been estimated at 0.22 to 1.9 per 100,000 inhabitants per year, although some of these cases may proceed directly from celiac disease, often undetected, to lymphoma without passing through a clinically apparent syndrome of RCD.[14,15]

Predisposing Factors

Whether patients with RCD have a particular genetic background differentiating them from those with uncomplicated CD is still debated. The small numbers of patients with RCD have had limited genetic investigations. However, severity of celiac disease was correlated with the number of HLA-DQ2 copies: homozygosity for HLA-DQ2 was observed in 25.5% of patients with RCDI, 44.1% of patients with RCDII, and 53.3% of patients with enteropathy-associated T-cell lymphoma (EATL), versus 20.7% of patients with uncomplicated celiac disease and 2.1% of controls.[16] Other genes involved in lymphocyte signaling [genes: *SH2B3* (12q34), *PTPN2* (18q11), *RGS1* (1q31)] are associated with celiac disease and could be involved in the risk of developing overt lymphoma.[17] Ongoing genomewide association studies suggest that the known celiac susceptibility variants may be not found in RCDII.[18]

Another important environmental factor is probably the exposure to gluten. Risk of lymphomatous complications was reported to be 4 times higher in patients not observing a GFD than in those who were compliant.[19] The amount of gluten consumption could be responsible for the differences in terms of severity of celiac disease. A recent study shows that the more severe outcome of celiac disease in southern compared with northern Europe is related to a higher gluten intake.[20]

Diagnosis

Diagnosis of RCD relies on persisting malabsorption and villous atrophy after 1 year of following a strict GFD typically confirmed by expert dietician review. An exception may be necessary for patients who present with severe malabsorption syndrome with ulcerative jejunitis who have strictly adhered to a GFD and are still experiencing an inexorable decline. These cases must be differentiated from the very severe presentation that can occasionally occur in regular celiac disease.[21] Initial endoscopic assessment includes standard or extended upper gastrointestinal endoscopy with biopsy. Sufficient biopsies must be taken to allow for a full assessment of the degree of mucosal injury and for special studies to determine the type of RCD or alternative diagnoses. Careful visual assessment for focal abnormalities that could indicate a prevalent malignancy is essential. Most will be situated in the proximal small intestine but may be beyond the reach of the standard or even an extended endoscopy. Double-balloon enteroscopy is a superior tool for identifying suspicious lesions for EATL or for a better assessment of ulcers, particularly for evidence of ulcerative jejunitis found in roughly 70% of patients with RCDII.[2,22] Capsule endoscopy is useful for showing the extent of lesions. Capsule endoscopy has superior sensitivity for predicting persistent villous atrophy compared with standard video endoscopy.[23] Furthermore, capsule endoscopy allows the visualization of ulcers all along the intestinal tract, which may suggest RCDII before diagnostic confirmation through direct biopsy sampling.[24] Moreover, the authors diagnosed 3 cases of overt lymphoma when capsule endoscopy showed very suspicious intestinal strictures and jejunal ulcers.[25] Double-balloon enteroscopy reaching the distal small bowel in the 3 cases provided histologic confirmation of the capsule findings.[25] One major although rare limitation of capsule endoscopy is the risk of retention, particularly in patients with RCDII who are particularly at risk of strictures (**Fig. 2**). Prior radiologic imaging of the small bowel is recommended to rule out stricturing disease and also diagnose extraintestinal lymphoma involvement of rarely giant cavitating lymph nodes (**Fig. 3**).[26] The second limitation is the need for biopsy during endoscopy (**Fig. 4**) for definitive diagnosis. In RCDI, histologic examination is similar to that found in active celiac disease with villous atrophy and increased normal IEL. No other diagnostic criteria have yet been defined for RCDI. In contrast, the hallmark abnormal IEL findings, detected using 3 combined techniques, make the diagnosis of RCDII more specific: more than 25% of the CD103+ or CD45 + IELs lacking surface CD3–T-cell receptor (TCR) complexes on flow cytometry (**Fig. 5**) or more than 50% IELs expressing intracellular CD3ε but not

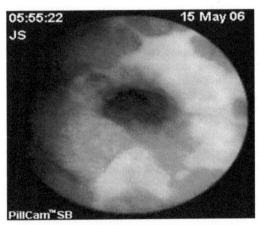

Fig. 2. Capsule endoscopy aspect of strictures in RCDII. (*Adapted from* Barret M, Malamut G, Rahmi G, et al. Diagnostic yield of capsule endoscopy in refractory celiac disease. Am J Gastroenterol 2012;107(10):1546–53; with permission.)

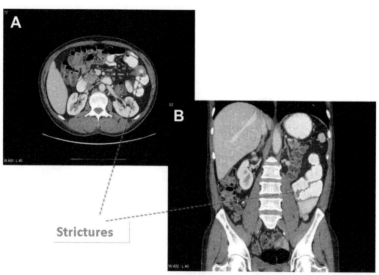

Strictures

Fig. 3. CT scan of small bowel strictures (*arrow*) of RCDII. (*A*) Axial plane. (*B*) Sagittal plane.

CD8 in formalin-fixed sections (**Fig. 6**), and/or the presence of a detectable clonal rearrangement of the gamma chain of the TCR in duodenal biopsies (**Fig. 7**).[2] Similar features allow detection of lymphocytic gastritis and colitis containing the same abnormal population in around 50% and 30% of patients with RCDII, respectively.[2] RCDII may be misdiagnosed when fluorescence-activated cell sorter analysis of freshly isolated IEL is lacking. Discrepancies in diagnostic tools are probably responsible for differences observed between European and North American countries.[1,27,28] Heterogeneity in detection of the clonal TCR rearrangement may also explain diagnostic differences. The authors showed that analysis of the delta chain rearrangement may be useful in patients with RCDII presenting with oligoclonal rearrangement of the gamma chain.[2] Other investigators have recently shown interest in detecting the beta chain of the TCR.[29] Nevertheless, evidence that abnormal IELs originate from immature T cells tempers interest in studying beta rearrangement, which occurs later in the

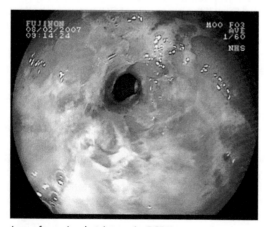

Fig. 4. Endoscopic view of proximal stricture in RCDII.

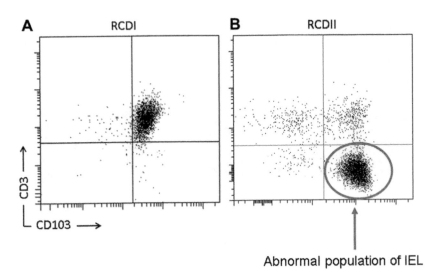

Fig. 5. Flow cytometry analysis of freshly isolated IEL from duodenum of patients with RCDI (*A*) and RCDII (*B*).

ontogeny. Finally, specificity of the PCR product must be shown through formation of homoduplexes.[2]

CLINICAL PRESENTATION AND PROGNOSIS

Celiac disease is primarily resistant to a GFD in roughly one-third and one-half of patients with RCDI and RCDII, respectively.[2] Besides the abnormal phenotype of IEL, RCDII has a generally more severe clinical presentation and is frequently associated with endoscopic ulcerative jejunitis responsible for severe protein-losing enteropathy. Symptoms are notably less severe in RCDI, and endoscopic and histologic features are similar to those found in active celiac disease.[2] RCDII is associated with poor prognosis, with 5-year survival rates of 44% to 58%.[1,2,30] The more severe malnutrition, as manifested by a low serum albumin level, combined with the higher risk of developing overt lymphoma explains the higher mortality associated with RCDII compared with RCDI.[2] Even if the prognosis of RCDI is much better than that of RCDII, the rates of complications and mortality have been reported to be much higher than those associated with uncomplicated celiac disease.[1,31]

No curative treatment yet exists for RCD. Steroids improved transient clinical symptoms in most patients with either type of RCD with inconstant histologic response.[2] Immunosuppressive drugs have only a poor effect on the histologic response and may predispose to overt lymphoma.[32] Of patients with RCDII, 33% to 52% develop EATL within 5 years after diagnosis.[2,30] Onset of EATL in RCDI is much lower than in RCDII, with a 5-year rate of 14% in the more pessimistic studies.[2] The high risk of transformation of RCDII may be because RCDII represents an intraepithelial lymphoma.[12] At this stage, clonal IELs are already engaged in malignant transformation, as attested by their clonality, the presence of their chromosomal abnormalities, the recurrent partial trisomy 1q22–q44, and their tendency to disseminate in and outside the intestine.[2,33] Abnormal IELs may be found in mesenteric lymph nodes, blood, bone marrow, and different epitheliums, such as lung and skin.[2] A high percentage of abnormal cells (up to 92%) is predictive of abnormal circulating cells

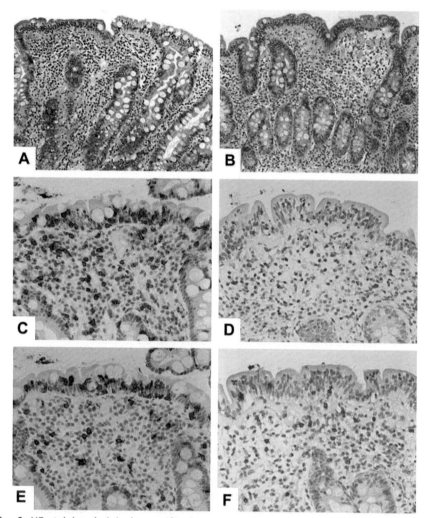

Fig. 6. HE staining (original magnification *A, B*: ×100) and immunohistochemistry performed on duodenal sections with anti-CD3 (original magnification *C, D*: ×200) and -CD8 (original magnification *E, F*: ×200) immunostaining in RCDI (*A, C, E*) and RCDII (*B, D, F*) patients. Subtotal villous atrophy with normal expression of CD3 and CD8 in RCDI and severe villous atrophy with less than 50% CD8 positive IEL in RCDII are seen.

in peripheral blood.[34] Extraintestinal RCDII lesions may be diagnosed through evidence of the same clonal TCRγδ chain rearrangements that present in duodenum (see **Fig. 6**), but also through immunohistochemistry showing CD103+, CD3i+, CD8– T cells.

EATL may develop in intestinal but also cutaneous lesions of RCDII, with expression of the same IEL-specific integrin CD103. The clonal association between RCDII IEL and EATL is demonstrated by the presence of TCRγ chain rearrangement.[12] Increase of abnormal IEL in RCDII correlates with the decrease of normal gamma-delta IEL, which is associated with a more frequent onset of overt T-cell lymphoma.[35] In clinical practice, regular follow-up, including control enteroscopy, CT scan, or MRI small-bowel

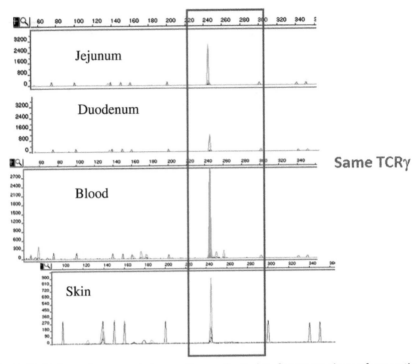

Fig. 7. Multiplex polymerase chain reaction performed in frozen specimens from patients with RCDII. Evidence of the same T-cell receptor gamma chain in all of the specimens tested.

follow-through, and positron emission tomography (PET) scan, is necessary to screen patients with RCDII to detect EATL as early as possible. However, no standard interval for follow-up has been established. Specialized investigations can be reasonably performed every year for patients with RCDI and every 6 months for those with RCDII.[2] PET scan is of particular interest because high intensity is correlated with location of proliferating overt lymphoma cells, contrasting with the lesser intensity of nonproliferating RCDII cells.[36] It can further guide radiologic-guided biopsy or explorative celioscopy. Moreover, findings may be indicative of treatment efficacy, showing significant decrease of signal intensity (**Fig. 8**).

PATHOGENESIS
Activation and Survival of IEL

Mechanisms of RCDI must be investigated. One plausible hypothesis is that the immunologic reaction initiated by gluten has evolved toward autoimmunity. Accordingly, symptoms improve with immunosuppressive treatments.[2,30] However, anti–tissue transglutaminase (anti-TG2) autoantibodies are often absent and, in contrast with autoimmune enteropathy from the lack of functional forkhead box P3 (FOXP3+) regulatory T cells, antienterocyte antibodies are not detected (Christophe Cellier, Nicole Brousse, Paris, France, personal data). Therefore the hypothesis/mechanism of intestinal autoimmunity remains to be substantiated.

More progress has been made recently in understanding the pathogenesis of RCDII. The phenotype is now well defined, with accumulation of small clonal IELs without

Baseline   **6 months**

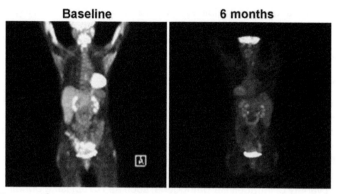

Fig. 8. PET scan of patient with RCDII before and after 6 months treatment with budesonide.

proliferation but with a defect in apoptosis.[37] The intestinal HLA-DQ2/8–restricted gliadin-specific response does not explain the loss of IEL homeostasis observed in celiac disease and RCDII. Ten years ago, in vitro and ex vivo experiments showed that the cytokine interleukin (IL)-15 could be the putative factor involved in resistance to apoptosis.[37] In active celiac disease and RCDII, an excess of IL-15 is produced by enterocytes and lamina propria mononuclear cells, and exerts potent antiapoptotic effects that prevent the elimination of activated IELs and promote their massive accumulation despite very low in situ proliferation.[37]

IELs are, in celiac disease and RCD, rich in cytolytic proteins (perforin, granzymes, FAS ligand) and produce large amounts of interferon gamma (IFN-γ), indicating their likely contribution to the prominent apoptosis observed in the flattened surface epithelium.[37–39] The granzyme-perforin cytotoxicity accounts for the severe epithelial lesions observed in RCDII but also probably in invasive EATLs expressing the cytotoxic markers granzyme B/TIA-1 (positivity in all of the authors' 31 tested EATLs, Georgia Malamut, Paris, France, personal data).

In addition, IL-15 is able to stimulate the expression of natural killer (NK) receptors (CD94 and NKG2D) on human IELs, and epithelial expression of one NKG2D ligand, the major histocompatibility complex (MHC) Ib molecule major histocompatibility complex class 1 homolog (MICA), enhanced in both active celiac disease and RCDII. NKG2D-MICA interactions can then activate a cytolytic attack of the epithelium.[40] Because of the presence of IL-15, the cytolytic attack of the epithelium may then be amplified and perpetuated via NKG2D independently of the TCR. The latter mechanism occurs in RCDII, in which abnormal IELs lacking a TCR can exert their cytotoxicity against epithelial cells.

Antiapoptotic Signaling Pathway of IL-15

In keeping with the observation that IL-15 transgenic mice develop CD8/NK lymphomas and leukemias,[41] the group of Nadine Cerf-Bensussan hypothesized that IL-15 played a significant role in the promotion of survival of these abnormal IELs. To test this hypothesis, they studied the IL-15–driven signaling pathway in normal and abnormal IELs. Using specific inhibitors and/or shRNA in IEL cell lines in vitro and experiments in situ in the small bowel of patients with RCDII, the group of Nadine Cerf-Bensussan showed that the survival signal delivered by IL-15 requires, through IL-15R$\beta\gamma$, activation of JAK, STAT5, and the antiapoptotic factor Bcl-xL.

Human anti–IL-15 antibodies inhibit ex vivo the IL-15–driven signaling pathway in intestinal organotypic cultures of patients with RCDII. In vivo, treatment with this antibody in mice overexpressing human IL-15 in the small bowel wiped out the IEL hyperplasia observed in these mice.[42]

Factors Explaining the High Production of IL-15

Mechanisms underlying intestinal overexpression of IL-15 in celiac disease and RCD remain to be elucidated. Gluten exposure[37] and other environmental factors, such as infections, may enhance production of IL-15. Epidemiologic factors argue that viral infections, such as rotavirus, may increase the risk of celiac disease autoimmunity in genetically predisposed individuals.[43] It can be hypothesized that viral infection triggers inflammation and autoimmunity through hyperproduction of IL-15. IL-15 is induced by a variety of intracellular pathogens, such as Toxoplasma gondii, Mycobacterium tuberculosis, Candida albicans, and herpesvirus 6 and 7.[44–47] The authors observed hepatitis B or C at the onset of refractoriness in 20% and 10% of patients with RCDI and RCDII, respectively.[2]

TREATMENT OF RCD: TOWARD NEW THERAPEUTIC STRATEGIES?

It has not yet been possible to design an effective treatment for RCDI or RCDII. Steroids, especially potent topically active steroids such as budesonide that undergo high first-pass inactivation by CYP3A4 in the liver, improve clinical symptoms in most patients with either type of RCD. However, a histologic response was observed only in 30% to 40% of cases.[2] To mitigate steroid-dependent side effects, immunosuppressors such as azathioprine, cyclosporine, or anti–tumor necrosis factor α were used, showing transient clinical response but rare mucosal improvement.[2] Absorption of oral systemic agents is unreliable and levels should be measured if possible.

In RCDII, immunosuppressive drugs have, as could be expected, no impact on the abnormal clonal IEL population and could enhance the risk of overt lymphoma, as observed with azathioprine and anti-CD52.[2,32] The bad prognosis of RCDII led to more aggressive treatments, such as chemotherapy. Contrary to EATL, which expressed Ki67, RCDII is characterized by the onset of IEL with abnormal phenotype CD3i+, CD8–, Ki67–, which massively accumulate without in situ–detectable proliferation.[37] The nonproliferative RCDII cells are thus difficult to eradicate through regular chemotherapy[2] and may represent a reservoir of cells susceptible to more aggressive transformation. Purine analogs, such as pentostatin or cladribine (2-CdA), showed moderate clinical, histologic, and hematologic efficacies.[48,49] In the authors' retrospective study of patients with RCDII,[2] 2-CdA induced clinical and histologic response. However, explosive onset of overt lymphoma was observed in the 2 treated patients within 3 to 8 weeks after treatment, precluding further use of these drugs, inasmuch as enhanced risk of transformation into overt lymphoma was previously observed in a series of 17 patients with RCDII treated with 2-CdA.[48] One possible alternative strategy is autologous hematopoietic stem cell transplantation, which induced clinical and histologic response but no sustained reduction of abnormal IEL in the 13 treated patients.[50,51] The use of chemotherapy before autologous hematopoietic stem cell transplant may probably increase hematologic response, and this strategy is being evaluated in a prospective phase II trial (ID-RCB: 2008-A01106-49). Establishing a targeted strategy seems necessary to complete the therapeutic armory for treating RCDII and to prevent overt lymphoma, the prognosis of which is even worse than for RCDII, with only 20% of patients alive 5 years after diagnosis.[14,52,53] Identification of the mechanisms underlying the onset of RCDII may help determine potential therapeutic targets. It was recently shown that IL-15 triggers an antiapoptotic pathway in human IEL in celiac disease and RCD, and seems to be a serious factor involved in the lymphomagenesis associated with celiac disease.[42] The work of Cerf-Bensussan et al shows how IL-15 is involved in the abnormal survival of IEL in RCDII, and highlights new possible therapeutic targets for treating RCDII and preventing EATL.[42]

Blocking IL-15 may therefore help reduce the numbers of clonal IEL and prevent epithelial damage. The recent development of a humanized anti–IL-15 antibody, which already has been used without any major side effects in a phase I/II trial in rheumatoid arthritis, suggests the feasibility of this therapeutic approach.[54] Another possibility is to block the downstream molecules activated by IL-15. Treatment of RCDII will probably involve a combination of conventional chemotherapy agents and targeted therapy with anti–IL-15 antibodies or JAK3 inhibitors in the next future.

SUMMARY

In conclusion, novel concepts of what RCD is have recently emerged and refer to 2 distinct entities sustained by 2 different pathogenic mechanisms. On one hand, RCDI is indistinguishable from uncomplicated active celiac disease except in its autonomy toward gluten exposure. Pathogenesis probably involves self-perpetuated inflammation from autoimmunity. On the other hand, RCDII resembles a low-grade lymphoma characterized by clonal expansion of small aberrant IEL. Diagnosis is based on specialized small bowel investigations (enteroscopy, videocapsule endoscopy) and techniques of IEL analyses (immunohistochemistry, molecular biology, flow cytometry). Survival of patients with RCDI has been described as inferior to that of those with celiac disease, and is associated with passage of RCDI to RCDII and onset of overt lymphoma.[1,2] Prognosis of RCDII is poor because of severe malnutrition and very high risk of overt lymphoma. Altogether, these rare but resistant and severe forms of celiac disease require efficient treatments. Recent advances in understanding of the pathogenesis of both forms of RCD offer new targeted strategies to cure RCD and prevent overt lymphoma.

ACKNOWLEDGMENTS

The authors thank Nadine Cerf-Bensussan and Bertrand Meresse (Inserm U989, Université Paris Descartes) for fluorescence-activated cell sorter analysis of normal and abnormal intraepithelial lymphocytes; Virginie Verkarre and Nicole Brousse (Pathology, Hôpital Necker Enfants Malades, Paris) for providing immunostainings of small bowel tissue sections; and Céline Callens and Elisabeth Macintyre (Biologic Hematology, Hôpital Necker Enfants Malades, Paris) for providing an example of multiplex polymerase chain reaction.

REFERENCES

1. Rubio-Tapia A, Kelly DG, Lahr BD, et al. Clinical staging and survival in refractory celiac disease: a single center experience. Gastroenterology 2009;136:99–107.
2. Malamut G, Afchain P, Verkarre V, et al. Presentation and long-term follow-up of refractory celiac disease: comparison of type I with type II. Gastroenterology 2009;136:81–90.
3. Rubio-Tapia A, Kyle RA, Kaplan EL, et al. Increased prevalence and mortality in undiagnosed celiac disease. Gastroenterology 2009;137:88–93.
4. Rubio-Tapia A, Ludvigsson J, Brantner TL, et al. The prevalence of celiac disease in the United States. Am J Gastroenterol 2012. [Epub ahead of print].

5. Murray JA, Van Dyke C, Plevak MF, et al. Trends in the identification and clinical features of celiac disease in a North American community, 1950-2001. Clin Gastroenterol Hepatol 2003;1:19–27.
6. Green PH, Cellier C. Celiac disease. N Engl J Med 2007;357:1731–43.
7. Vahedi K, Mascart F, Mary JY, et al. Reliability of antitransglutaminase antibodies as predictors of gluten-free diet compliance in adult celiac disease. Am J Gastroenterol 2003;98:1079–87.
8. Akram S, Murray JA, Pardi DS, et al. Adult autoimmune enteropathy: Mayo Clinic Rochester experience. Clin Gastroenterol Hepatol 2007;5:1282–90.
9. Khokhar N, Gill ML. Tropical sprue: revisited. J Pak Med Assoc 2004;54:133–4.
10. Malamut G, Verkarre V, Suarez F, et al. The enteropathy associated with common variable immunodeficiency: the delineated frontiers with celiac disease. Am J Gastroenterol 2010;105:2262–75.
11. Cellier C, Patey N, Mauvieux L, et al. Abnormal intestinal intraepithelial lymphocytes in refractory sprue. Gastroenterology 1998;114:471–81.
12. Cellier C, Delabesse E, Helmer C, et al. Refractory sprue, coeliac disease, and enteropathy-associated T-cell lymphoma. French Coeliac Disease Study Group. Lancet 2000;356:203–8.
13. West J, Holmes G. Celiac disease and its complications: a time traveller's perspective. Gastroenterology 2009;136:32–4.
14. Egan LJ, Walsh SV, Stevens FM, et al. Celiac-associated lymphoma. A single institution experience of 30 cases in the combination chemotherapy era. J Clin Gastroenterol 1995;21:123–9.
15. Askling J, Linet M, Gridley G, et al. Cancer incidence in a population-based cohort of individuals hospitalized with celiac disease or dermatitis herpetiformis. Gastroenterology 2002;123:1428–35.
16. Al-Toma A, Goerres MS, Meijer JW, et al. Human leukocyte antigen-DQ2 homozygosity and the development of refractory celiac disease and enteropathy-associated T-cell lymphoma. Clin Gastroenterol Hepatol 2006;4:315–9.
17. Smyth DJ, Plagnol V, Walker NM, et al. Shared and distinct genetic variants in type 1 diabetes and celiac disease. N Engl J Med 2008;359:2767–77.
18. Wijmenga C. Genetics and risk for associated autoimmune disorders and refractory coeliac disease (abstract). Mastering the coeliac condition. 2012; Florence, Italy.
19. Holmes GK, Prior P, Lane MR, et al. Malignancy in coeliac disease–effect of a gluten free diet. Gut 1989;30:333–8.
20. Biagi F, Corazza GR. Mortality in celiac disease. Nat Rev Gastroenterol Hepatol 2011;7:158–62.
21. Jamma S, Rubio-Tapia A, Kelly CP, et al. Celiac crisis is a rare but serious complication of celiac disease in adults. Clin Gastroenterol Hepatol 2010;8:587–90.
22. Daum S, Cellier C, Mulder CJ. Refractory coeliac disease. Best Pract Res Clin Gastroenterol 2005;19:413–24.
23. Murray JA, Rubio-Tapia A, Van Dyke CT, et al. Mucosal atrophy in celiac disease: extent of involvement, correlation with clinical presentation, and response to treatment. Clin Gastroenterol Hepatol 2008;6:186–93.
24. Daum S, Wahnschaffe U, Glasenapp R, et al. Capsule endoscopy in refractory celiac disease. Endoscopy 2007;39:455–8.
25. Barret M, Malamut G, Rahmi G, et al. Diagnostic yield of capsule endoscopy in refractory celiac disease. Am J Gastroenterol 2012, in press.
26. Huppert BJ, Farrell MA, Kawashima A, et al. Diagnosis of cavitating mesenteric lymph node syndrome in celiac disease using MRI. AJR Am J Roentgenol 2004;183:1375–7.

27. Roshan B, Leffler DA, Jamma S, et al. The incidence and clinical spectrum of refractory celiac disease in a North American referral center. Am J Gastroenterol 2011;106:923–8.

28. Malamut G, Cellier C. Is refractory celiac disease more severe in old Europe? Am J Gastroenterol 2010;106:929–32.

29. Perfetti V, Brunetti L, Biagi F, et al. TCRβ clonality improves diagnostic yield of TCRγ clonality in refractory celiac disease. J Clin Gastroenterol 2012;46(8):675–9.

30. Al-Toma A, Verbeek WH, Hadithi M, et al. Survival in refractory coeliac disease and enteropathy associated T cell Lymphoma: retrospective evaluation of single centre experience. Gut 2007;56:1373–8.

31. Daum S, Ipczynski R, Schumann M, et al. High rates of complications and substantial mortality in both types of refractory sprue. Eur J Gastroenterol Hepatol 2009;21:66–70.

32. Goerres MS, Meijer JW, Wahab PJ, et al. Azathioprine and prednisone combination therapy in refractory coeliac disease. Aliment Pharmacol Ther 2003;18: 487–94.

33. Verkarre V, Romana SP, Cellier C, et al. Recurrent partial trisomy 1q22-q44 in clonal intraepithelial lymphocytes in refractory celiac sprue. Gastroenterology 2003;125:40–6.

34. Malamut G, Verkarre V, Meresse B, et al. High rate of abnormal intestinal intraepithelial lymphocytes is predictive of extra-digestive diffusion in refractory coeliac disease [abstract]. Gut 2008;57(Suppl II):A30.

35. Malamut G, Meresse B, Verkarre V, et al. A low rate of gamma-delta intraepithelial lymphocytes is predictive of onset of overt lymphoma in refractory celiac disease of type II [abstract]. Presented at 14th International Celiac Disease Symposium; 2011; Oslo, Norway.

36. Hoffmann M, Vogelsang H, Kletter K, et al. 18F-fluoro-deoxy-glucose positron emission tomography (18F-FDG-PET) for assessment of enteropathy-type T cell lymphoma. Gut 2003;52:347–51.

37. Mention JJ, Ben Ahmed M, Begue B, et al. Interleukin 15: a key to disrupted intraepithelial lymphocyte homeostasis and lymphomagenesis in celiac disease. Gastroenterology 2003;125:730–45.

38. Ciccocioppo R, Di Sabatino A, Parroni R, et al. Increased enterocyte apoptosis and Fas-Fas ligand system in celiac disease. Am J Clin Pathol 2001;115:494–503.

39. Di Sabatino A, Ciccocioppo R, D'Alo S, et al. Intraepithelial and lamina propria lymphocytes show distinct patterns of apoptosis whereas both populations are active in Fas based cytotoxicity in coeliac disease. Gut 2001;49:380–6.

40. Hue S, Mention JJ, Monteiro RC, et al. A direct role for NKG2D/MICA interaction in villous atrophy during celiac disease. Immunity 2004;21(3):367–77.

41. Fehniger TA, Suzuki K, Ponnappan A, et al. Fatal leukemia in interleukin 15 transgenic mice follows early expansions in natural killer and memory phenotype CD8 + T cells. J Exp Med 2001;193:219–31.

42. Malamut G, El Machhour R, Montcuquet N, et al. IL-15 triggers an antiapoptotic pathway in human intraepithelial lymphocytes that is a potential new target in celiac disease-associated inflammation and lymphomagenesis. J Clin Invest 2010;120:2131–43.

43. Stene LC, Honeyman MC, Hoffenberg EJ, et al. Rotavirus infection frequency and risk of celiac disease autoimmunity in early childhood: a longitudinal study. Am J Gastroenterol 2006;101:2333–40.

44. Doherty TM, Seder RA, Sher A. Induction and regulation of IL-15 expression in murine macrophages. J Immunol 1996;156:735–41.

45. Flamand L, Stefanescu I, Menezes J. Human herpesvirus-6 enhances natural killer cell cytotoxicity via IL-15. J Clin Invest 1996;97:1373–81.

46. Vazquez N, Walsh TJ, Friedman D, et al. Interleukin-15 augments superoxide production and microbicidal activity of human monocytes against candida albicans. Infect Immun 1998;66:145–50.

47. Waldmann TA, Tagaya Y. The multifaceted regulation of interleukin-15 expression and the role of this cytokine in NK cell differentiation and host response to intracellular pathogens. Annu Rev Immunol 1999;17:19–49.

48. Dray X, Joly F, Lavergne-Slove A, et al. A severe but reversible refractory sprue. Gut 2006;55:1210–1.

49. Al-Toma A, Goerres MS, Meijer JW, et al. Cladribine therapy in refractory celiac disease with aberrant T cells. Clin Gastroenterol Hepatol 2006;4:1322–7.

50. Al-Toma A, Visser OJ, van Roessel HM, et al. Autologous hematopoietic stem cell transplantation in refractory celiac disease with aberrant T-cells. Blood 2006;34:27.

51. Tack GJ, Wondergem MJ, Al-Toma A, et al. Auto-SCT in refractory celiac disease type II patients unresponsive to cladribine therapy. Bone Marrow Transplant 2011;46:840–6.

52. Gale J, Simmonds PD, Mead GM, et al. Enteropathy-type intestinal T-cell lymphoma: clinical features and treatment of 31 patients in a single center. J Clin Oncol 2000;18:795–803.

53. Daum S, Ullrich R, Heise W, et al. Intestinal non-Hodgkin's lymphoma: a multicenter prospective clinical study from the German Study Group on Intestinal non-Hodgkin's Lymphoma. J Clin Oncol 2003;21:2740–6.

54. Waldmann TA. Targeting the interleukin-15 system in rheumatoid arthritis. Arthritis Rheum 2005;52:2585–8.

Celiac Disease in the Developing World

Kassem Barada, MD[a], Hussein Abu Daya, MD[a],
Kamran Rostami, MD, PhD[b], Carlo Catassi, MD[c,d],*

KEYWORDS

- Celiac disease • Developing world • Prevalence • Presentation • Diagnosis
- Genetics • Treatment • Gluten-free diet

KEY POINTS

- The prevalence of celiac disease (CD) in developing countries may be underestimated because of lack of awareness and low suspicion of the disease.
- Physicians must learn to recognize the variable clinical presentations of CD including the classic, atypical, and silent forms. Screening for the disease should be done among at-risk groups for early identification of patients with CD.
- Gluten-free diet represents a challenge for patients and their physicians, especially in these regions of the world, although it remains the only effective and safe therapy available.
- Large prospective studies are needed to assess the incidence, the clinical course, the efficacy of treatment modalities used, patient compliance, disease complications, and response to treatment in developing countries.

INTRODUCTION

Celiac disease (CD) is an autoimmune disorder that occurs in genetically predisposed individuals on ingestion of gluten. It has a prevalence of 0.8% to 2.67% in the Western world.[1–3] However, it is still underdiagnosed because of lack of specificity of clinical symptoms, and the diagnosis is often made after considerable delay.[4] First thought to be uncommon in developing countries, recent studies from the Middle East (ME), North Africa (NA), south and east Asia (SEA), and Latin America (LA) suggest it is almost equally prevalent in those regions.[5–15] The true prevalence of the disease, its

Competing interest: The authors declare no competing interest.
[a] Division of Gastroenterology, Department of Internal Medicine, American University of Beirut Medical Center, Riad-El-Solh Beirut 1107 2020, Lebanon; [b] College of Medical and Dental Sciences, University of Birmingham, Birmingham, UK; [c] Department of Pediatrics, Università Politecnica delle Marche, 60121 Ancona, Italy; [d] Center for Celiac Research, Mucosal Biology Research Center, University of Maryland School of Medicine, Baltimore, MD, USA
* Corresponding author.
E-mail address: catassi@tin.it

genetic background, its clinical features, and response to treatment are still not fully explored in many parts of the developing world. Contributing to the lack of studies are different factors including limited knowledge of the disease and limited funds available for research.

A literature review was performed using the electronic databases PubMed and Medline (1950–2012) as search engines, and celiac disease was used as a MeSH (medical subject headings) term. The search was limited to ME, SEA, Africa, and LA. This article compares the parameters of CD with those in Western countries, its epidemiology in low-risk and high-risk populations, its genetic background, its most common clinical presentations, and the diagnostic tests used and their reported sensitivity and specificity. The efficacy of the treatment modalities used and compliance with a gluten-free diet (GFD) are determined.

HISTORY

The discovery 10,000 years ago in the Neolithic age of ways to produce and store food was the greatest revolution humankind ever experienced. Passage from collection to production originated the first system in which human labor was transferred into activities, which produced income for long periods of time. The principle of property was consolidated, and fortifications to protect the land and food stores were developed.[16] The origin of farming practices was in the Fertile Crescent, the wide belt of southeast Asia.[16] Domestication of ancient grasses began in Neolithic settlements from wild progenitors *Triticum monococcum bocoticcum* and *Triticum monococcum uratru* in the northeastern region (Turkey, Iran, and Iraq) and *Triticum turgidum dicoccoides* in the southwestern region (Palestine, Syria, and Lebanon) of the Fertile Crescent. This region extends from the Mediterranean coast on its western extreme to the great Tigris-Euphrates plain eastward.[17,18] Cultivation of wheat and barley, first exploited and intensively developed in the Levant and western Zagros, slowly spread westward across northern Europe to reach Britain by circa 4000 BC.[16,19] The major lifestyle and dietary changes caused by the agriculture revolution led to the appearance of new diseases, such as CD.

The first description of this disorder comes from Aretaeus of Cappadocia, a contemporary of the Roman physician Galen living in the second half of the second century AD. The Greek word koiliakos, used by Aretaeus, originally meant suffering in the bowels. Later, Samuel Gee in 1888 published the first complete modern description of the clinical picture of CD and theorized on the importance of diet in its control. His contribution led to the eponym Gee disease under cyclic vomiting syndrome.[20] In the 1940s and 1950s, Willem-Karel Dicke went on to formally establish the GFD, changing treatment methods and clinical outcomes of children suffering from CD. By 1952, Dicke recognized that the disease is caused by the ingestion of wheat proteins, not carbohydrates. In the past, CD was considered typical of subjects of European origin.

During the 1980s, Simoons theorized that the previously described pattern of the spreading of agriculture could explain the higher CD incidence in some Western countries, particularly Ireland. According to this theory, the spreading of wheat consumption exerted a negative selective pressure on CD-predisposing genes, such as HLA-B8. Higher B8 frequency in northeastern Europe, and consequently higher CD frequency, might therefore be attributable to a lack of exposure to cereals in some countries. The Simoons theory has been challenged by recent epidemiologic data showing that Fertile Crescent countries, such as Turkey, now rank among the countries with the highest frequency of CD.[21] HLA-related CD-predisposing genotypes DQ2 and DQ8 are common in both Europe and the ME, probably because of some protective role conferred by these genotypes against human infections and parasites. However, genetic predisposition does not lead to disease without the proper environmental trigger(s). Until 500 years ago, humankind mostly consumed wheat varieties containing less toxic gluten (einkorn and emmer) than current varieties (the hexaploid *Triticum aestivum*). Furthermore, the techniques of bread making have greatly changed over time, with current leavening agents (baker's yeast and chemical products) degrading immunodominant gluten peptides much less than the natural sourdough that was used for thousands of years. The prevalence of CD, as well as other autoimmune disorders like type 1 diabetes, has greatly increased in recent years, for reasons that are currently unclear but are likely related to environmental changes.[22]

CD EPIDEMIOLOGY

Until a few years ago, celiac disease was thought to be a rare disorder affecting almost exclusively people of European origin. Typical gastrointestinal symptoms were the main clue for diagnosis at that time, and confirmation was accomplished by small intestinal biopsy. The availability of highly sensitive and specific serologic tests, such as the antiendomysium (EMA), and the antitransglutaminase (t-TG) antibodies, made it possible to evaluate the prevalence of CD in the general unselected populations of the Western world.

The introduction of serologic tests in the screening process in the developing world revealed that there is a wide variation in the prevalence across continents and regions. In unselected (low-risk) populations, it ranges from 0.5% to 1.8% in the ME, 0.32% to 1.04% in SEA, 0.14% to 5.6% in NA, and 0.15% to 2.7% in LA (**Table 1**). The low prevalence reported in some studies probably reflects the use of low-sensitivity assays.[23,24] In at-risk populations, it varies from the lowest reported 1.2% in Mexico to the highest reported 54.6% in Indian children strongly suspected to have CD (**Table 2**). These variations can be attributed to the heterogeneity of the studied populations, subject selection, diagnostic tests used, and whether or not histologic confirmation of the diagnosis was done. For example, 2 studies from Brazil reported a 12-fold difference in CD prevalence, probably caused by the use of different screening methods.[15,24]

CD in Low-Risk Populations

The prevalence of CD among low-risk adults and children ranges from 0.14% to 5.7% (see **Table 1**). Biopsy-proven CD prevalence varies from a low of 0.32% in Indian children to a high of 1.9% in Brazilian children,[5,7,10,12,15,25–27] whereas in adults it varies from 0.15% in Brazil to 1.2% in Turkey[6,10,11,14,24] (Barada and colleagues, unpublished data, 2011). CD seroprevalence reached 2.7% in Mexican adults[13] and 5.6% in western Saharan children.[8] Most studies screened healthy blood donors,[6,13,23,24,28–30] of whom young men represented more than 68%. Several studies from Iran, India, and Mexico screened healthy individuals, of whom 30% to 50% were women, and reported similar disease prevalence among men and women.[10,13,31]

In studies from the ME and NA, CD prevalence seems to be similar to that of Western countries. In the ME, it varies between 0.5% and 1.8% as reported by 8 studies from Lebanon, Jordan, Turkey, Israel, and Iran.[6,12,14,28,29,31] In North African countries, mainly Egypt, Algeria (Saharawi refugee camps), Libya, and Tunisia, it ranged from the lowest 0.14% to the highest 5.6%.[5,8,23,25,27,30] The Saharawi population living in Algeria has the highest CD prevalence (5.6%) among all world populations, which might be explained by heavy gluten ingestion, high levels of

Table 1
Prevalence of CD in the developing world among low-risk populations

	Country	Population	Method	Confirmation by Duodenal Biopsy	Result
ME					
Barada (unpublished data, 2011)	Lebanon	1000 adult patients presenting for EGD	t-TG/DGP,[a,b] t-TG,[a,b] EMA[a]	Yes	1.8% by histology and 1.5% by serology and histology combined
Saberi-Firouzi et al,[14] 2008	Iran	1440 healthy adults	Total IgA, EMA,[a] t-TG[a]	Yes	0.5%
Bahari et al,[6] 2010	Iran	1600 healthy adult blood donors	Total IgA, t-TG[a,b]	Yes	0.88%
Nuseir 2010	Jordan	1985 school children	t-TG,[a] EMA[a]	No	0.8%
Tatar et al,[29] 2004	Turkey	2000 healthy blood donors	t-TG[a,b]	Yes (incomplete)	1.38% by serology and 1.17% by histology
Akbari et al,[31] 2006	Iran	2799 healthy individuals	t-TG,[a] EMA[a]	Yes	0.96%
Shamir et al,[28] 2002	Israel	1571 healthy blood donors	t-TG,[a] EMA[a]	Yes (incomplete)	0.63%
Khuffash et al,[44] 1987	Kuwait	60,000 newborns (incidence study)	NR	Yes	1 in 3000 births
Mokhallalaty et al,[105] 2002	Lebanon	42,600 hospitalized children	AGA, EMA	Yes	0.5%
South and East Asia					
Bhattacharya et al,[7] 2009	India	400 children attending care center	t-TG[a]	Yes	1%
Makharia et al,[10] 2011	India	10,488 healthy individuals	Questionnaire, t-TG[a]	Yes	By serology 1.44% and by histology 1.04%
Sood et al,[26] 2006	India	4347 school children	t-TG	Yes (incomplete)	0.48% by serology and 0.32% by histology

Africa

Study	Country	Population	Antibodies	Biopsy	Prevalence
Abu-Zekry et al,[25] 2008	Egypt	1500 healthy children	t-TG,[a,b] EMA[a]	Yes	0.53%
Catassi et al,[8] 1999	Sahara (Algeria)	989 Saharawi children	t-TG,[a] EMA	No	5.6%
Alarida et al,[5] 2011	Libya	2920 school children	t-TG,[a] EMA[a]	Yes	0.79%–1.13%
Ben Hariz et al,[27] 2007	Tunisia	6286 school children	t-TG,[a] EMA[a]	Yes (incomplete)	0.64%
Mankai et al,[30] 2006	Tunisia	2500 healthy blood donors	AGA,[a,b] EMA[a]	No	0.3%
Bdioui et al,[23] 2006	Tunisia	1418 healthy blood donors	EMA[a]	Yes	0.14%
Latin America					
Remes-Troche et al,[13] 2006	Mexico	1009 healthy adult blood donors	t-TG[a]	No	2.7%
Gomez et al,[9] 2001	Argentina	2000 healthy individuals	Total IgA, AGA,[a,b] EMA[a]	Yes	0.6%
Gandolfi et al,[24] 2000	Brazil	2045 healthy adult blood donors	Total IgA, AGA,[a,b] EMA[a]	Yes	0.15%
Pratesi et al,[42] 2003	Brazil	4405 healthy individuals	Total IgA, AGA,[a] EMA[a]	Yes	0.36% by serology and 0.34% by histology
Trevisiol et al,[15] 2004	Brazil	1030 children and adolescents attending the hospital	t-TG,[a,b] EMA, and HLA studies	Yes	1.9%
Melo et al,[11] 2006	Brazil	3000 adult blood donors	t-TG,[a] EMA[a]	Yes (incomplete)	0.33%

Abbreviations: AGA, antigliadin antibodies; DGP, deamidated gliadin peptide antibodies; EMA, antiendomysial antibodies; NR, not reported; t-TG, tissue transglutaminase.
[a] IgA.
[b] IgG.

Table 2
Prevalence of CD in the developing world among high-risk populations

Country		Population	Method	Confirmation by Duodenal Biopsy	Prevalence
ME					
Rahimi 2010	Iran	316 adults with nonalcoholic fatty liver disease	Total IgA, EMA, t-TG[a]	Yes	2.2%
Emami et al,[90] 2008	Iran	350 patients suspected of having CD	t-TG[a]	Yes	6%
Hashemi et al,[92] 2008	Iran	104 children with idiopathic short stature	AGA,[a] t-TG[a]	Yes	33.6%
Zamani et al,[85] 2008	Iran	206 patients with iron deficiency anemia	Total IgA, EMA,[a] t-TG[a]	Yes	14.6%
Rostami Nejad et al,[82] 2009	Iran	450 dyspeptic patients	Total IgA, t-TG[a]	Yes	6.2%
Rostami Nejad et al,[82] 2009	Iran	670 with GI symptoms	Total IgA, t-TG[a,b]	No	3.7%
Shakeri 2009	Iran	247 patients with recurrent aphthous stomatitis	Total IgA, EMA,[a] t-TG[a]	Yes	2.8%
Emami et al,[90] 2008	Iran	108 patients with epilepsy	t-TG[a]	Yes	3.7%
Zamani et al,[85] 2008	Iran	288 patients with Behçet disease	Total IgA, EMA,[a] t-TG[a]	Yes	1.3%
Mirzaagha 2010	Iran	100 patients with autoimmune liver disease	t-TG[a]	Yes	5%
Jadallah and Khader,[91] 2009	Jordan	742 adults with irritable bowel syndrome	t-TG[a]	Yes	3.23%
Al-Ashwal et al,[46] 2003	Saudi Arabia	123 patients with IDDM	AGA,[a] ARA[a]	Yes (incomplete)	4.9%–8.1%
Mansour et al,[98] 2005	Iraq	40 patients with IDDM	NR	Yes	15%
Aygun et al,[96] 2005	Turkey	122 patients with IDDM	Total IgA, EMA[a]	Yes	2.45%
Guliter et al,[48] 2007	Turkey	136 patients with autoimmune thyroiditis	t-TG[a]	Yes (incomplete)	5.9%

South and East Asia

				Capsule endoscopy	
Jiang et al,[36] 2009	China	62 adults with chronic diarrhea	Total IgA, EMA, t-TG[a,b]	Yes	6.5%
Wang et al,[37] 2011	China	118 children with chronic diarrhea	Total IgA, AGA,[b] t-TG[a]	Yes	11.9%
Wu et al,[38] 2010	China	78 adults with IBS-D or IDDM	NR	No	9%
Kaur et al,[64] 2002	India	117 children with high clinical suspicion	NR	Yes	30%
Poddar et al,[50] 2006	India	549 children with high clinical suspicion	EMA,[a] t-TG,[a] AGA[a]	Yes	54.6%
Ahmad et al,[76] 2010	India	112 children with severe short stature	t-TG[a]	No	20.5%

Africa

Mohammed et al,[78] 2006	Sudan	80 children with high clinical suspicion	AGA,[a,b] EMA	Yes (incomplete)	38%–55% by serology and 22.5% by histology
El-Shabrawi 2011	Egypt	26 children with autoimmune hepatitis	t-TG,[a] EMA[a]	Yes	15.4% by serology and 11.5% by histology
Laadhar 2006	Tunisia	261 patients with IDDM	Total IgA, AGA,[a,b] t-TG,[a,b] EMA[a]	No	3.4%–5.4%
Mankai et al,[80] 2007	Tunisia	205 children with IDDM	EMA	Yes (incomplete)	8.3% by serology and 5.3% by histology
Al-Tawati 1998	Libya	243 children with high clinical suspicion	NR	Yes	31.6%
Ben Abdelghani 2011	Tunisia	24 adults with SLE	AGA, t-TG	Yes	8.3% by serology and 4.1% by histology
Abu-Zekri 2008	Egypt	150 children with diarrhea and failure to thrive	t-TG,[a,b] EMA[a]	Yes	4.7%
Ashabani 2003	Libya	234 patients with IDDM	AGA, ARA, t-TG, EMA	Yes	10.3%
Boudraa et al,[45] 1996	Algeria	116 children with IDDM	AGA,[a,b] EMA[a]	Yes	20% by serology and 16.4% by histology

(continued on next page)

Table 2
(continued)

Country		Population	Method	Confirmation by Duodenal Biopsy	Prevalence
Latin America					
Blanco Rabassa 1981	Cuba	519 children with high clinical suspicion	NR	Yes	8.8%
Castillo-Ortiz 2011	Mexico	85 adults with rheumatoid arthritis	AGA, t-TG	No	1.2%
Remes-Troche et al,[13] 2006	Mexico	84 adults with IDDM	t-TG[a]	Yes (incomplete)	10.7% by serology and 5.9% by histology
Sugai et al,[84] 2010	Argentina	679 patients with GI symptoms (518 low risk and 161 high risk)	t-TG,[a,b] a-DGP,[a,b] AAA	Yes	3.3% in low risk and 33.1% in high risk by histology
Tenure 2006	Brazil	236 children with IDDM	Total IgA, AGA,[a,b] EMA[a]	Yes	2.6%
Modelli 2010	Brazil	214 children with high clinical suspicion	Total IgA, AGA,[a,b] t-TG,[a] EMA[a]	Yes	2.3%

Abbreviations: AAA, IgA antiactin antibodies; a-DGP, antibodies reacting with deamidated gliadin-derived peptides; AGA, antigliadin antibodies; ARA, antireticulin antibody; EMA, antiendomysial antibodies; GI, gastrointestinal; IBS-D, diarrhea-predominant irritable bowel syndrome; IDDM, insulin-dependent diabetes mellitus; NR, not reported; t-TG, tissue transglutaminase.
[a] IgA.
[b] IgG.

consanguinity, and high frequencies of HLA-DQ2.[8] Data are not available from sub-Saharan African countries except for a case series of 20 CD cases from South Africa in 1981 in which 55% were female, all were adults, most did not present with the classic features of CD, and all were diagnosed by histology.[32] Two other case series from Djibouti and Sudan included 8 and 7 cases respectively, all of whom were children, with a female preponderance.[33,34] Reasons for the rarity of this disease in those countries might include the type of staple cereals, which are mostly gluten free (eg, rice and millet), the lesser prevalence of the genes predisposing for HLA-DQ2 and HLA-DQ8,[35] underdiagnosis, or underreporting.

Only 3 studies screening for CD in low-risk populations were reported from the region of SEA and all were from India.[7,10,26] No studies were found from China or other Far Eastern countries except for 3 studies on high-risk populations from China[36-38] and 2 case report/series for 23 patients from Japan.[39,40] CD has historically been considered to be absent in the Far East. However, CD might not be rare in countries like China, particularly in provinces such as Jiangsu with its increasing gluten intake and an appreciable presence of HLA-DQ2/DQ8 alleles.[38,41]

Studies from Central and South America suggested a variation in CD prevalence, ranging from 0.15% to 1.9%. There are 6 studies screening for CD in low-risk populations in 3 countries in LA: Mexico, Argentina, and Brazil.[9,11,13,15,24,42] A seventh study from Argentina determined the prevalence of CD using secondary databases from electronic medical records in a tertiary medical center and reported a 0.22% prevalence among 128,748 individuals, of whom 80% were female.[43] The 4 studies from Brazil reported a prevalence ranging from 0.15% to 0.34% in adults to 1.9% in children.[11,15,24,42] The study from Mexico screened healthy adult blood donors using t-TG immunoglobulin (Ig) A antibodies and found a prevalence of 2.7%; however, the diagnosis was not confirmed by biopsy. The investigators explained this high prevalence by the studies from Brazil and Argentina not reflecting the ethnic diversity of LA, and their results cannot be projected to the Mexican population because it is mostly composed of Mexican Mestizo individuals who have 56% Native American Indian genes, 40% white genes, and 4% African genes.[13] As expected, prevalence was higher in symptomatic individuals attending hospital clinics than in asymptomatic individuals.

Several factors play a role in underestimating the disease prevalence in the developing world, including exclusion of subjects with iron deficiency anemia (IDA), abnormal liver function tests (LFTs), and the low percentage of participating women. In addition, low suspicion among physicians and selection bias toward patients presenting with severe symptoms may have contributed to the low reported incidence of CD by missing asymptomatic and mildly symptomatic individuals.[27,44]

CD in High-Risk Populations

High-risk populations include patients with 1) positive family history of CD; (2) insulin-dependent diabetes mellitus (IDDM); (3) autoimmune disorders; (4) liver disorders, particularly autoimmune hepatitis and primary biliary cirrhosis; (5) skin disorders, mainly dermatitis herpetiformis, (6) those with symptoms of malabsorption such as chronic diarrhea, refractory IDA, and weight loss; (7) patients with genetic disorders (particularly Down and Turner syndromes); and (8) IgA deficiency.[35] Among these, the prevalence of CD in the developing world ranges from 1.2% to 55% (see **Table 2**).

CD prevalence among patients with IDDM is 1% to 12% assessed by serologic markers and 1% to 11% by histology in Western countries.[3] It is more common in children than in adults with IDDM. In 10 reports from Saudi Arabia, Iraq, Turkey, Tunisia, Libya, Algeria, China, Mexico, and Brazil, the prevalence of CD among patients with

IDDM was 2.45% to 20% assessed by serologic tests and 2.4% to 16.4% by histology (see **Table 2**). In this respect, the highest CD prevalence among patients with IDDM (16.4%) has been detected in Algeria.[45] Small sample size and a high rate of consanguinity may have contributed to this high prevalence. CD and IDDM share many genetic factors including HLA DR3-DQ2 and HLA DR4-DQ8 haplotype.[46,47] Autoimmune thyroiditis and CD share a common genetic background.[48] In a Turkish study, 5.9% of patients with autoimmune thyroiditis had CD.[48] This compares well with the 3% to 5% prevalence reported in Western countries.[3,49] The highest reported prevalence (54.6%) in a high-risk population of 549 children with a high clinical suspicion of CD was in India.[50] A study on severely symptomatic hospitalized children in Kuwait suggested an incidence of 1 in 3000 births over 5 years.[44]

Prevalence of CD in Relatives

In the United States and Europe, the prevalence of CD was 4.5% to 20% among first-degree relatives.[1] The National Institutes of Health (NIH) estimates the prevalence of CD among first-degree relatives to be 4% to 12%, assessed by biopsy.[51] Similar results have been reported from developing countries, including recent reports from the Punjab region of India, Turkey, Algeria, Brazil, Chile, and Argentina.[45,52–56] Teresi and colleagues[52] screened 763 first-degree relatives of patients with CD in Sahrawi refugee camps and showed a serologic prevalence of 8.5%. Another study from Brazil showed a biopsy-defined CD prevalence of 6.7%.[54] A prevalence of 20% in first-degree relatives of patients with biopsy-proven CD was reported from Punjab. Also, clustering of CD within families has been reported from Jordan and Algeria.[51] The high rate of consanguinity in these countries might contribute to a higher CD prevalence and provides an opportunity for studying genotype-phenotype correlations.

GENETIC BACKGROUND

The familial clustering of celiac disease indicates that the genetic background is important in the pathogenesis of this condition.[3] This genetic predisposition is primarily related to the HLA genes, mainly the HLA-DQ2 and HLA-DQ8 alleles. The HLA-DQ2 allele is identified in more than 90% of the patients with CD, and HLA-DQ8 is identified in most of the remaining patients, with both alleles accounting for 40% of the total genetic predisposition to CD.[2] However, these alleles occur in 30% of the general population and several non-HLA genes that may influence the susceptibility to the disease have been identified.[51] One such gene is the CTLA-4 gene, which is thought to regulate T-cell immune function.[57] Other predisposing genes, including the IL12A, IL18RAP, and SH2B3 genes, have also been identified.[58]

The strong association between CD and HLA-DQ2 has been confirmed in developing countries mainly in the ME, NA, and India (**Table 3**). The HLA-DQ2 (DQA1*0501-DQB1*0201) haplotype frequency in patients with CD ranged from 11% in Chile to 100% in Israeli Bedouins.[55,59] However, most studies reported a frequency of more than 79%.[54,60–65] HLA-DQ8 (DQA1*0301-DQB1*0302) is less associated with CD, with a frequency of 5% to 15%.[61,62,66] Two studies from Chile reported a predominance of the DQ8 compared with the DQ2 haplotype,[55,67] although a more recent study involving patients with CD of the same country detected a change in the predominant HLA haplotypes, from DQ8 to DQ2.[68] Alarida and colleagues[69] reported a higher prevalence of DQ2 and DQ8 genotypes in unselected Libyan children compared with European populations (57.1% vs 30%). Moreover, another study showed that the overall prevalence of HLA-DQ2 and DQ8 in the Saharawi general population is 41.6%; one of the highest in the world.[52] Wu and colleagues[38] showed that

Table 3
CD genetics in patients diagnosed in the developing world

Country		Population	HLA Haplotypes (%)	HLA Alleles (%)
ME				
El-Akawi et al,[60] 2010	Jordan	44 patients with CD	DQA1*0501- DQB1*0201 (80)	DQB1*0201 (100) DQA1*0501 (80)
Eller et al,[59] 2006; Neuhausen et al,[62] 2002	Israel	Bedouin patients with CD	DRB1*03- DQA1*0501- DQB1*0201 (100%) DQA1*0301- DQB1*0302 (14%)	DQB1*0201 (93–100) DQA1*0501 (79–100) DRB1*03 (100) DQA1*0301 (14) DQB1*0302 (14)
Tumer et al,[71] 2000; Kuloglu et al,[61] 2008	Turkey	Children with CD	DQA1*0501- DQB1*0201 (52–81) DQA1*0301- DQB1*0302 (15)[a] DR3–DQ2 (30) DR3–DR4 (21) DR7–DQ2 (21)	A2 (42), B8 (39–41), B13 (14.7), CW7 (45–48), DR3 (70), DR7 (30–41), DR17 (54.7)
South and East Asia				
Kaur et al,[64] 2002	India	35 children with CD	DQA1*0501- DQB1*0201 (97.1) A26-B8-DR3 (34.3)	DQB1*0201 (100) DQA1*0501 (97.1) B*08 (71.4) DRB1*03 (94.2)
Africa				
Afredj 2009	Algeria	9 patients with CD with BCS	NR	DQB1*02 (66) DQB1*03 (33)
Alarida et al,[69] 2010; Bouguerra et al,[63] 1997; Bouguerra et al,[63] 1999	Libya, Tunisia	Children with CD	DQA1*0501- DQB1*0201 (84.5) DQ2 and/or DQ8 (97) DR53 (15)	DQB1*0201 (84–97) DQA1*0501 (84.5) DQB1*03 (13) DRB4 (15–55.3)
Lopez-Vazquez et al,[66] 2004	Algeria (Sahrawi)	125 patients with CD	DQA1*0501- DQB1*0201 (88) DQA1*0301- DQB1*0302 (5)[a] B8-DR3-DQ2 (52)[a]	DR3 (80)[a] DQB1*0201 (88) DQA1*0501 (88)
Latin America				
Cintado et al,[65] 2006; Castro-Antunes 2011; Martins et al,[54] 2010; Araya et al,[55] 2000; Parada et al,[68] 2011	Cuba, Brazil, Chile	Patients with CD	DQA1*0501- DQB1*0201 (11–88) DQA1*0301- DQB1*0302 (10–26)	DQB1*0201 (25–93) DQA1*0501 (48–89) DQB1*03 (25–43) DRB1 (27) (only 1 study)

(continued on next page)

Table 3 (continued)			HLA Haplotypes	
Country		Population	(%)	HLA Alleles (%)
Pérez-Bravo 1999	Chile	62 children with CD	DQB1*0302-DQA1*0301/ DQB1*0302-DQA1*0301 (26) DQB1*0201-DQA1*0501/ DQB1*02 01-DQA1*0501 (11)	DQB1*0201 (50) DQA1*0501 (95) DQB1*03 (85) DQA1*0301 (66)[a]

Abbreviation: BCS, Budd-Chiari syndrome.
[a] Not significant compared with the general population.

CD might exist in China, especially in the Jiangsu province; this is one of the main wheat-producing areas, where the HLA-DQ2 haplotype frequency among its Han inhabitants is 7.2% and that of DQ8 is 4.7%.

Other HLA and non-HLA genes are also associated with increased risk of CD. HLA-DRB4, A2, A25(10), A26, B8, B13, CW7, DR3, DR7, and DR17, have been reported to be associated with CD in developing countries (see **Table 3**) A Turkish study suggested that the HLA-A25(10) is a common allele in Turkish children with CD.[70] No such association has been described in Western countries. HLA-B8, a gene expressed in major histocompatibility complex (MHC) I antigen presenting cells, is found to be associated with CD in Turkey,[61,70,71] Algeria,[66] Iraq,[72] and India.[64] In addition, Saharawi patients with atypical CD were found to overexpress the MHC class I chain-related gene A (MICA) allele 5.1, similarly to what is reported in Western countries.[66] In contrast, the association between the CTLA-4 gene and CD found in Western countries was not found in Tunisian children with CD.[73]

Recent genome-wide association studies (GWASs) on CD in the West have led to the discovery of new CD-associated non-HLA loci including IL12A, IL18RAP, IL2/IL21, SH2B3, rs6441961,[3(p21)] and the CCR1/CCR3 cluster focus.[58,74] Most of these genes are shared with other autoimmune disorders. No GWASs with a primary end point of finding CD-associated non-HLA loci have been performed in the developing world.

CLINICAL PRESENTATION

Until the 1990s, the predominant CD presentation was with villous atrophy and malabsorption symptoms. However, with the availability of reliable serologic tests and with increasing awareness among physicians and patients, the frequency of atypical and silent/subclinical forms increased significantly.[2,3,50] There is limited information on atypical or silent CD in most of the developing countries compared with developed countries. A study comparing American and Turkish patients found that the former presented mostly with atypical symptoms such as fatigue, abdominal pain, and bloating, and the latter with diarrhea and anemia.[75]

Classic/Typical CD

This form is characterized by villous atrophy and malabsorptive symptoms. It is more prevalent among younger children with chronic diarrhea, impaired growth/failure to thrive, abdominal distension, muscle wasting, anorexia, and behavioral changes.[35] In contrast with Western countries, this form is still the most common presentation of CD in SEA, Africa, and, to a lesser extent, ME and Latin America.

In India, China, South Africa, Sudan, Libya, and Tunisia, typical CD was reported to occur in 68% to 100% of diagnosed patients.[32,37,50,64,76–79] However, a Tunisian screening study in children with IDDM reported that all patients diagnosed with CD had the atypical or silent form.[80] Possible explanations for the rarity of atypical/silent CD in some parts of the developing world include lack of awareness, shortage of pediatric gastrointestinal experts, and the nonavailability of laboratory support for celiac serology.[50] Some countries in the developing world may therefore still recognize the classic form of CD.[43]

In the ME and Latin America, the picture is mixed, with some countries reporting substantial or even predominant presentations with atypical and/or silent forms among patients with CD.[6,9,81–85] In contrast, 5 reports from Kuwait, Turkey, Brazil, and Chile reported that 80% to 100% of their diagnosed patients had typical CD.[44,55,86–88] Most of these studies involved children with CD.

Among the 16 studies reporting a predominance of the typical presentation among patients with CD in the developing world, 50% to 100% presented with diarrhea, 43% to 100% had weight loss/failure to thrive, and 9% to 100% had abdominal pain, distention, or flatulence (**Table 4**). Diarrhea and abdominal distension were significantly more common in younger children, whereas abdominal pain, growth retardation, and failure to thrive were more common among those who were older. This finding is ascribed to the preponderance of classic CD among younger children versus atypical CD seen among older children.[87] In China and Egypt, CD was one of the most common causes of chronic diarrhea with a frequency of 4.7% to 11.9%.[25,36,37] The study from Egypt included 150 children presenting with diarrhea and failure to thrive.[25,36,37] In addition, 7 more studies screened for CD in patients with high clinical suspicion in Iran, India, Sudan, Libya, Cuba, and Argentina. The reported prevalence of CD in these studies was between 6% and 54.6%.[50,64,77,78,84,89,90] Moreover, Jadallah and Khader[91] found a 3.23% CD prevalence among 742 Jordanian patients with irritable bowel syndrome. This finding is in accordance with the observation that 36% of American patients with CD are being diagnosed initially as having irritable bowel syndrome.[51]

Atypical CD

Atypical CD is usually seen in older children and adults lacking classic malabsorptive features. Atypical gastrointestinal symptoms include recurrent abdominal pain, bloating, constipation, nausea, and vomiting. Extraintestinal manifestations include dental enamel defects, recurrent aphthous stomatitis, anemia, short stature, osteopenia/osteoporosis, hypertransaminasemia, dermatitis herpetiformis, headache, neurologic symptoms, epilepsy, amenorrhea, and infertility.[35] In this review, 13 studies reported a significantly increased frequency of the atypical form among patients with CD ranging mainly between 25% and 93%; 5 were from the ME, 1 from India, 3 from Africa, and 4 from LA.[6,9,32,68,76,78,80–85]

Short stature is seen in about one-third of children with CD in Western countries.[51] In children with short stature and no gastrointestinal symptoms, 2% to 8% have CD.[35] In the developing world, it is the presenting symptom in 6% to 61% of patients with atypical CD, and in 7% to 72% of patients in all studies irrespective of the dominant form of presentation (see **Table 4**). The highest prevalence of short stature (72%) was reported from Chile. In accordance, 2 studies from India and Iran indicated that 20.5% to 33.6% of children with idiopathic short stature have CD.[76,92] The

Table 4
Clinical presentation of patients with CD in the developing world

Country		Population	Classic CD (%)	Atypical CD (%)	Silent CD (%)	Abdominal Pain/ Distention/ Flatulence (%)	Weight Loss/ Failure to Grow (%)	Diarrhea (%)	Short Stature (%)	Anemia (%)
ME										
Zamani et al,[85] 2008	Iran	30 CD + patients with IDA	0	100	0	20	NR	7	0	100
Rostami Nejad et al,[82] 2009	Iran	25 patients with CD with GI symptoms	8	92	0	60	20	8	NR	NR
Bahari et al,[6] 2010	Iran	14 adults with CD by screening	29	35	36	43	NR	29	7	7
Assiri et al,[94] 2008; Saadah,[83] 2011; Khuffash et al,[44] 1987; Demir et al,[87] 2000	Saudi Arabia, Kuwait, Turkey	62 children with CD	NR or 49–100	NR or 0–51	NR or 0	33–80	35–100	40–100	18–45	40–66
Barada (unpublished data, 2011)	Lebanon	18 adults with CD by screening	28	72	0	56	50	28	NR	44
South and East Asia										
Wang et al,[37] 2011	China	14 children with CD + chronic diarrhea	100	0	0	43	43	100	22	29
Kaur et al,[64] 2002; Poddar et al,[50] 2006	India	Children with CD	84–90	10–16	0	NR or 48	81–91	84–90	60–71	84–90
Sood et al,[79] 2003	India	96 adults with CD	68	NR	NR	9	NR	68	NR	19

Reference	Country	Population								
Ahmad et al,[76] 2010	India	23 children with CD with severe short stature	74	26	0	NR	70	74	100	52
Africa										
Kavin,[32] 1981	South Africa	20 adults with CD	75	25	0	25–60	60	75	NR	50
Mohammed et al,[78] 2006; Al-tawaty and Elbargathy,[77] 1998; Kallel 2009	Sudan, Libya, Tunisia	Children with CD with high suspicion (except Kallel et al)	NR or 50–100	NR or 0–50	NR or 0	6–78	50–100	48–50	NR or 30–61	20–100
Mankai et al,[80] 2007	Tunisia	11 children with CD with IDDM	0	27	73	18	9	0	0	18
Latin America										
Sugai et al,[84] 2010; Gomez et al,[9] 2001	Argentina	patients with CD by screening	8–66	25.5	8–67	NR	NR or 25	NR or 8	NR	NR or 25
Tenure 2006	Brazil	6 CD + children with IDDM by screening	100	0	0	100	NR	50	NR	NR
Arevalo et al,[99] 2010	Peru	10 adults with CD	80	20	0	100	NR	80	NR	56
Kotze et al,[86] 2011	Brazil	14 elderly patients with CD	100	0	0	93	93	100	NR	82
Galvao et al,[81] 2004	Brazil	50 children with CD	56	44	0	56	88	56	32	NR
Araya et al,[55] 2000; Mancilla et al,[95] 2005; Parada et al,[68] 2011	Chile	patients with CD	NR or 74–100	NR or 0–26	NR or 0	38–85	38–77	74–100	NR or 6–72	29–70

pathogenesis of CD-associated short stature is still uncertain, but some speculate a role for zinc deficiency impairing the production of IGF-1, which, combined with other deficiencies that are characteristically found in patients with CD, is detrimental for bone growth.[35]

Anemia is a frequent presenting feature in patients with CD in the West, where its prevalence at the time of CD diagnosis is 12% to 69%.[93] In developing countries, anemia occurs in 7% to 100% of patients with CD and most cases are attributable to iron deficiency (see **Table 4**). In 9 out of 23 studies, more than 60% of patients with CD presented with anemia.[44,50,55,64,77,78,83,85,86] IDA is the most common form in the setting of CD, with a higher prevalence in adults compared with children. Worldwide prevalence of CD among patients with IDA is 2.8% to 8.7% and may be as high as 15%.[51] Zamani and colleagues[85] found that 14.6% of Iranian patients with IDA had also CD. However, the anemia seen in patients with CD can also result from vitamin B_{12} and folic acid deficiencies, and some have anemia from chronic disease.[93]

Osteopenia and osteoporosis are common complications of CD, occurring in 40% and 3.4% to 26% of patients, respectively.[35] Seven studies from Brazil, Chile, India, Saudi Arabia, and Turkey reported CD-associated bone metabolism disorders and hypocalcemia in up to 27% of patients.[44,68,83,86,87,94,95] In Brazil, 86% of elderly patients with CD had osteoporosis,[86] whereas in Chile it was found in 6% of children and young adults with CD.[68] Rickets was found in only 1.3% of children in India, and in 10% and 25% of patients in Saudi Arabia and Kuwait, respectively.[44,50,94] In the pediatric population, a prompt initiation of a GFD is essential for recovery from CD-associated osteoporosis. However, in adults, spontaneous recovery is more difficult even with treatment, an observation that highlights the need for a timely diagnosis as a preventive measure.[35]

Liver involvement in CD is manifested early by hypertransaminasemia. Between 5% and 10% of patients with unexplained increase of serum aminotransferases have CD.[51] Liver biopsy may reveal lesions ranging from reactive hepatitis to cirrhosis, which may be partially or totally reversed with a GFD. Only 3 studies from Chile, India, and Turkey reported abnormal LFTs among patients with CD.[50,87,95] The studies from Turkey and Chile reported high transaminases in 38% of patients, whereas the Indian study reported a frequency of 43%. Transaminase levels normalized on the GFD in all Turkish patients except those with cirrhosis.[87]

Recurrent aphthous stomatitis was reported in 2% of Turkish children, 1% of Indian children, and 7% of Iranian adults with CD.[6,50,87] Khoshbaten and colleagues reported a CD seroprevalence of 6.5% among 100 Iranian couples with unexplained infertility, whereas histologic prevalence was at least 1.5% (histologic diagnosis was attempted in only 25% of patients).[41] These results indicate a higher seroprevalence of CD in those with infertility compared with those with normal fertility.

Subclinical CD

Similar to the case of atypical CD, the introduction of reliable serologic tests has led to increased recognition of silent/subclinical CD. A thorough evaluation may reveal a low-grade illness in many of these individuals.[35] In this review, 4 studies from Iran, Lebanon, Tunisia, and Argentina reported silent CD prevalence of more than 36% (range 8%–73%).[6,9,80,84] Most of these patients were adults who were diagnosed with CD by population screening. Mankai and colleagues[80] reported the highest frequency of silent CD (73%) among children with CD with IDDM.

Associated Diseases

Several disorders are associated with CD, including autoimmune diseases (IDDM, thyroiditis, and liver disease); IgA deficiency; and Down, Williams, and Turner syndromes. About 30% of patients with CD have IDDM and/or autoimmune thyroiditis.[45,48] In developing countries, the prevalence of autoimmune diseases among patients with CD was shown to be as low as 1% in Indian children, and as high as 40% in Saudi Arabian children.[50,83] However, these studies did not have determination of autoimmune disease prevalence in CD as a primary end point. In Western countries, the prevalence of CD among children with IDDM is 4.5%.[35] This was within the 2.6% to 16.4% range reported in developing countries.[13,38,45,46,80,88,96] The highest CD prevalence among children with IDDM was in Algeria (16.4%–20%[45]), and the lowest in Brazil (2.6%[88]), although a low-sensitivity serologic test was used in the latter, thus underestimating the true prevalence. Aygun and colleagues[96] reported an even lower prevalence of 2.45% among Turkish adult patients with IDDM. The prevalence of IDDM in patients with CD is as low as 0.33% in Indian children[50] and as high as 29% in Saudi Arabian children.[83] This high prevalence in the Saudi Arabian study is probably caused by more than 50% of the patients included in this study having been identified during screening of high-risk individuals including children with IDDM. A 7-fold increase in CD prevalence has been reported in patients with autoimmune thyroid disease in Western countries.[35] Guliter and colleagues[48] reported a 5.9% frequency of CD among Turkish patients with autoimmune thyroiditis.

DIAGNOSIS

With all the recent advancements in CD diagnosis using serologic, histologic, and genetic tools, many screening algorithms have been developed. However, all algorithms start with serologic tests and include testing for IgA IgG tissue transglutaminase (t-TG), and IgA and IgG antiendomysial antibodies (EMA) and, most recently, antigliadin antibodies (AGA) to deamidated synthetic gliadin peptides (DGP).[2,3] The specificity of EMA determination is nearly 100%; however, this determination is expensive and operator dependent. The American Gastroenterological Association has recommended that anti–t-TG should be used as a first-line test in the primary care setting.[97] Duodenal biopsy remains the standard diagnostic test.[3]

In our review, 34 out of 41 studies of CD prevalence in the developing world used initial serologic screening confirmed by duodenal biopsy in those testing positive (see **Tables 1** and **2**). However, in one-third of these 34 studies, confirmation by biopsy was incomplete. Intestinal biopsies were the sole mode of diagnosis in 5 studies because of the unavailability of serologic tests.[36,44,64,77,89,98] Serologic marker sensitivity and specificity vary widely across the developing world. The sensitivity of IgA AGA is 45% to 100%,[9,30,45,87,99,100] whereas that of IgG AGA is 73% to 100%.[45,56,87,100] EMA had a sensitivity of 64% to 80% in LA[56,88,100]; from 72% to 95% in NA, ME, and India[50,85,87]; and a specificity reaching 91% to 100% in all studies.[28,31,45,50,56,85,88,100] However, very low EMA sensitivity (19%–20%) was reported from Peru, Iran, and Israel.[28,31,99] These results may be caused by improper intestinal mucosal sampling, poor performance of EMA in the presence of milder villous atrophy, and low power in detecting early CD.[28,101] IgA t-TG sensitivity is 72% to 100%, and specificity is 97% to 100%, being superior to other serologic tests.[29,31,50,85,100] Moreover, the positive and negative predictive values for EMA were 70% to 96% and 88 to 99.5%, respectively, whereas those for t-TG were 44.8% to 98% and 93% to 99.5%, respectively.[50,56,88,92] The sensitivity and specificity of different combinations of these serologic tests proved to be superior to those of a single test.[56]

These wide variations in sensitivity and specificity are attributed to population differences, bias in patient selection, and the methodology used, including number of biopsy specimens and choice of gold standard. Other problems with serologic tests include lower performance in the clinical setting compared with research laboratories and differences in test kit sensitivity and specificity.[51]The process of case finding focused on at-risk groups is currently the best approach to improve the diagnostic rates. This procedure minimizes costs and is ethically appropriate.[35]

TREATMENT

A GFD remains the mainstay of CD treatment. Supportive nutritional care is also recommended in the case of vitamin, iron, and calcium deficiencies. GFD usually results in clinical, serologic, and histologic remission.[2,3] In the long term, it reduces the risk of malignant complications, and protects against developing autoimmune diseases such as IDDM, hematologic disorders, and inflammatory bowel diseases.[102] Adherence to a GFD in Western countries is reported to be generally less than 50%, but it can increase to 81% in children.[83,103,104] Sixteen studies from all over the developing world reported a GFD adherence of 45% to 100%, with 91% to 100% improvement in symptoms and general well-being.[8,10,44,46,52,64,68,78,80,83,85,86,90,91,104,105] This wide variation in compliance partially depends on the patients' age group, because it has been shown that those who start a GFD at an age of less than 10 years are 1.3 to 2 times more compliant.[104] Moreover, this higher level of adherence in comparison with Western countries may be caused by the limited number of patients studied and the use of different parameters to assess adherence, including dietary history and whether or not repeated serologic testing was done.

Maintaining a strict long-term GFD is challenging in both developing and developed countries, especially in children and adolescents. In these age groups, noncompliance may occur because of several factors including ignorance about the diet, social/peer pressure, nonavailability of GFD, disliking the taste of alternative food, increased outdoor activities, increased risk-taking behavior, and conflicts with parents.[104] Moreover, wheat and barley are major diet constituents with few acceptable alternatives, and it can be difficult to convince parents that bread is the cause of diarrhea.[44] Also, patients with atypical or silent CD are hard to convince because of lack of immediate feedback when adhering to a GFD and their beliefs of lack of benefit from such a diet.[51,106] Chauhan and colleagues[104] reported that Indian children with CD, who have to follow strict diets and are mainly not compliant, may have problems of adaptation to the social life. These children may also be prone to psychological problems such as depression, anxiety, and feeling of isolation. Moreover, adherence to a GFD is lower in patients who are diagnosed through a population mass screening in which subjects have minimal or even absent symptoms, than in those referred because of clinical suspicion.[52] In addition, more than 30% of those who think that they are adhering to a GFD are consuming gluten-contaminated food daily.[106]

The benefits of adherence to a GFD have been well documented in developing countries. Demir and colleagues[87] reported improvement in growth rate in Turkish children with CD adhering to a GFD. Moreover, diabetic children with CD adhering to a GFD have fewer hypoglycemic episodes and better diabetic control.[83] Zamani and colleagues[85] found that Iranian patients with CD with IDA who are on a GFD had spontaneous recovery of their anemia even without iron supplementation. In addition, a Saudi Arabian study of 80 children with CD reported a significant improvement in growth parameters and spontaneous recovery of anemia, hypoalbuminemia, and hypertransaminasemia in those who were on a GFD after 1-year follow-up.[83]

There are no studies regarding refractory CD or its treatment from developing countries, and no trials of immunosuppressive or immune-modulator drugs have been described.

SUMMARY

Recent studies indicate that CD is a common disease in both the developed and the developing worlds. It affects not only people of European descent but also native populations of Latin America, south and east Asia, the ME, and Africa, with prevalence similar to that of Western populations.

The prevalence of CD in these regions may be underestimated because of lack of awareness and low suspicion of the disease. Physicians must learn to recognize the variable clinical presentations of CD, including the classic, atypical, and silent forms. Screening for the disease should be done among at-risk groups for early identification of patients with CD. The GFD represents a challenge for both patients and their physicians, especially in these regions of the world, although it remains the only effective and safe therapy available.

Large prospective studies are needed to assess the incidence, the clinical course, the efficacy of treatment modalities used, patient compliance, disease complications, and response to treatment in developing countries. The association of CD with other autoimmune diseases and the presence of specific genetic markers may be areas of future research. The high rate of consanguinity in some areas of the developing world might provide an opportunity for establishing genotype-phenotype correlations in CD.

REFERENCES

1. Fasano A, Berti I, Gerarduzzi T, et al. Prevalence of celiac disease in at-risk and not-at-risk groups in the United States: a large multicenter study. Arch Intern Med 2003;163:286–92.
2. Green PH, Cellier C. Celiac disease. N Engl J Med 2007;357:1731–43.
3. Rostom A, Murray JA, Kagnoff MF. American Gastroenterological Association (AGA) Institute technical review on the diagnosis and management of celiac disease. Gastroenterology 2006;131:1981–2002.
4. Green PH. Where are all those patients with Celiac disease? Am J Gastroenterol 2007;102:1461–3.
5. Alarida K, Harown J, Ahmaida A, et al. Coeliac disease in Libyan children: a screening study based on the rapid determination of anti-transglutaminase antibodies. Dig Liver Dis 2011;43:688–91.
6. Bahari A, Karimi M, Sanei-Moghaddam I, et al. Prevalence of celiac disease among blood donors in Sistan and Balouchestan province, southeastern Iran. Arch Iran Med 2010;13:301–5.
7. Bhattacharya M, Dubey AP, Mathur NB. Prevalence of celiac disease in north Indian children. Indian Pediatr 2009;46:415–7.
8. Catassi C, Ratsch IM, Gandolfi L, et al. Why is coeliac disease endemic in the people of the Sahara? Lancet 1999;354:647–8.
9. Gomez JC, Selvaggio GS, Viola M, et al. Prevalence of celiac disease in Argentina: screening of an adult population in the La Plata area. Am J Gastroenterol 2001;96:2700–4.
10. Makharia GK, Verma AK, Amarchand R, et al. Prevalence of celiac disease in the northern part of India: a community based study. J Gastroenterol Hepatol 2011;26:894–900.

11. Melo SB, Fernandes MI, Peres LC, et al. Prevalence and demographic characteristics of celiac disease among blood donors in Ribeirao Preto, State of Sao Paulo, Brazil. Dig Dis Sci 2006;51:1020–5.

12. Nusier MK, Brodtkorb HK, Rein SE, et al. Serological screening for celiac disease in schoolchildren in Jordan. Is height and weight affected when seropositive? Ital J Pediatr 2010;36:16.

13. Remes-Troche JM, Ramirez-Iglesias MT, Rubio-Tapia A, et al. Celiac disease could be a frequent disease in Mexico: prevalence of tissue transglutaminase antibody in healthy blood donors. J Clin Gastroenterol 2006;40: 697–700.

14. Saberi-Firouzi M, Omrani GR, Nejabat M, et al. Prevalence of celiac disease in Shiraz, southern Iran. Saudi J Gastroenterol 2008;14:135–8.

15. Trevisiol C, Brandt KG, Silva GA, et al. High prevalence of unrecognized celiac disease in an unselected hospital population in north-eastern Brasil (Recife, Pernambuco). J Pediatr Gastroenterol Nutr 2004;39:214–5.

16. Furon R. Manuel de Prehistorie Generale. Paris: Payor; 1958.

17. Feldman M, Sears ER. The wild gene resources of wheat. Sci Am 1981;244: 102–12.

18. Lewin R. A revolution of ideas in agriculture origins. Science 1988;240:984–6.

19. Cambel HB, Braidwood RJ. An old farmer's village in Turkey. Le Scienze 1970; 22:96–103.

20. Gee S. On fitful or recurrent vomiting. In: Saint Bartholomew's Hospital Reports; 1882. p. 1–6 as cited by Online 'Mendelian Inheritance in Man' (OMIM) 500007.

21. Dalgic B, Sari S, Basturk B, et al. Prevalence of celiac disease in healthy Turkish school children. Am J Gastroenterol 2011;106:1512–7.

22. Catassi C. Editorial: celiac disease in Turkey: lessons from the Fertile Crescent. Am J Gastroenterol 2011;106:1518–20.

23. Bdioui F, Sakly N, Hassine M, et al. Prevalence of celiac disease in Tunisian blood donors. Gastroenterol Clin Biol 2006;30:33–6.

24. Gandolfi L, Pratesi R, Cordoba JC, et al. Prevalence of celiac disease among blood donors in Brazil. Am J Gastroenterol 2000;95:689–92.

25. Abu-Zekry M, Kryszak D, Diab M, et al. Prevalence of celiac disease in Egyptian children disputes the east-west agriculture-dependent spread of the disease. J Pediatr Gastroenterol Nutr 2008;47:136–40.

26. Sood A, Midha V, Sood N, et al. Prevalence of celiac disease among school children in Punjab, North India. J Gastroenterol Hepatol 2006;21:1622–5.

27. Ben Hariz M, Kallel-Sellami M, Kallel L, et al. Prevalence of celiac disease in Tunisia: mass-screening study in schoolchildren. Eur J Gastroenterol Hepatol 2007;19:687–94.

28. Shamir R, Lerner A, Shinar E, et al. The use of a single serological marker underestimates the prevalence of celiac disease in Israel: a study of blood donors. Am J Gastroenterol 2002;97:2589–94.

29. Tatar G, Elsurer R, Simsek H, et al. Screening of tissue transglutaminase antibody in healthy blood donors for celiac disease screening in the Turkish population. Dig Dis Sci 2004;49:1479–84.

30. Mankai A, Landolsi H, Chahed A, et al. Celiac disease in Tunisia: serological screening in healthy blood donors. Pathol Biol (Paris) 2006;54:10–3.

31. Akbari MR, Mohammadkhani A, Fakheri H, et al. Screening of the adult population in Iran for coeliac disease: comparison of the tissue-transglutaminase antibody and anti-endomysial antibody tests. Eur J Gastroenterol Hepatol 2006;18: 1181–6.

32. Kavin H. Adult coeliac disease in South Africa. An analysis of 20 cases emphasizing atypical presentations. S Afr Med J 1981;59:628–32.
33. Coton T, Grassin F, Maslin J, et al. Celiac disease: special features in Africa. Description of 8 cases in Djibouti (Horn of Africa). Med Trop (Mars) 2008;68:144–8 [in French].
34. Suliman GI. Coeliac disease in Sudanese children. Gut 1978;19:121–5.
35. Lionetti E, Catassi C. New clues in celiac disease epidemiology, pathogenesis, clinical manifestations, and treatment. Int Rev Immunol 2011;30:219–31.
36. Jiang LL, Zhang BL, Liu YS. Is adult celiac disease really uncommon in Chinese? J Zhejiang Univ Sci B 2009;10:168–71.
37. Wang XQ, Liu W, Xu CD, et al. Celiac disease in children with diarrhea in 4 cities in China. J Pediatr Gastroenterol Nutr 2011;53:368–70.
38. Wu J, Xia B, von Blomberg BM, et al. Coeliac disease: emerging in China? Gut 2010;59:418–9.
39. Makishima H, Komiyama Y, Asano N, et al. Peripheral T-cell lymphoma following diffuse large B-cell lymphoma associated with celiac disease. Intern Med 2008;47:295–8.
40. Shaoul R, Marcon MA, Okada Y, et al. Gastric metaplasia: a frequently overlooked feature of duodenal biopsy specimens in untreated celiac disease. J Pediatr Gastroenterol Nutr 2000;30:397–403.
41. Khoshbaten M, Rostami Nejad M, Farzady L, et al. Fertility disorder associated with celiac disease in males and females: fact or fiction? J Obstet Gynaecol Res 2011;37:1308–12.
42. Pratesi R, Gandolfi L, Garcia SG, et al. Prevalence of coeliac disease: unexplained age-related variation in the same population. Scand J Gastroenterol 2003;38:747–50.
43. Begue C, Beratarrechea AG, Varela E, et al. Celiac disease: diagnosis prevalence in a community hospital. Acta Gastroenterol Latinoam 2010;40:317–22 [in Spanish].
44. Khuffash FA, Barakat MH, Shaltout AA, et al. Coeliac disease among children in Kuwait: difficulties in diagnosis and management. Gut 1987;28:1595–9.
45. Boudraa G, Hachelaf W, Benbouabdellah M, et al. Prevalence of coeliac disease in diabetic children and their first-degree relatives in west Algeria: screening with serological markers. Acta Paediatr Suppl 1996;412:58–60.
46. Al-Ashwal AA, Shabib SM, Sakati NA, et al. Prevalence and characteristics of celiac disease in type I diabetes mellitus in Saudi Arabia. Saudi Med J 2003;24:1113–5.
47. Elsurer R, Tatar G, Simsek H, et al. Celiac disease in the Turkish population. Dig Dis Sci 2005;50:136–42.
48. Guliter S, Yakaryilmaz F, Ozkurt Z, et al. Prevalence of coeliac disease in patients with autoimmune thyroiditis in a Turkish population. World J Gastroenterol 2007;13:1599–601.
49. Collin P, Salmi J, Hallstrom O, et al. Autoimmune thyroid disorders and coeliac disease. Eur J Endocrinol 1994;130:137–40.
50. Poddar U, Thapa BR, Singh K. Clinical features of celiac disease in Indian children: are they different from the West? J Pediatr Gastroenterol Nutr 2006;43:313–7.
51. Barada K, Bitar A, Mokadem MA, et al. Celiac disease in Middle Eastern and North African countries: a new burden? World J Gastroenterol 2010;16:1449–57.
52. Teresi S, Crapisi M, Vallejo MD, et al. Celiac disease seropositivity in Saharawi children: a follow-up and family study. J Pediatr Gastroenterol Nutr 2010;50:506–9.

53. Nass FR, Kotze LM, Nisihara RM, et al. Serological and clinical follow-up of relatives of celiac disease patients from southern Brazil. Digestion 2011;83:89–95.

54. Martins Rde C, Gandolfi L, Modelli IC, et al. Serologic screening and genetic testing among Brazilian patients with celiac disease and their first degree relatives. Arq Gastroenterol 2010;47:257–62.

55. Araya M, Mondragon A, Perez-Bravo F, et al. Celiac disease in a Chilean population carrying Amerindian traits. J Pediatr Gastroenterol Nutr 2000;31:381–6.

56. Vazquez H, Sugai E, Pedreira S, et al. Screening for asymptomatic celiac sprue in families. J Clin Gastroenterol 1995;21:130–3.

57. Djilali-Saiah I, Schmitz J, Harfouch-Hammoud E, et al. CTLA-4 gene polymorphism is associated with predisposition to coeliac disease. Gut 1998;43:187–9.

58. Zhernakova A, Elbers CC, Ferwerda B, et al. Evolutionary and functional analysis of celiac risk loci reveals SH2B3 as a protective factor against bacterial infection. Am J Hum Genet 2010;86:970–7.

59. Eller E, Vardi P, Babu SR, et al. Celiac disease and HLA in a Bedouin kindred. Hum Immunol 2006;67:940–50.

60. El-Akawi ZJ, Al-Hattab DM, Migdady MA. Frequency of HLA-DQA1*0501 and DQB1*0201 alleles in patients with coeliac disease, their first-degree relatives and controls in Jordan. Ann Trop Paediatr 2010;30:305–9.

61. Kuloglu Z, Doganci T, Kansu A, et al. HLA types in Turkish children with celiac disease. Turk J Pediatr 2008;50:515–20.

62. Neuhausen SL, Weizman Z, Camp NJ, et al. HLA DQA1-DQB1 genotypes in Bedouin families with celiac disease. Hum Immunol 2002;63:502–7.

63. Bouguerra F, Dugoujon JM, Babron MC, et al. Susceptibility to coeliac disease in Tunisian children and GM immunoglobulin allotypes. Eur J Immunogenet 1999;26:293–7.

64. Kaur G, Sarkar N, Bhatnagar S, et al. Pediatric celiac disease in India is associated with multiple DR3-DQ2 haplotypes. Hum Immunol 2002;63:677–82.

65. Cintado A, Sorell L, Galvan JA, et al. HLA DQA1*0501 and DQB1*02 in Cuban celiac patients. Hum Immunol 2006;67:639–42.

66. Lopez-Vazquez A, Fuentes D, Rodrigo L, et al. MHC class I region plays a role in the development of diverse clinical forms of celiac disease in a Saharawi population. Am J Gastroenterol 2004;99:662–7.

67. Perez-Bravo F, Araya M, Mondragon A, et al. Genetic differences in HLA-DQA1* and DQB1* allelic distributions between celiac and control children in Santiago, Chile. Hum Immunol 1999;60:262–7.

68. Parada A, Araya M, Perez-Bravo F, et al. Amerindian mtDNA haplogroups and celiac disease risk HLA haplotypes in mixed-blood Latin American patients. J Pediatr Gastroenterol Nutr 2011;53:429–34.

69. Alarida K, Harown J, Di Pierro MR, et al. HLA-DQ2 and -DQ8 genotypes in celiac and healthy Libyan children. Dig Liver Dis 2010;42:425–7.

70. Erkan T, Kutlu T, Yilmaz E, et al. Human leukocyte antigens in Turkish pediatric celiac patients. Turk J Pediatr 1999;41:181–8.

71. Tumer L, Altuntas B, Hasanoglu A, et al. Pattern of human leukocyte antigens in Turkish children with celiac disease. Pediatr Int 2000;42:678–81.

72. Jabbar AA. HLA and disease associations in Iraq. Dis Markers 1993;11:161–70.

73. Clot F, Fulchignoni-Lataud MC, Renoux C, et al. Linkage and association study of the CTLA-4 region in coeliac disease for Italian and Tunisian populations. Tissue Antigens 1999;54:527–30.

74. Moore JK, West SR, Robins G. Advances in celiac disease. Curr Opin Gastroenterol 2011;27:112–8.

75. Palabykoglu M, Botoman VA, Coban S, et al. A tale of two cities: typical celiac sprue presenting symptoms are significantly more common in Turkish than in US patients. J Clin Gastroenterol 2008;42:62–5.

76. Ahmad F, Alam S, Shukla I, et al. Screening children with severe short stature for celiac disease using tissue transglutaminase. Indian J Pediatr 2010;77:387–90.

77. al-Tawaty AI, Elbargathy SM. Coeliac disease in north-eastern Libya. Ann Trop Paediatr 1998;18:27–30.

78. Mohammed IM, Karrar ZE, El-Safi SH. Coeliac disease in Sudanese children with clinical features suggestive of the disease. East Mediterr Health J 2006; 12:582–9.

79. Sood A, Midha V, Sood N, et al. Adult celiac disease in northern India. Indian J Gastroenterol 2003;22:124–6.

80. Mankai A, Ben Hamouda H, Amri F, et al. Screening by anti-endomysium anti-bodies for celiac disease in Tunisian children with type 1 diabetes mellitus. Gastroenterol Clin Biol 2007;31:462–6.

81. Galvao LC, Brandao JM, Fernandes MI, et al. Clinical presentation of children with celiac disease attended at a Brazilian specialized university service, over two periods of time. Arq Gastroenterol 2004;41:234–8 [in Portuguese].

82. Rostami Nejad M, Rostami K, Pourhoseingholi MA, et al. Atypical presentation is dominant and typical for coeliac disease. J Gastrointestin Liver Dis 2009;18: 285–91.

83. Saadah OI. Celiac disease in children and adolescents at a singe center in Saudi Arabia. Ann Saudi Med 2011;31:51–7.

84. Sugai E, Moreno ML, Hwang HJ, et al. Celiac disease serology in patients with different pretest probabilities: is biopsy avoidable? World J Gastroenterol 2010; 16:3144–52.

85. Zamani F, Mohamadnejad M, Shakeri R, et al. Gluten sensitive enteropathy in patients with iron deficiency anemia of unknown origin. World J Gastroenterol 2008;14:7381–5.

86. da Silva Kotze LM, Nisihara RM, Kotze LR, et al. Celiac disease in older Brazilians. J Am Geriatr Soc 2011;59:1548–50.

87. Demir H, Yuce A, Kocak N, et al. Celiac disease in Turkish children: presentation of 104 cases. Pediatr Int 2000;42:483–7.

88. Tanure MG, Silva IN, Bahia M, et al. Prevalence of celiac disease in Brazilian children with type 1 diabetes mellitus. J Pediatr Gastroenterol Nutr 2006;42:155–9.

89. Rabassa EB, Sagaro E, Fragoso T, et al. Coeliac disease in Cuban children. Arch Dis Child 1981;56:128–31.

90. Emami MH, Karimi S, Kouhestani S, et al. Diagnostic accuracy of IgA anti-tissue transglutaminase in patients suspected of having coeliac disease in Iran. J Gastrointestin Liver Dis 2008;17:141–6.

91. Jadallah KA, Khader YS. Celiac disease in patients with presumed irritable bowel syndrome: a case-finding study. World J Gastroenterol 2009;15:5321–5.

92. Hashemi J, Hajiani E, Shahbazin HB, et al. Prevalence of celiac disease in Iranian children with idiopathic short stature. World J Gastroenterol 2008;14: 7376–80.

93. Harper JW, Holleran SF, Ramakrishnan R, et al. Anemia in celiac disease is multifactorial in etiology. Am J Hematol 2007;82:996–1000.

94. Assiri AM, El Mouzan MI, Al Sanie A, et al. Pattern of celiac disease in infants and children. Trop Gastroenterol 2008;29:217–20.

95. Mancilla AC, Madrid SA, Valenzuela EJ, et al. Adult celiac disease: clinical experience. Rev Med Chil 2005;133:1317–21 [in Spanish].

96. Aygun C, Uraz S, Damci T, et al. Celiac disease in an adult Turkish population with type 1 diabetes mellitus. Dig Dis Sci 2005;50:1462–6.

97. Green PH, Rostami K, Marsh MN. Diagnosis of coeliac disease. Best Pract Res Clin Gastroenterol 2005;19:389–400.

98. Mansouri A, Makris DP, Kefalas P. Determination of hydrogen peroxide scavenging activity of cinnamic and benzoic acids employing a highly sensitive peroxyoxalate chemiluminescence-based assay: structure-activity relationships. J Pharm Biomed Anal 2005;39:22–6.

99. Arevalo F, Roe E, Arias-Stella-Castillo J, et al. Low serological positivity in patients with histology compatible with celiac disease in Peru. Rev Esp Enferm Dig 2010;102:372–5.

100. Piaggio MV, Demonte AM, Sihufe G, et al. Serological diagnosis of celiac disease: anti-gliadin peptide antibodies and tissue anti-transglutaminase. Medicina (B Aires) 1999;59:693–7 [in Spanish].

101. Abrams JA, Diamond B, Rotterdam H, et al. Seronegative celiac disease: increased prevalence with lesser degrees of villous atrophy. Dig Dis Sci 2004; 49:546–50.

102. Cosnes J, Cellier C, Viola S, et al. Incidence of autoimmune diseases in celiac disease: protective effect of the gluten-free diet. Clin Gastroenterol Hepatol 2008;6:753–8.

103. Leffler DA, Edwards-George J, Dennis M, et al. Factors that influence adherence to a gluten-free diet in adults with celiac disease. Dig Dis Sci 2008;53: 1573–81.

104. Chauhan JC, Kumar P, Dutta AK, et al. Assessment of dietary compliance to gluten free diet and psychosocial problems in Indian children with celiac disease. Indian J Pediatr 2010;77:649–54.

105. Mokhallalaty MD, Naja Z, Ziedeh F, et al. Celiac disease at Makassed General Hospital (8 years of experience). Revue Medicale Libanaise 2002;14:49–53.

106. Rostami K, Malekzadeh R, Shahbazkhani B, et al. Coeliac disease in Middle Eastern countries: a challenge for the evolutionary history of this complex disorder? Dig Liver Dis 2004;36:694–7.

Nutrition Assessment in Celiac Disease

Suzanne Simpson, RD[a],*, Tricia Thompson, RD, MS[b]

KEYWORDS

- Celiac disease • Gluten-free diet • Nutrition assessment

KEY POINTS

- Nutrition assessment is the first step in the nutrition care process.
- Assessment of typical dietary intake in celiac disease must be thorough.
- The only treatment for celiac disease is a strict, lifelong gluten-free diet.

According to the Academy of Nutrition and Dietetics Evidence Analysis Library, "medical nutrition therapy provided by a registered dietitian is strongly recommended for individuals with celiac disease."[1] Therefore, consultation with a dietitian/nutritionist who has expertise in celiac disease should be mandatory for all patients with celiac disease at diagnosis as well as during follow-up (**Box 1**). The gluten-free diet is currently the only treatment for celiac disease; patients with celiac disease must be monitored closely by a dietitian to assess the healthfulness of the gluten-free diet as well as to discuss motivation, quality of life, symptom improvement, and barriers to compliance.

Nutrition assessment is the first step in the nutrition care process. During the assessment pertinent data are gathered and compared with normal values. A nutrition diagnosis is determined, and a nutrition care plan developed and prescribed. The nutrition intervention should include goals that are quantifiable, achievable, time defined, and negotiated with the patient so as to improve dietary intake and reduce risk factors. The assessment continues at each patient visit. A complete nutrition assessment includes a review of dietary intake, anthropometric measures, biochemical data, medical tests, and procedures (**Box 2**). Communication with the referring physician/gastroenterologist is advisable for optimal patient care. During the assessment, the dietitian may determine that a diagnosed patient with gastrointestinal symptoms, not related to gluten intake, could be related to another food-intolerance or medical issue that the physician must investigate. Similarly, the dietitian may determine that a micronutrient deficiency or weight loss is not caused by inadequate caloric intake. Dietitians can also recommend that the physician screen for celiac disease in

[a] Celiac Disease Center at Columbia University, Suite 956, 180 Fort Washington Avenue, New York, NY 10032, USA; [b] Gluten Free Watchdog, LLC, 348 Summer Street, Manchester, MA 01944, USA
* Corresponding author.
E-mail address: Sms2246@columbia.edu

Gastrointest Endoscopy Clin N Am 22 (2012) 797–809
http://dx.doi.org/10.1016/j.giec.2012.07.010
1052-5157/12/$ – see front matter © 2012 Elsevier Inc. All rights reserved.

> **Box 1**
> **When to refer patients with celiac disease to a dietitian**
>
> At diagnosis: initial assessment followed by 2 to 3 more visits within the first year of diagnosis as well as annual visits thereafter (minimally)
>
> Suspicion of gluten ingestion (positive serologies after 1 or more years on a gluten-free diet)
>
> Lactose intolerance
>
> Fructose intolerance
>
> Food allergies
>
> Constipation/diarrhea/gastroesophageal reflux disease
>
> Fluctuations in body mass index: weight gain or loss
>
> Micronutrient deficiencies or toxicities
>
> Gastroparesis
>
> Hypercholesterolemia
>
> Type 1 diabetes
>
> Refractory celiac disease

patients who do not have a diagnosis but exhibit symptoms, significant medical history or family history, or unexplained nutrient deficiencies.

ASSESSMENT OF DIETARY INTAKE

Assessment of typical dietary intake in celiac disease must be thorough. All food and beverages consumed on weekdays and weekends should be reviewed, including name brands of products and frequency of food eaten away from the home (restaurants, social events, other people's homes, travel). It is helpful for the patient to complete a food diary for the dietitian to review. Dietary restrictions such as food intolerances, food allergies, religious observances, and self-imposed restrictions are considered. Patients should be queried about their compliance to a strict gluten-free diet and the frequency of gluten ingestion (purposely or inadvertently). It is important to assess patients' knowledge and understanding of the diet by reviewing their label-reading skills, how they order foods in restaurants, and what cross-contamination procedures are used in shared kitchens. Patients may have obtained information about the gluten-free diet elsewhere, and it is important to assess the source for its accuracy (Internet, other nutritionists, books, peers, magazines). Medications, vitamins, and dietary supplements must be reviewed for their possible gluten status, their purpose, and whether they meet or exceed the Dietary Reference Intake. It is important to assess quality of life, social history/social support, sufficiency of income, and ability to access gluten-free food. Inquiry should be made as to who prepares food at home, particularly in a shared kitchen. A review of gastrointestinal symptoms (such as type, frequency, and volume of bowel movements, abdominal pain, bloating, nausea or vomiting, delayed gastric emptying, reflux, flatulence) is required. Compliance with a strict gluten-free diet usually reduces gastrointestinal symptoms in celiac disease[2–13] and should always be encouraged.

Anthropometric Assessment

Assess age, height, weight, body mass index, growth parameters in children, weight history, physical activity, and disordered eating and/or diets (currently or in the past).

Box 2
Nutrition assessment checklist

Dietary history: foods and beverages consumed at all meals and snacks, including name brands

Adequate calories, protein, micronutrient intake (the typical gluten-free diet can increase the risk of calcium, iron, fiber, vitamin D, folate, niacin, zinc, and vitamin B12 deficiencies because of lack of fortification of gluten-free packaged foods including breads and pastas)

Foods away from the home: restaurant frequency, fast food, take out, order in, cafeteria, other people's homes, social and work events

Travel: foods consumed, frequency of travel

Supplements: herbal remedies, over-the-counter diet aids

Vitamins and minerals: check if gluten-free and check amounts of micronutrients compared with recommended intake

Prescription medications: must be gluten-free

Cross-contamination prevention measures

Medical history, family history, symptoms, laboratory measures, review of all tests and procedures

Anthropometrics: height, weight, body mass index

Social support: family, work, peers

Quality of life: work, family, exercise, risk of depression

Physical activity level

Assess knowledge of gluten-free diet food labels: knowing how to identify gluten in an ingredient list; understanding the meaning of nutrition food claims such as no gluten, gluten-free, wheat-free, made in the same factory that processes wheat, low gluten

Readiness for change: assess the patient's willingness to change diet and the patient's goals for learning and meeting with the dietitian

Family history: other family members with celiac disease; family members tested for celiac disease

Potential nutrition diagnoses: follows a strict gluten-free diet, ingesting gluten inadvertently in restaurants, ingesting gluten on purpose monthly, inadequate calcium/vitamin D intake, inadequate fiber intake, risk of iron deficiency, constipation due to inadequate fiber intake, excessive caloric intake resulting in weight gain, at risk of overweight

---

Medical Procedures

Review all medical procedures including: endoscopy report (classification of Marsh score, number and location of segments biopsied); bone mineral density; breath tests (bacterial overgrowth, fructose intolerance, lactose intolerance); gastric emptying study; colonoscopy; and surgery. Review medical history (eg, gastrointestinal, immune, neurologic, and psychological); other health conditions; autoimmune diseases; family history of celiac disease; allergies; muscle stores; and fat stores. Inquire about appetite, current gastrointestinal symptoms, and symptoms prior to the diagnosis of celiac disease.

Physical

Assess appearance of hair, skin, nails, and body shape.

NUTRITION INTERVENTION AND EDUCATION

The gluten-free diet is the medical and nutritional treatment for celiac disease. A gluten-free diet is discussed in later sections of this article. Gluten must be removed from the diet completely and permanently. **Box 3** includes a list of items that must be included in the nutrition education for patients with celiac disease. It is important to answer questions the patient may have, establish trust, and set goals with the patient that can be addressed during follow-up.

FOLLOW-UP

Celiac disease is a lifelong systemic disease with a burdensome treatment that requires regular follow-up visits with the expert dietitian and gastroenterologist; patients must be monitored for compliance, symptoms, well-being, and medical issues. **Box 4** lists items that need to be monitored during follow-up visits.

If a patient with celiac disease is not treated with the gluten-free diet, there can be serious consequences. The intake of gluten may result in gastrointestinal symptoms, malabsorption and micronutrient deficiencies, villous atrophy and the development of neurologic complications, fertility problems, reduced quality of life, intestinal lymphoma, and reduced bone mineral density. The dietitian must assess compliance during follow-up, particularly in patients with symptoms. If gluten exposure is determined not to be the cause of symptoms, other potential causes could be lactose, fructose, and carbohydrate intolerances, bacterial overgrowth, refractory celiac disease, related cancers, and other gastrointestinal diseases and conditions. These conditions would require investigation by a gastroenterologist.

Box 3
Nutrition education for the gluten-free diet

Label reading: list of ingredients that must be avoided, review of labeling laws, surprising sources of gluten, cross-contamination procedures, nutrition claims (eg, gluten-free, wheat-free, low gluten, made in the same facility as wheat), sources of important nutrients such as calcium, vitamin D, iron, fiber

Recommendations for portions and variety of foods from all food groups

Heart-healthy recommendations to prevent high cholesterol

High fiber, as tolerated, to prevent weight gain and constipation

Review of gluten-free grains: 50% of grains consumed should be whole grains

Discuss risk of vitamin deficiencies

Encourage healthful gluten-free food choices

Discuss risks associated with ingesting gluten

Discuss vitamin supplementation as needed

Discuss use of supplements such as probiotics, over-the-counter remedies

Discuss family testing

Discuss restaurant eating, social situations, menu planning, recipes, grocery shopping

Coordinate care with other providers as needed

Discuss other dietary restrictions within the confines of the gluten-free diet: lactose-free diet, low-fructose diet, diabetes meal plan/carbohydrate counting

Implement weight-centered guidelines as needed: weight control or high calorie

---

| **Box 4** |
| **Nutrition items to monitor at follow-up visits** |
| Implementation of nutrition goals |
| Factors affecting the quality of life |
| Medical status (eg, gastrointestinal, immune, neurologic, psychological) |
| Social supports |
| Body mass index |
| Compliance with the gluten-free diet |
| Label reading |
| Restaurant habits |
| Diet history and gluten-free dietary pattern with specific focus on intake of nutrients at risk of deficiency (iron, calcium, vitamin D, B vitamins, fiber, folate, niacin, zinc), intake compared with recommendations, excessive sugar and fat from prepared gluten-free foods, caloric intake |
| Vitamin intake |
| Medications and supplements |
| Antibody levels, potential exposure to cross-contamination, hidden sources of gluten in foods |
| Answer patient's questions |

Individuals with celiac disease have been found to show improved quality of life after compliance with a gluten-free diet for at least 1 year.[12,13] However, they may not attain the same level of quality of life as the general population; this has been reported more frequently by women than men, and particularly by those who continue to have gastrointestinal symptoms despite adherence to a gluten-free diet.[14,15]

For most patients with celiac disease, compliance with a gluten-free dietary pattern results in significant improvements in hematological parameters including anemia and iron deficiency.[15–19] Iron supplementation in a gluten-free multivitamin with iron or additional therapeutic doses of iron may be required.

THE GLUTEN-FREE DIET

The only treatment for celiac disease is a strict, lifelong gluten-free diet. The gluten-free diet is free of all but very small amounts of gluten, defined in celiac disease as specific sequences of amino acids found in wheat, barley, and rye. All foods containing these grains as ingredients or through contamination must be removed from the diet. The gluten-free diet should be based on gluten-free whole grains (eg, whole corn, brown rice, millet, sorghum, wild rice, teff, buckwheat, amaranth, and quinoa), plain low-fat milk and milk products (or milk alternatives such as soy milk), unprocessed lean protein (meat, poultry, fish, legumes), fruits, and vegetables.

Labeled Gluten-Free Foods

There is an abundance of food products labeled gluten-free, including breads, pastas, breakfast cereals, and baking mixes. Under the US Food and Drug Administration (FDA) proposed rule for labeling of food as gluten-free, food labeled gluten-free must meet all of the following criteria[20]:

- It cannot include an ingredient that is a prohibited grain. Prohibited grains include wheat, barley, rye, and triticale (a cross between wheat and rye).

- It cannot include an ingredient derived from a prohibited grain that has not been processed to remove gluten. Examples of these types of ingredients include wheat flour, hydrolyzed wheat protein, wheat germ, malt, and barley malt flavoring.
- It can include an ingredient derived from a prohibited grain that has been processed to remove gluten as long as use of the ingredient does not result in the final food product containing 20 parts per million (ppm) or more gluten. Examples of these types of ingredients are wheat starch and modified food starch made from wheat.
- It must contain less than 20 ppm gluten.

The definition of gluten-free differs slightly from the Codex Standard for Foods for Special Dietary Use for Persons Intolerant to Gluten.[21] Under this standard, gluten-free foods are dietary foods that fit one of the following two definitions:

- Foods that are made only from ingredients that do not contain wheat, barley, rye, oats (under Codex, the use of oats uncontaminated with wheat, barley, and rye may be determined at a national level), or their cross-bred varieties, and with a gluten content not greater than 20 ppm.
- Foods made using one or more ingredients from wheat, barley, rye, oats, or their cross-bred varieties, which have been specially processed to remove gluten and with a gluten content not greater than 20 ppm.

Reading Labels of Foods Not Labeled Gluten-Free

If a food product sold in the United States is not labeled gluten-free, consumers must be educated as to how to read labels carefully and look for sources of wheat, barley, and rye. The ingredients list (and in the case of wheat, the "Contains" statement) should be read for the words and ingredients that follow. If any of these words or ingredients are included on the label of a food not labeled gluten-free, the product should be avoided by individuals with celiac disease.

- "Wheat." Under the FDA Food Allergen Labeling and Consumer Protection Act (FALCPA), if an ingredient in a packaged food product regulated by the FDA includes protein from wheat, the word wheat must be included on the food label either in the ingredients list or "Contains" statement.[22] As a result, consumers do not need to be concerned about ingredients such as modified food starch and dextrin if wheat is not named on the food label.
- "Barley"
- "Rye"
- "Oats." Only oats and products containing oats labeled gluten-free should be eaten by individuals with celiac disease.[23] Although oats are considered inherently gluten-free, they also are highly likely to be contaminated with wheat, barley, or rye.[24,25]
- "Malt." The single word malt in an ingredients list refers to barley malt.[26] If another source of malt is used, such as corn, the ingredients list will read "corn malt."
- "Brewer's yeast." This type of yeast may be a product of the beer-brewing process (ie, spent brewer's yeast).[27] As a result it may be contaminated with malt and grain.

Foods regulated by the United States Department of Agriculture

Although the labeling of most food in the United States is under the jurisdiction of the FDA, some foods are regulated by the United States Department of Agriculture

(USDA). These foods are meat products, poultry products, egg products (defined as liquid, dried, and frozen, whole eggs, egg yolks, and egg whites with or without added ingredients), and mixed food products containing in general more than 3% raw meat or 2% or more cooked meat or poultry meat.[28–30] Whereas the FDA has mandatory allergen labeling under FALCPA, the USDA does not. Manufacturers are encouraged to voluntarily follow FALCPA-like allergen labeling, and the USDA believes 80% to 90% of product labels are in voluntary compliance.[28] There are a few additional ingredients consumers must look for in the ingredients lists of foods regulated by the USDA if the manufacturer is not voluntarily complying with FALCPA. If any of the ingredients that follow (this is in addition to the ingredients already listed) are included on the label of a USDA-regulated food not in voluntarily compliance with FALCPA-like allergen labeling, the food should be avoided until the manufacturer is contacted and it is confirmed that the source of the ingredient is not wheat.

- "Modified food starch." Modified food starch in a food regulated by the USDA may be derived from wheat, and "wheat" may not be included on the food label if the manufacturer is not voluntarily complying with FALCPA-like allergen labeling.[31] Although wheat can be the source of modified food starch, the source is most likely corn if the ingredient is manufactured in the United States.
- "Dextrin." Dextrin in a food regulated by the USDA may be derived from wheat, and "wheat" may not be included on the food label if the manufacturer is not voluntarily complying with FALCPA-like allergen labeling.[31] Although wheat can be the source of dextrin, the source is most likely corn if the ingredient is manufactured in the United States.
- "Starch." The single word starch in the ingredients list of a food product regulated by the USDA may refer to either corn starch or wheat starch.[32] If the starch is derived from wheat, the word "wheat" may not be included on the food label if the manufacturer is not voluntarily complying with FALCPA-like allergen labeling.[31] Although the starch may be wheat, it is most likely corn if the ingredient is manufactured in the United States.

It is important to emphasize that the vast majority of manufacturers of USDA-regulated foods are in voluntary compliance with FALCPA-like allergen labeling, and in most cases modified food starch, dextrin, and starch are derived from corn, not wheat.

Contamination

Inherently gluten-free grains and flours may become contaminated with wheat, barley, or rye any time they are grown, harvested, transported, or processed in the same area. A study by Thompson and colleagues[33] found that of 22 samples of naturally gluten-free grains and flours sold in the United States, 9 contained mean levels of gluten ranging from 8.5 to 2925.0 ppm of gluten. Seven of these samples contained mean levels of gluten at or above 20 ppm gluten and would not be considered gluten-free under the FDA's proposed gluten-free labeling rule. Because of the possible risk of cross-contamination, the Academy of Nutrition and Dietetics Celiac Disease Toolkit recommends that individuals with celiac disease buy naturally gluten-free grains and flours that are labeled gluten-free.[34] It is also recommended that products that are predominantly grain-based be labeled gluten-free.[34] A comparison of the gluten content of labeled versus nonlabeled gluten-free millet, rice, soy, and sorghum flours is provided in **Table 1**. On testing, labeled gluten-free brands contained lower amounts of gluten than the brands not labeled gluten-free.[33,35]

Table 1
Content of labeled versus nonlabeled gluten-free flours

Flour	Labeled Gluten-Free?	Mean Gluten Content (ppm)[a]
Millet	No	305.0
Millet	No	327.0
Millet	Yes	15.5
Rice	No	8.5
Rice	Yes	<5
Sorghum	No	234.0
Sorghum	Yes	<5[b]
Soy	No	2925.0
Soy	No	92.0
Soy	Yes	<5[c]

Abbreviation: ppm, parts per million.
[a] Flours not labeled gluten-free: 1 sample tested in duplicate (mean of 2 extractions); flours labeled gluten-free: 3 samples of same brand tested in duplicate (6 extractions).
[b] Five extractions tested at less than 5 ppm gluten; 1 extraction tested at 7 ppm gluten.
[c] Five extractions tested at less than 5 ppm gluten; 1 extraction tested at 6 ppm gluten.
Data from Thompson T, Lee AR, Grace T. Gluten contamination of grains, seeds, and flours in the United States: a pilot study. J Am Diet Assoc 2010;110:937–40; and Gluten-free watchdog, LLC. Available at: http://www.glutenfreewatchdog.org/. Accessed August 14, 2012.

Nutritional Quality of the Gluten-Free Diet

As with any eating plan, a gluten-free diet may be healthy or unhealthy, depending in large part on food choice. According to the Academy of Nutrition and Dietetics Evidence Analysis Library, "adherence to the gluten-free dietary pattern may result in a diet that is high in fat and low in carbohydrates and fiber, as well as low in iron, folate, niacin, vitamin B12, calcium, phosphorus and zinc."[36] As a result, the Academy's Evidence-Based Nutrition Practice Guideline for Celiac Disease recommends the consumption of whole and enriched gluten-free grains and products.[23] The addition of a gluten-free age-specific and gender-specific multivitamin and mineral supplement is advised if "usual food intake shows nutritional inadequacies that cannot be alleviated through improved eating habits."[23]

There are several possible reasons for this macronutrient and micronutrient profile of the gluten-free diet. Individuals with celiac disease may not consume the recommended number of servings of grain foods. A study conducted by Thompson and colleagues[37] found that only 21% of adult female participants in the United States consumed the minimum recommended number of grain food servings. A retrospective review of diet histories of patients with celiac disease at a United States celiac disease center found that 38% of meals and snacks eaten by study participants did not contain a grain or starch component.[38] Low overall grain consumption can result in diets that are low in carbohydrates and fiber and proportionally higher in fat.[39] It also can result in diets that are low in iron, folate, niacin, and zinc.[39]

Individuals with celiac disease may consume grain foods made primarily from refined gluten-free grains and starch. One study found that of 268 gluten-free breads, pastas, and breakfast cereals for sale in the United States and reviewed for ingredients, 73% listed a refined grain or starch as the first ingredient.[40] Of these refined grain foods, only 16% were enriched or fortified with B vitamins and iron. These data are in stark contrast to those of refined wheat-based breads, pastas, and breakfast cereals, most of which are enriched or fortified. Since the time this study was conducted there appears to have been an increase in products incorporating gluten-free whole grains, such as amaranth, buckwheat, sorghum, quinoa, millet, teff, wild rice, brown rice, whole corn, and gluten-free oats. However, the number of manufacturers of refined grain foods enriching or fortifying their products has remained roughly the same. An overreliance on refined grain-based foods (vs whole grains) that are not enriched or fortified can result in diets that are low in fiber, iron, folate, niacin, vitamin B12, and zinc.[39]

Individuals with celiac disease also may consume grain-based foods that are high in fat. Gluten-free versions of foods that are typically thought of as low-fat or fat-free, such as pretzels, may contain large amounts of fat, because manufacturers of gluten-free foods may add extra fat to their products to improve the taste and texture.

In addition, many individuals with celiac disease are lactose intolerant when they are newly diagnosed. As a result, they may limit their intake of milk-based products, which may result in decreased intakes of calcium, vitamin B12, and phosphorus.[39]

To help ensure a healthy gluten-free diet, individuals should be:

- Referred to a dietitian well-versed in celiac disease as soon as possible after diagnosis
- Encouraged to consume foods made from gluten-free whole grains (eg, quinoa, gluten-free oats, teff) and to choose these products over refined gluten-free grains (eg, white rice, milled corn)
- Counseled to choose enriched or fortified refined grain foods over refined grain foods that are not enriched
- Advised to use the Nutrition Facts panel to compare the fat and fiber content of gluten-free grain foods and to choose products with more fiber and less fat whenever possible
- Eat or drink calcium rich foods such as calcium-fortified soy milk, calcium fortified orange juice, and calcium-processed plain tofu

Weight Gain and the Gluten-Free Diet

According to the Academy of Nutrition and Dietetics Evidence Analysis Library, "a small number of studies in adults show a trend toward weight gain after diagnosis; further research is needed in this area."[36] There are reasons why individuals with celiac disease might gain weight after diagnosis. Before diagnosis, increased amounts of calories may have been necessary to prevent or slow weight loss caused by malabsorption. Once a diagnosis is made, a gluten-free diet is started, and the intestine heals, fewer calories may be needed. Individuals may have to adjust their caloric intake and relearn appropriate portion control to prevent unwanted weight gain.

Unintentional Gluten Ingestion

If gluten ingestion is suspected but the patient appears to be following a strict gluten-free diet, gluten contamination should be considered. To help ferret out possible sources of contamination, the following areas should be investigated.

Contaminated food at point of purchase
- What types of grains (eg, rice, buckwheat, quinoa) are eaten? What specific brands are purchased? Are they labeled gluten-free?
- What types of foods not labeled gluten-free are purchased? Are any of these predominantly grain-based (eg, breakfast cereals, rice pastas, buckwheat noodles, taco shells, rice crackers, and so forth)?

- What types of labeled gluten-free foods are eaten? Do any brands have a history of contamination?
- Are any grains or flours purchased from bulk bins? Gluten-free grains and flours from bulk bins may be contaminated with wheat, barley, or rye, owing to the use of shared scoops.
- Are any grains or flours purchased from co-operatives that buy products in bulk and repackage in smaller containers? If so, they may be contaminated with gluten-containing grains if wheat, barley, and/or rye are repackaged in the same area.
- Are any grains or flours purchased from ethnic food stores? These grains and flours may not be labeled gluten-free.

Contaminated food at home
- Is the home completely gluten-free?
- If not, are gluten-free foods stored separately or on a higher shelf from gluten-containing foods? Doing so will prevent gluten-containing crumbs from raining down on the gluten-free food.
- Are products such as peanut butter, jelly, and mayonnaise used on both gluten-free and gluten-containing bread? If so, these products may be contaminated with gluten-containing crumbs due to "double-dipping."
- Are separate cooking and serving utensils used to prepare both gluten-free and gluten-containing meals?
- Are shared plates, pots, and so forth well cleaned after use with gluten-containing food?
- Are microwaves, toaster ovens, counter tops, silverware drawers, and so forth kept clean and free of wheat-containing crumbs?
- Is there shared use of a traditional pop-up toaster? This type of toaster is very hard to clean. If it has to be shared, the use of toaster bags is recommended.

Contaminated food at a restaurant
- How often are meals eaten away from home?
- Is wait staff queried about gluten-free options?
- Is wait staff informed about the need for the meal to be gluten-free and free of cross-contamination (eg, cleaned section of grill, separate pans, preparation tools) to the extent possible?
- Are French fries and/or tortilla chips frequent choices? These foods may be cooked in oil previously used to prepare breaded foods, such as onion rings.
- Is soup a frequent choice? Soup may be thickened with wheat flour or contain a wheat-based commercial broth/bouillon.
- Is rice pilaf a frequent choice? This rice dish typically contains wheat noodles and could contain a wheat-based broth/bouillon.
- What sauces or dressings are eaten? These products may contain wheat or barley ingredients.

Learning all of this dietary information may be overwhelming to patients, especially at first. Referral to a dietitian well versed in celiac disease and the gluten-free diet is essential.

REFERENCES

1. Academy of nutrition and dietetics evidence analysis library celiac disease evidence-based nutrition practice guideline. Available at: http://www.adaevidencelibrary.com/default.cfm?auth=1. Accessed August 14, 2012.

2. Cucchiara S, Bassotti G, Castellucci G, et al. Upper gastrointestinal motor abnormalities in children with active celiac disease. J Pediatr Gastroenterol Nutr 1995; 21:435–42.

3. Usai P, Bassotti G, Usai Satta P, et al. Oesophageal motility in adult coeliac disease. Neurogastroenterol Motil 1995;7:239–44.

4. Chiarioni G, Bassotti G, Germani U, et al. Gluten-free diet normalizes mouth-to-cecum transit of a caloric meal in adult patients with celiac disease. Dig Dis Sci 1997;42:2100–5.

5. Fine KD, Meyer RL, Lee EL. The prevalence and causes of chronic diarrhea in patients with celiac sprue treated with a gluten-free diet. Gastroenterology 1997;112:1830–8.

6. Benini L, Sembenini C, Salandini L, et al. Gastric emptying of realistic meals with and without gluten in patients with coeliac disease. Effect of jejunal mucosal recovery. Scand J Gastroenterol 2001;36:1044–8.

7. Cuomo A, Romano M, Rocco A, et al. Reflux oesophagitis in adult coeliac disease: beneficial effect of a gluten free diet. Gut 2003;52:514–7.

8. Midhagen G, Hallert C. High rate of gastrointestinal symptoms in celiac patients living on a gluten-free diet: controlled study. Am J Gastroenterol 2003;98:2023–6.

9. Tursi A, Brandimarte G, Giorgetti G. High prevalence of small intestinal bacterial overgrowth in celiac patients with persistence of gastrointestinal symptoms after gluten withdrawal. Am J Gastroenterol 2003;98:839–43.

10. Murray JA, Watson T, Clearman B, et al. Effect of a gluten-free diet on gastrointestinal symptoms in celiac disease. Am J Clin Nutr 2004;79:669–73.

11. Hopper AD, Leeds JS, Hurlstone DP, et al. Are lower gastrointestinal investigations necessary in patients with coeliac disease? Eur J Gastroenterol Hepatol 2005;17:617–21.

12. Viljamaa M, Collin P, Huhtala H, et al. Is coeliac disease screening in risk groups justified? A fourteen-year follow-up with special focus on compliance and quality of life. Aliment Pharmacol Ther 2005;22:317–24.

13. Green PH, Stavropoulos SN, Panagi SG, et al. Characteristics of adult celiac disease in the USA: results of a national survey. Am J Gastroenterol 2001;96: 126–31.

14. Lee SK, Lo W, Memeo L, et al. Duodenal histology in patients with celiac disease after treatment with a gluten-free diet. Gastrointest Endosc 2003;57:187–91.

15. Rashid M, Cranney A, Zarkadas M, et al. Celiac disease: evaluation of the diagnosis and dietary compliance in Canadian children. Pediatrics 2005;116:e754–9.

16. Rea F, Polito C, Marotta A, et al. Restoration of body composition in celiac children after one year of gluten-free diet. J Pediatr Gastroenterol Nutr 1996;23:408–12.

17. O'Leary C, Wieneke P, Healy M, et al. Celiac disease and the transition from childhood to adulthood: a 28-year follow-up. Am J Gastroenterol 2004;99:2437–41.

18. Masjedizadeh R, Hajiani E, Hashemi J, et al. Celiac disease in South-West of Iran. World J Gastroenterol 2006;12:4416–9.

19. Poddar U, Thapa BR, Singh K. Clinical features of celiac disease in Indian children: are they different from the West? J Pediatr Gastroenterol Nutr 2006;43:313–7.

20. US Food and Drug Administration. Federal Register Proposed Rule - 72 FR 2795, January 23 2007: Food labeling; gluten-free labeling of foods. Available at: http://www.fda.gov/Food/LabelingNutrition/FoodAllergensLabeling/GuidanceCompliance RegulatoryInformation/ucm077926.htm. Accessed August 14, 2012.

21. Codex Alimentarius Commission. Standard for Gluten-free Foods (Stan 118) Revised 2008. Available at: http://www.codexalimentarius.net/web/more_info. jsp?id_sta=291. Accessed August 14, 2012.

22. US Food and Drug Administration. Center for Food Safety and Applied Nutrition. Food Allergen Labeling and Consumer Protection Act of 2004 (Title II of Public Law 108-282). 2004. Available at: http://www.fda.gov/food/labelingnutrition/Food AllergensLabeling/GuidanceComplianceRegulatoryInformation/ucm106187.htm. Accessed August 14, 2012.

23. Academy of Nutrition and Dietetics Evidence Analysis Library. Celiac disease evidence-based nutrition practice guideline. Available at: http://www. adaevidencelibrary.com/. Accessed August 14, 2012.

24. Thompson T. Gluten contamination of commercial oat products in the United States. N Engl J Med 2004;351:2021–2.

25. Koerner TB, Cleroux C, Poirier C, et al. Gluten contamination in the Canadian commercial oat supply. Food Addit Contam Part A Chem Anal Control Expo Risk Assess 2011;28:705–10.

26. US Food and Drug Administration. Code of Federal Regulations. Malt. 21CFR184.1443a. Revised April 2009. Available at: http://www.accessdata. fda.gov/scripts/cdrh/cfdocs/cfcfr/CFRSearch.cfm?fr=184.1443a&SearchTerm= malt. Accessed August 14, 2012.

27. Thompson T. Is marmite gluten-free? 2010. Available at: glutenfreedietitian.com; http://www.glutenfreedietitian.com/newsletter/is-marmite-gluten-free/. Accessed August 14, 2012.

28. Thompson T. Labeling of USDA-regulated foods. 2009. Available at: glutenfreedietitian.com; http://www.glutenfreedietitian.com/newsletter/?s=labeling +of+USDA+regulated+foods. Accessed August 14, 2012.

29. US Department of Agriculture. A guide to federal food labeling requirements for meat and poultry products. 2007. Available at: http://www.fsis.usda.gov/pdf/ labeling_requirements_guide.pdf. Accessed August 14, 2012.

30. US Department of Agriculture. Food Safety and Inspection Service. Definition egg product. 9 CFR 590.5. Available at: http://edocket.access.gpo.gov/cfr_2008/ janqtr/pdf/9cfr590.5.pdf. Accessed August 14, 2012.

31. US Department of Agriculture. Food Safety and Inspection Service. Questions and answers related to ingredients of public health Concern. Available at: http://www.fsis.usda.gov/regulations/FAQs_for_Notice_45-05/index.asp. Accessed August 14, 2012.

32. US Department of Agriculture. Food Safety and Inspection Service. Food safety. Food standards and labeling policy book. 2005. Available at: http://www.fsis.usda.gov/ OPPDE/larc/Policies/Labeling_Policy_Book_082005.pdf. Accessed August 14, 2012.

33. Thompson T, Lee AR, Grace T. Gluten contamination of grains, seeds, and flours in the United States: a pilot study. J Am Diet Assoc 2010;110:937–40.

34. Academy of nutrition and dietetics celiac disease toolkit. Chicago: American Dietetic Association; 2011.

35. Gluten-free watchdog, LLC. Available at: www.glutenfreewatchdog.org. Accessed August 14, 2012.

36. Academy of Nutrition and Dietetics Evidence Analysis Library. Celiac Disease Evidence Analysis Library Project. Available at: http://www.adaevidencelibrary. com/. Accessed August 14, 2012.

37. Thompson T, Dennis M, Higgins LA, et al. Gluten-free diet survey: are Americans with coeliac disease consuming recommended amounts of fibre, iron, calcium and grain foods? J Hum Nutr Diet 2005;18:163–9.

38. Lee AR, Ng DL, Dave E, et al. The effect of substituting alternative grains in the diet on the nutritional profile of the gluten-free diet. J Hum Nutr Diet 2009;22: 359–63.

39. Thompson T. ADA pocket guide to gluten-free strategies for clients with multiple dietary restrictions. Chicago (Illinois): American Dietetic Association; 2011.
40. Thompson T. Thiamin, riboflavin, and niacin contents of the gluten-free diet: is there cause for concern? J Am Diet Assoc 1999;99:858–62.

Nondietary Therapies for Celiac Disease

Rupa Mukherjee, MD[a],*, Ciaran P. Kelly, MD[a],
Detlef Schuppan, MD, PhD[a],[b]

KEYWORDS

- Gluten-free diet • Nondietary therapies • Tissue transglutaminase
- Gluten vaccination • TNF-α • Interferon-γ • Gliadin • Immunity

KEY POINTS

- Currently, the only available therapy for celiac disease is strict lifelong adherence to a gluten-free diet.
- Based on the current understanding of celiac disease pathogenesis, several potential targets of therapeutic intervention exist.
- These novel strategies provide promise of alternative, adjunctive treatment options but also raise important questions regarding safety, efficacy, and monitoring of long-term treatment effect.
- The development of surrogate markers for celiac disease activity should be a concomitant priority along with ongoing drug development.

INTRODUCTION

Celiac disease is a common cause of chronic small intestinal inflammation and is one of the most common autoimmune disorders in the developed world. The prevalence of this disease ranges from 1:70 to 1:200 based on antibody screening and confirmatory intestinal biopsy data from North and South America and Western European and Middle Eastern countries.[1–3] Factors critical in precipitating celiac disease have been well established, including a defined trigger, specifically gluten proteins from

Financial Disclosures: Rupa Mukherjee: None; Detlef Schuppan: None.
Ciaran Kelly: Has received funds for consultancy, advisory board membership, or travel from: Alba Therapeutics Corporation, Alvine Pharmaceuticals, Inc., and ImmusanT, Inc; and received research funding support from Alba Therapeutics Corporation, Alvine Pharmaceuticals, Inc., SQI Diagnostics, and Shire.
[a] Department of Medicine, Division of Gastroenterology, The Celiac Center, Beth Israel Deaconess Medical Center, Harvard Medical School, 330 Brookline Avenue, Boston, MA 02215, USA; [b] Division of Molecular and Translational Medicine, Department of Medicine I, Johannes Gutenberg University, Langenbeckstr.1, Mainz 55131, Germany
* Corresponding author.
E-mail address: rmukherj@bidmc.harvard.edu

wheat and related cereal proteins; the presence of HLA class II genes DQ2 or DQ8; and the generation of autoantibodies to tissue transglutaminase 2 (TG2).[4-6] TG2 plays a pivotal role in immune activation by deamidating specific gliadin peptides, which increases their affinity for HLA-DQ2 or HLA-DQ8.[7] The deamidated gliadin peptide–TG2 complexes presented by antigen-presenting cells can elicit a vigorous adaptive immune response characterized by activation of CD4+ T-helper 1 (Th1) cells.[6] Apart from this adaptive immune response, wheat protein also triggers innate immunity, which is not restricted to patients with celiac disease. The dual activation of both the adaptive and innate immune responses enhances intestinal mucosal inflammation, which is manifested clinically with a variable spectrum of disease presentations, ranging from asymptomatic disease to severe malabsorption.[8]

PATHOGENESIS OF CELIAC DISEASE
Genetic and Environmental Factors

The interplay of genetic and environmental factors contributes to the enteropathy of celiac disease. The central role of HLA class II genes and to a lesser extent non-HLA genes as predisposing hereditary factors has been validated.[4] Most patients with celiac disease carry a variant of HLA-DQ2 (DQ2.5; DQA1*05/DQB1*02), whereas the remaining patients carry HLA-DQ8 (DQA1*03/DQB1*0302).[9] These class II molecules are expressed on antigen-presenting cells, predominantly macrophages, dendritic cells, and B cells. The HLA genes play a critical role in disease pathogenesis by preferentially presenting gluten peptides to CD4+ Th1 cells in the lamina propria. The T cells become activated on recognition of the gluten peptides, and subsequently function as central effector cells of inflammation by releasing different cytokines, notably, interferon (IFN)-γ, a key marker of the inflammatory Th1 response.[5] The release of these cytokines precipitates a cascade of immune, mesenchymal, and epithelial cell activation in the small intestine, resulting in the hallmark lesions of crypt hyperplasia, villous atrophy, and increased intraepithelial lymphocytes. Recent genome-wide association studies and linkage analyses have identified several non-HLA loci implicated in celiac disease susceptibility, putatively through their effects on T-cell regulation and inflammation.[10,11] However, the overall increased genetic risk conveyed by these polymorphisms is likely modest, estimated at 3% to 4% compared with a 30% to 35% contribution by HLA-DQ2 and/or HLA-DQ8.[12]

In addition to genetics, environmental factors play an important role in celiac disease pathogenesis. Gluten is the most significant identified factor. Dietary gluten contains several distinct T-cell epitopes rich in proline and glutamine residues. The high proline content of dietary gluten leads to peptides that are not easily degraded by gastrointestinal proteases, leading to an elevated concentration of potentially immunogenic epitopes in the small intestine. IgA-TG2, a ubiquitous intracellular and facultative extracellular enzyme that can associate with the extracellular matrix, plays a central role in celiac disease pathogeneis.[13,14] TG2 targets certain glutamine residues found in dietary gluten and deamidates them to negatively charged glutamic acid residues. The negatively charged gluten peptides are able to bind with greater affinity to HLA-DQ2 or HLA-DQ8, leading to enhanced gluten-specific CD4+ Th1 cell activation.[15] TG2 also deamidates a 33-amino-acid (33-mer) peptide from α2-gliadin, considered to be a prominent celiac disease antigen.[16] The exact mechanism through which the immunogenic gluten peptides reach the lamina propria from the intestinal lumen is debatable, and several theories have been proposed. The release of zonulin, a gluten-induced mediator of tight junctional disassembly and leakage by intestinal epithelial cells, was suggested as a major mechanism,[17,18] whereas others showed that enhanced transport of gluten into the lamina propria may occur via epithelial transcytosis.[19] A third possibility, shown in a murine model of celiac disease, is that dendritic cells residing in the lamina propria preferentially bind gluten peptides through projecting protrusions between intestinal epithelial cells, reaching and thus sampling the intestinal lumen. Another hypothesis is that specialized intestinal epithelioid cells (M cells, an integral part of the follicle-associated mucosal lymphoid tissue) may preferentially process gluten peptides (**Fig. 1**).[20] A more detailed description of the pathophysiology of celiac disease is discussed elsewhere in this issue by Kupfer and Jabri.

A NEED FOR NONDIETARY THERAPIES

Currently, the only available therapy for celiac disease is strict lifelong adherence to a gluten-free diet (GFD). Although the GFD is proven to be a safe and effective therapy, it is not ideal. One problem is that gluten-free labeling laws in the United States and some European countries only include food products that contain less than 20 parts per million of gluten,[21] whereas the threshold for what is considered safe or clinically acceptable exposure to gluten can vary widely for patients.[22] Moreover, the GFD is expensive, not readily available in many countries, and may be lower in its nutritional value, which can significantly impact patient adherence and quality of life. Even with strict adherence to the diet, some patients can have progressive or unresponsive disease that requires combination therapy for management. Studies have also shown

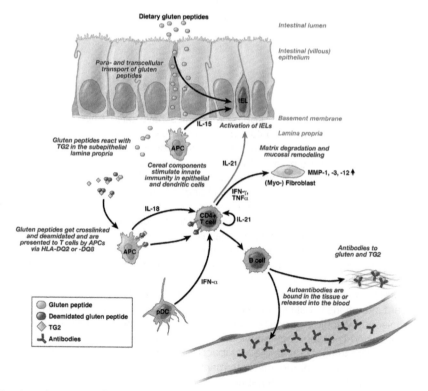

Fig. 1. Pathogenesis of celiac disease. (*From* Schuppan D, Junker Y, Barisani D. Celiac disease: from pathogenesis to novel therapies. Gastroenterology 2009;137(6):1912–33; with permission.)

that histologic improvement does not necessarily correlate with improved clinical response or strict adherence to the GFD.[23] In a recent survey study from the United Kingdom, 40% of patients with celiac disease expressed dissatisfaction with the GFD.[24] Important reasons for this included dietary and social restrictions imposed by having to avoid all possible hidden sources of gluten, but also the higher costs and often lower palatability of gluten-free foods. All 300 patients expressed interest in novel therapies, with a vaccine being the preferred choice, followed by an anti-zonulin agent or peptidase therapy. The survey found that nearly 20% of patients use complementary or alternative medicine in their management of celiac disease. Generally, the initial goal for any nondietary therapy for celiac disease is to neutralize low doses of gluten ingested through unintentional or unavoidable gluten exposure.

It is anticipated that nondietary therapy for celiac disease will have to meet stringent criteria regarding safety and toxicity given that the current modality, the GFD, can be considered mostly safe. The expectation is that topical or luminal agents should have very low potential for toxicity. Consequently, approaches that alter the immune system may be considered only for severe cases given the potential for greater toxicity secondary to immunosuppression. To determine efficacy, subjective and objective outcome measures would be required. The U.S. Food and Drug Administration has produced guidelines on the use of patient-reported outcomes, and these are likely to be valuable in celiac disease.[21] A need also exists for surrogate markers of disease activity as an objective measure of efficacy. Based on the current understanding of celiac disease pathogenesis, several potential targets of therapeutic intervention exist. This article discusses the therapeutic strategies that have been studied in preclinical models of celiac disease and/or show promise in phase I and II clinical trials (**Fig. 2** and **Table 1**).

INTRALUMINAL THERAPIES
Food Modification

Wheat strains can be selected for lower immunogenicity or engineered to decrease or eliminate immunogenic T-cell epitopes. Strategies have used RNA interference to silence the gluten genes that contain celiac disease immunogenic epitopes[25] or to engineer wheat strains with reduced immunogenic epitope content. Hexaploid wheat strains have been bred from ancient diploid and tetraploid wheat species over thousands of years. These ancient wheat strains have been shown to confer significantly less immunogenicity,[4] a property that goes hand in hand with reduced α, β, γ, and ω gliadins.[26,27] Psyllium has recently been studied as a replacement for gluten because it has minimal effects on food odor or texture while still retaining desired baking properties.[28] Bread prepared from psyllium was rated highly among patients with celiac disease and nonceliac controls for its texture and taste. Studies have also evaluated the genetic modification of wheat through the deletion of key gliadin genes. Specifically, the deletion of the α-gliadin locus on chromosome 6 in the hexaploid modern wheat strain *Triticum aestivum* led to a decrease in T-cell stimulatory epitopes without significant alterations in baking properties.[29] The deleted gliadin genes will likely need to be replaced by nonimmunogenic gliadin variants or avenins to approximate normal dough elasticity. This approach remains in preclinical investigation.

Lactic acid bacteria, such as the lactobacilli of sourdough, possess several peptidases. When added to sourdough for fermentation, lactobacilli are able to proteolyze the proline/glutamine-rich gluten peptides, including the highly immunogenic 33-mer peptide from α2-gliadin.[30,31] A pilot double-blind study of 17 patients with celiac disease investigated symptomatic response to 2 types of bread containing 2 g of

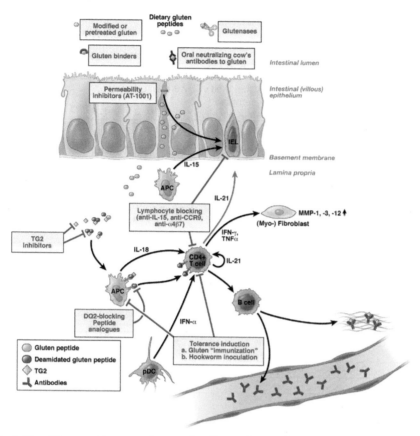

Fig. 2. Novel therapeutic approaches to celiac disease. (*From* Schuppan D, Junker Y, Barisani D. Celiac disease: from pathogenesis to novel therapies. Gastroenterology 2009;137(6):1912–33; with permission.)

gluten: bread produced with baker's yeast and bread produced with lactobacilli. Most patients who ingested the bread made from baker's yeast developed enhanced intestinal permeability, as measured by the excretion of carbohydrates lactulose and L-rhamnose, whereas the patients who ingested the bread pretreated with lactobacilli did not show any intestinal permeability changes. However, patients were challenged for only 2 days in this study, and therefore firm conclusions cannot be drawn[31] and doubt remains if immunogenic gluten peptidase will be completely inactivated. Another interesting finding is the presence of gluten-degrading proteases produced during germination of wheat.[32] Unfortunately, bread made from flour of germinating wheat, rye, or barley leads to elimination of the major gliadin and glutenin proteins, resulting in unpalatable and crumbly bread.[4] Another therapeutic approach in preclinical testing is to incubate gliadin with TG2 and lysine methyl ester. Lysine-modified gliadins lose their affinity for HLA-DQ2, leading to diminished activation of intestinal T cells. Pretreatment of whole wheat flour with lysine methyl ester and microbial transglutaminase (TG) derived from *Streptomyces mobaraensis* greatly diminished the stimulatory effect of the flour on the T-cell response.[33] Flour pretreated with microbial TG also improves the texture and volume of bread. However, the use of microbial TG

Table 1
Nondietary therapies for celiac disease

Target	Compound	State of Development	References
Gluten modification			
Engineered grains	Genetically modified wheat variants with lower immunogenicity	Preclinical	26–29
Pretreated flour	Pretreatment with lactobacilli	Preclinical	30–32
	Pretreatment with microbial TG and *N*-methyl-lysine	Preclinical	33
Oral proteases	Prolyl endopeptidases, AN-PEP, STAN-1	Phase I and II clinical trial	34,38–40
	ALV003	Phase II clinical trial	42,43
Intraluminal therapies			
Gluten-sequestering polymers	Polymer resin, P(HEMA-co-ss)	Preclinical	44,45
Neutralizing gluten antibodies	Cow's milk antigluten antibodies	Preclinical	46
Gluten tolerization and immune modulation			
Hookworm infection	*Necator americanus*	Phase II clinical trial	47–50
Mucosal tolerance	Genetically modified *Lactococcus lactis*	Preclinical	51–54
Gluten vaccination	Nexvax2	Phase II clinical trial	4
Modulation of intestinal permeability			
Zonulin receptor antagonists	AT-1001	Phase IIb clinical trial	60
Rho kinase inhibition	Fasudil	Approved drug	64,65
RhoA inhibition	BA-210	Phase II clinical trial	63
Mitogen for intestinal epithelium	R-spondin 1	Phase III clinical trial for Crohn disease	66
Downregulation of the adaptive immune response			
Tissue transglutaminase 2 inhibitors	ZED-101	Preclinical	67–69
Inhibitory gluten peptides	Innate immunity inhibitory decapeptide, QQPQDAVQPF	Preclinical	71,72
HLA-DQ2 inhibitors	DQ2-blockers	Preclinical	74,75
Immune cell–targeted therapies			
CCR9 antagonists	Ccx282-B, CCX025	Phase II clinical trials planned	77,78
Anti–integrin α4β7	Vedolizumab (also known as LDP-02, MLN02, MLN0002)	Phase II clinical trial for Crohn disease	80
Anti–α4 integrin	Natalizumab	Phase II trial in Crohn disease	79
Inhibition of CD40-CD40L	Anti–CD40-CD40L	Preclinical	83

(*continued on next page*)

Table 1 (continued)			
Target	**Compound**	**State of Development**	**References**
Anti–IFN-γ	Fontolizumab	Phase II clinical trial for Crohn disease, discontinued	86
Anti–TNF-α	Infliximab, adalimumab	Infliximab for RCD	87,88
IL-15 antagonists	AMG714	Phase II clinical trial in rheumatoid arthritis and psoriasis	9,89
IL-10 agonist	Recombinant human IL-10	Phase I clinical trial	90–92
Anti-CD3	Visilizumab, teplizumab, otelixizumab	Visilizumab: phase II in UC, GvHD Teplizumab: phase II in T1D Otelixizumab: phase III in T1D	93–95
Anti-CD20	Rituximab, tositumomab, ibritumomab	Approved drug	96,97
Bone marrow transplantation		Clinical trial in patients with EATL	101–103
Mesenchymal stem cell therapy		Phase II clinical trial for Crohn disease	104

Abbreviations: GvHD, graft-versus-host disease; IL, interleukin; T1D, type 1 diabetes; TG, transglutaminase; TNF, tumor necrosis factor; UC, ulcerative colitis.

in food preparation remains a matter of debate. Further studies are required to develop and validate nonimmunogenic flours and to produce bread and other baked products with good consistency and adequate nutritional value.

Oral Proteases for Gluten Detoxification

Gluten proteins have a high proline and glutamine content, making them partly resistant to proteolysis by gastric, pancreatic, and intestinal brush border endopeptidases and exopeptidases, which have poor affinity for peptide bonds adjacent to proline and glutamine residues.[9] This resistance results in incomplete proteolysis of gluten with the accumulation of long oligopeptides, such as the gliadin 33-mer and 26-mer peptide fragments, which can potently elicit an HLA-DQ2– or HLA-DQ8–restricted T-cell inflammatory response in patients with celiac disease. One strategy to prevent these peptides from reaching the lamina propria is to use prolyl endopeptidases (PEPs) expressed in various microorganisms, such as *Flavobacterium meningosepticum* or *Aspergillus niger*, that can cleave and thus inactivate these immunodominant, proline-rich peptides.[34–36] In a randomized, double-blind, cross-over study involving 20 asymptomatic patients with biopsy-proven celiac disease in remission, patients consumed 5 g of gluten for 14 days and were subsequently crossed-over to consume gluten pretreated with PEP derived from *F meningosepticum* for an additional 14 days. The study found that pretreatment of gluten with PEP mitigated the development of fat or carbohydrate malabsorption in most patients who developed these abnormalities after the 2-week gluten challenge.[37]

However, the use of PEP therapy can be limited by the length of the substrate and, except for the *A niger* enzyme, usually requires near-neutral pH for maximum activity and a long period (>1 h) to completely digest the immunogenic gliadin peptides. The ability of *A niger* PEP (AN-PEP) to degrade gluten was studied in a dynamic system closely mimicking the gastrointestinal tract, where it accelerated the degradation of gluten in the stomach compartment to such an extent that hardly any immunogenic gluten reached the duodenal compartment.[38] In addition, the proenzyme of barley endoprotease B (EP-B2) is effective at digesting gluten in rat stomach in a dose- and time-dependent manner.[39] Consequently, combination therapy with EP-B2 and PEP from *Sphingomonas capsulata* has been shown to effectively break down whole wheat gluten in vitro and in a rat model.[40] PEPs and EP-B2 can be administered as lyophilized powders in capsules or tablets, and these formulations are currently in phase I/II clinical trials. Another enzyme cocktail, called STAN1, has been developed with modest capacity to detoxify gluten.[41] This cocktail is undergoing phase II evaluation.

An additional drug candidate, ALV003, is being developed as an orally administered, fixed-dose (1:1 ratio by weight) mixture of 2 glutenases (ALV001 and ALV002).[42] ALV001 is a modified recombinant version of the proenzyme form of cysteine endo-protease, EP-B2, from barley.[43] ALV002 is a modified recombinant version of a PEP from the bacterium *S capsulata* (SC-PEP). To date, ALV003 has been evaluated in 3 phase I and IIa clinical studies. In general, ALV003 was found to be safe and well tolerated, with no dose-limiting toxicities. Moreover, it was found to be highly effective in degrading gluten primarily in the stomach before it reached the duodenal compartment. In a study of 20 patients with biopsy-proven celiac disease who were randomly assigned to gluten (16 g daily for 3 days) pretreated with ALV003 or placebo, no significant improvements were seen in clinical response with ALV003, although predigestion of gluten with ALV003 did improve immune responses.[43] In other words, biopsy data showed less small intestinal mucosal injury in patients treated with ALV003 compared with those treated with placebo. The percentage of intraepithelial lymphocytes was essentially unchanged in the ALV003-treated patients but significantly increased in the placebo-treated patients. ALV003 is currently being investigated in further phase II studies with the goal of establishing its efficacy and safety in preventing gluten-related symptoms and immune responses in patients with celiac disease.

The major foreseeable problem with oral enzyme therapy is that whether the quantity of enzyme and the time available for it to act will be sufficient to degrade the immunotoxic gluten peptides in a daily gluten load (10–20 g) is unclear. However, oral enzyme therapy may eliminate the detrimental side effects from smaller gluten exposures and therefore may benefit patients' sensitivity to low-level gluten exposure, and reduce the incidence of refractory celiac disease type I (RCD I) from inadvertent low-level gluten ingestion.

Gluten-Sequestering Polymers

Sequestration of gliadin intraluminally using an oral polymeric resin, poly(hydroxyethyl methacrylate-co-styrene sulfonate) [P(HEMA-co-ss)], was suggested as a strategy to block access of the immunotoxic gluten peptides to the mucosal immune cell compartment.[44] In vitro studies showed that this polymer bound gliadin in a specific manner and prevented its digestion to immunogenic peptides. In vivo studies in HLA-DQ8+ transgenic mice sensitized with gliadin showed that the polymer reduced mucosal injury.[45] Potential problems with this strategy include lack of specificity for gliadin and potential binding of other nutrient proteins. Moreover, which dose of gluten can be effectively bound in vivo by a given dose of polymer is unclear.

Neutralizing Gluten Antibodies

Orally acting IgG antibodies can be used to specifically bind and inactivate luminal antigens.[46] Cows are a readily available source of large quantities of milk (colostrum)-derived antibodies. The large-scale production of cow's milk gluten-neutralizing antibodies for oral use has been proposed as a safe therapeutic option. These antibodies could be labeled as food additive and used as adjunctive therapy to the GFD when trace ingestion of gluten is unavoidable, such as during travel, social, and business events. National Institutes of Health–sponsored preclinical testing is underway, with plans for a phase I trial in the United States in the near future.

GLUTEN TOLERIZATION AND IMMUNOMODULATION
Hookworm Infection

It has been proposed that chronic helminthiasis, such as hookworm infection, may alter pathogenic Th1-weighted immune responses in diseases such as inflammatory bowel disease and possibly celiac disease.[47,48] A pilot, randomized, double-blinded, placebo-controlled study was performed over 21 weeks in 20 healthy helminth-naïve adults with celiac disease on a strict GFD who were infected with the hookworm *Necator americanus.* In general, hookworm administration in patients with celiac disease did not result in a clinically significant suppression of intestinal pathology although there was a trend toward reduced mucosal inflammation after wheat challenge.[49,50] This study confirmed the safety and feasibility of using hookworm infection as a model to study immune responses in celiac disease and other intestinal inflammatory disorders.

Mucosal Tolerance Induction

Mucosal tolerance to gluten has been demonstrated in murine models of celiac disease.[51,52] In both wild-type and HLA-DQ8 transgenic mice, intranasal administration of α-gliadin diminished T-cell proliferation and IFN-γ secretion after peripheral immunization.[51,53] Based on these results, a strategy to induce gluten-specific tolerance was devised through the active delivery of immunogenic gliadin peptides to the intestinal mucosa by genetically modified *Lactococcus lactis* (LL). LL expresses a deamidated, HLA-DQ8-restricted immunodominant gliadin epitope (LL-eDQ8d).[54] In a DQ8 transgenic mouse model, oral administration of LL-eDQ8d induced suppression of local and system T-cell responses to gliadin peptide and induced production of interleukin (IL)-10, transforming growth factor β, and Foxp3+ regulatory T cells. It will be important to know if T-cell responses to other gluten epitopes can be suppressed via this approach. Moreover, this approach has not been validated in any human study.

Gluten Vaccination

Protein-based desensitization is the cornerstone of therapy for various allergic diseases. The most likely mode of action is the induction of CD4+ regulatory T cells to suppress T-cell–mediated inflammation. In celiac disease, the aim of this therapy is to shift the T-cell response from proinflammatory to regulatory; in other words, to tolerance to gluten. Three select immunogenic 16-mer peptides derived from α-gliadin, ω-gliadin, and hordein that account for 60% of the overall gluten T-cell response have been identified in a remarkable effort and studied in a TCR/DQ2 transgenic murine model.[4] Gluten vaccination using these 3 peptides via subcutaneous injection induced enhanced tolerance in this celiac murine model through the suppression of CD4+ T-cell proliferation and IL-2 and IFN-γ production, and through increased expression of regulatory T cells. This gluten vaccine (ImmusanT, Nexvax2

[Cambridge, MA]), developed initially in Australia, has passed phase I clinical trials and is slated to begin phase II clinical trials. The vaccine is only suited for patients with celiac disease who possess the HLA-DQ2 haplotype (most patients with celiac disease) because the peptides are only presented by HLA-DQ2; a separate vaccine would have to be formulated for HLA-DQ8–positive patients. The vaccine is administered as a weekly or monthly subcutaneous injection with the goal of allowing patients with celiac disease to resume eating regular or near-normal levels of gluten-containing food without experiencing adverse effects. During the phase I trial, patients who received the highest dose of gluten peptides experienced gastrointestinal distress, inadvertently serving as positive controls, thus confirming that the peptides in the vaccine formulation include key gluten-derived targets. The vaccine is currently in phase II trials.

MODULATION OF INTESTINAL PERMEABILITY
Modulation of Enterocyte Tight Junctions

In healthy individuals, the tight junctions between epithelial cells control the exposure of submucosal tissues to macromolecules and bacterial components that could elicit an inflammatory response. Patients with active celiac disease have a defect in these tight junctions, which may increase permeability for immunodominant gluten peptides to enter the lamina propria, where they enhance the T-cell inflammatory response.[55,56] Zonulin, a precursor of prehaptoglobin-2 that has been suggested as a regulator of epithelial permeability, is overexpressed in the intestinal tissue of patients with celiac disease.[17] Although zonulin was initially believed to facilitate opening of the intestinal epithelial tight junctions via the ZOT receptor,[57,58] a recent study showed that it instead acts via modulation of intestinal epithelial signal transduction. AT-1001 is an octapeptide that regulates enterocyte tight junctions and may reduce paracellular permeability.[59] This therapeutic agent has undergone pilot testing in 14 subjects with celiac disease in remission versus 7 control patients, all of whom had intact intestinal permeability without increased cytokine production even after gluten challenge.[60] In a follow-up randomized, double-blinded, placebo-controlled phase II trial, AT-1001 was studied for its safety and tolerability in patients with celiac disease in remission who were challenged with a large dose of gluten. This proof of concept study showed that AT-1001, when compared with placebo, was safe and well tolerated, reduced proinflammatory cytokine production, and reduced gastrointestinal symptoms in patients receiving a daily 2.5-g dose of gluten. In a phase IIb dose escalation study, AT-1001 was given to 184 patients with celiac disease in remission who were challenged with 3 g of daily gluten over 42 days.[61] Patients treated with AT-1001 had significantly improved gastrointestinal symptom scores and lower celiac antibody titers compared with those treated with placebo. However, the primary end point, reduction in the lactulose to mannitol ratio as a measure of intestinal permeability, was not reached. Further phase IIb clinical trials are underway to assess the efficacy of 3 different doses of AT-1001 (0.5, 1.0, and 2.0 mg three times daily) versus placebo for treatment in adults with celiac disease as an adjunct to the GFD.

Rho Kinase Inhibition

The ability of IFN-γ to increase intestinal permeability is facilitated by Rho kinase (ROCK-1 and ROCK-2).[62] Therefore, blocking Rho kinase could represent a therapeutic target in celiac disease.[63] RhoA, a microfilament regulator, and ROCK modulate the structure and function of epithelial tight junctions and axon growth.[9] The benefit of blocking ROCK has been studied for the treatment of spinal cord injuries.

The ROCK-1 and -2 inhibitor fasudil is an approved drug in Japan for the treatment of cerebral vasospasm, and the RhoA inhibitor (BA-120) is in phase II clinical trials for spinal cord injuries.[64,65] However, the toxicity profile of the ROCK or RhoA inhibitors makes them unlikely candidates for chronic long-term use in patients with celiac disease. Next-generation, more specific ROCK-1 or ROCK-2 inhibitors are currently being investigated for other indications, such as pulmonary hypertension and multiple sclerosis, and could hold promise as a therapeutic target for celiac disease in the future.

R-Spondin 1

R-spondin 1, an epithelial mitogen that can induce regeneration of the intestinal mucosa, was recently studied in a murine model of drug-induced enteropathy and colitis.[66] R-spondin 1 ameliorated both the enteropathy and colitis in this model. This agent could have a future therapeutic role in inflammatory bowel or celiac disease.

DOWNREGULATION OF THE ADAPTIVE IMMUNE RESPONSE
Inhibitors of TG2

TG2 plays a pivotal role in celiac disease pathogenesis through modifying and thereby potentiating the toxicity of gliadin peptides. Therefore, another therapeutic strategy is to inhibit the deamidation of gliadin peptides using TG2 inhibitors, which should reduce the peptides' binding affinity for HLA-DQ2 and HLA-DQ8 and thus diminish their T-cell stimulatory function.[67] Several nonselective transglutaminase inhibitors (that also inhibit at least 7 transglutaminases) have been tested in vitro. These agents can function as competitive, reversible, and irreversible inhibitors of these enzymes. Cystamine, a competitive inhibitor, has been examined ex vivo in cultures of duodenal tissue from patients with celiac disease, and was found to block the proliferative capacity of gluten-responsive T cells.[68] KCC009, an irreversible inhibitor and a dihydroisoxazole derivative with increased affinity for human TG2, was tested in healthy mice and showed good oral bioavailability, a short serum half-life, efficient TG2 inhibition in small intestinal tissue, and a low toxicity profile.[69] However, despite their efficacy in preclinical testing, transglutaminase inhibitors should be used with caution because of their ubiquitous expression and their important biologic roles.[13] Mice deficient in TG2 do not develop overt abnormalities except for mild autoimmunity at older age, which makes locally acting, highly specific inhibitors of TG2 attractive. Consequently, a new generation of TG2 inhibitors engineered with a high-affinity thiol binding group has been developed, which has up to 70- to 225-fold increased specificity for TG2 versus the other transglutaminases based on in vitro testing.[4] How far these oral and locally acting TG2-inhibitors can neutralize the immunogenicity of ingested gliadin peptides must be shown. A clinical study is in the planning stages.

Inhibitory Gluten Peptides

A 10-mer "innate inhibitory" decapeptide (sequence QQPQDAVQPF) has been isolated by affinity chromatography and gel filtration from the alcohol-soluble protein fraction of durum wheat.[70] The ability of this peptide to inhibit cell apoptosis was shown in duodenal biopsy samples from patients with celiac disease challenged with peptic-tryptic (PT) digests of gliadin in vitro.[71] The authors described that the decapeptide induced a switch from a Th1 to Th2 phenotype because it downregulated IFN-γ and up-regulated IL-10 production in intestinal T cells in patients with celiac disease.[72] Other studies have investigated modification of certain proline residues found in "toxic" gliadin peptides, such as A-gliadin residues 31–49, to induce T-cell inhibition.[73] However, these modified peptides have not been tested rigorously and further research is required to propose a viable therapeutic agent.

Inhibitors of HLA-DQ2

The presentation of gliadin peptides on HLA-DQ2 in most patients and of HLA-DQ8 in the minority of patients with celiac disease drives the adaptive immune response. Therefore, the ability to block HLA-DQ2– or HLA-DQ8–mediated presentation of gluten peptides would be attractive in a therapeutic target to prevent immune activation. This method has been previously explored for other HLA-associated diseases and autoimmune conditions but has largely been ineffective primarily because of difficulty in delivering the blocking compounds into the affected organs. In contrast, the topical delivery of HLA blockers through the oral route should facilitate easier drug delivery in patients with celiac disease.[74] Several peptides with high affinity for HLA-DQ2 have been engineered by amino acid substitution and dimerization or placement of aldehyde groups.[4] These peptide antagonists have shown moderate efficacy in inhibiting IFN-γ production by peripheral blood mononuclear cells in patients with celiac disease, thereby demonstrating some potential for dampening gluten-induced T-cell activation. A major drawback with the use of these inhibitors is that they retain partial agonistic effects when tested on gliadin-specific T-cell lines. In addition, the binding affinity for most of these engineered peptides was not strong enough to effectively and completely block access of the stimulatory gliadin peptides to HLA-DQ2. As a result, there has been renewed effort to identify optimal HLA-DQ2 binders with 50-fold greater binding affinity to HLA-DQ2 than the current immunodominant gluten epitope, DQ2-a-I.[75] However, the current peptide-based HLA-DQ2 blockers pose several challenges. In particular, how the modified peptides would reach their target cells in the lamina propria while competing with the luminal, immunogenic gliadin peptides is unclear. Also, concern exists about the side-effect profile of this approach, notably the potential for immunosuppression and hypersensitivity reactions. The inhibition of HLA-DQ2 remains in preclinical testing, with ongoing research to identify a highly specific, nontoxic, high-affinity, nonimmunogenic HLA-DQ blocker to be used in preclinical testing before any testing in human subjects.

IMMUNE CELL–TARGETED THERAPIES: RCD AND EATL

Therapeutic options for RCD I and II and EATL are discussed in further detail in a separate article elsewhere in this issue by Malamut et al. The following sections provide a brief overview of available immune cell–targeted therapies for celiac disease and its complicated (RCD I), premalignant (RCD II), or malignant (EATL) variants.

CCR9/CCL25 and Integrin α4β7 Antagonists

Circulating leukocytes are selectively recruited to intestinal tissue via chemokines and their chemokine receptors, and tissue-specific adhesion molecules. The effector and memory T lymphocytes that mainly home to the small intestine express the chemokine receptor, CCR9, and the integrin α4β7 adhesion molecule.[4] CCR9 mediates homing by binding to its ligand, CCL25, whereas integrin α4β7 facilitates attachment to the intestinal mucosa via the mucosal vascular addressin, MadCam-1.[76] Preclinical testing in a murine model of inflammatory bowel disease showed that blocking CCR9/CCL25 minimized histologic damage in ileitis.[77] Further study showed that the orally bioavailable CCR9 inhibitor, Ccx282-B, attenuated the severity of inflammation in a murine model of chronic ileitis. This agent was also studied in a phase II clinical trial in patients with moderate to severe Crohn disease who showed improvement in their Crohn Disease Activity Index score.[78] A second oral CCR9 inhibitor, CCX025, has completed a phase I clinical trial and is currently undergoing phase II testing.[4] MAdCAM-1, which mediates binding of integrin $\alpha 4\beta 7$ to the intestinal mucosa and is upregulated in patients with active celiac disease, is also a potential therapeutic target. Natalizumab, a monoclonal antibody against $\alpha 4$ integrin, has shown efficacy in Crohn disease.[79] A humanized monoclonal antibody against $\alpha 4\beta 7$ integrin, vedolizumab (formerly called MLN0002, MLN02, LDP-02), has been studied in a phase II clinical trial for ulcerative colitis and Crohn disease, but currently no studies are planned using this agent in celiac disease.[80] The true benefit of blocking lymphocyte homing and adhesion to the intestinal mucosa remains unclear because the mode of action is not antigen-specific, locally activated lymphocytes are not excluded, and beneficial suppressor regulatory T cells are likely also inhibited in the process.[81]

CXCL10/CXCR3

CXCL10 is another T-cell–specific chemokine that binds to its receptor CXCR3, which is primarily expressed by Th1 cells that drive inflammation in celiac disease. Recent studies have shown that stimulation of human monocytes by a gliadin extract increased CXCL10 expression.[82] This finding suggests that CXCL10 may play a role in T-cell recruitment as part of the innate immune response. The ability to block CXCL10 may represent a future therapeutic target in celiac disease.

Inhibition of the CD40–CD40L Interaction

A critical costimulatory signal in T-cell activation is the interaction between CD40 on antigen-presenting cells and the CD40 ligand (CD40L) on T cells. The effect of CD40L and colocalization of CD40 with the dendritic cell activation markers CD11c and CD123 was studied using duodenal biopsy samples from patients with celiac disease before and after treatment with the GFD, patients with RCD, and nonceliac controls. CD40 and CD40L expression was higher in untreated patients and those with RCD than in controls; expression normalized after treatment with the GFD. Furthermore, the addition of the anti-CD40L antibody to celiac biopsies inhibited gliadin-induced production of IFN-γ and IL-17.[83] These data suggest that disruption of the CD40–CD40L interaction may offer an important therapeutic option in RCD.

Anti–IFN-γ and Anti–Tumor Necrosis Factor α

IFN-γ is one of the main proinflammatory cytokines produced by CD4+ T cells in response to gluten, and tumor necrosis factor (TNF)-α has been shown to mediate secretion of matrix metalloproteinases (MMPs) from intestinal myofibroblasts, which results in unfavorable architectural remodeling of the intestinal mucosa.[84,85] Blockade of these cytokines could help control the inflammatory cascade and prevent activation of proteolytic MMPs. The anti–IFN-γ antibody, fontolizumab, was developed for the management of inflammatory bowel disease and is well tolerated by patients.[86] However, further product development has stopped and no clinical trials are planned for its use in celiac disease. Monoclonal antibodies against TNF-α (infliximab and adalimumab) are commonly used in the treatment of inflammatory bowel disease, and case reports describe their utility in patients with severe, RCD.[87,88]

IL-15 Antagonists

The cytokine IL-15 seems to be mainly induced via the innate immune response in celiac disease and may play a critical role in the development and exacerbation of RCD. IL-15 antibodies have been shown to reverse intestinal damage in a transgenic mouse model of immune-mediated enteropathy resulting from the targeted overexpression of IL-15 in enterocytes.[89] IL-15 is a potential therapeutic option for RCD II and EATL, especially given that the expansion of premalignant and malignant lymphocytes may be driven by IL-15. Although a phase II clinical trial has addressed the utility of an anti–IL-15 monoclonal antibody (AMG714) in patients with rheumatoid arthritis and psoriasis,[9] currently no clinical trials are investigating the use of an IL-15 antagonist for the treatment of RCD.

IL-10 Agonists

The cytokine IL-10 suppresses proinflammatory cytokine secretion from Th1 cells. In theory, an IL-10 agonist could be used to manage Th1-mediated autoimmune disorders, such as celiac disease or inflammatory bowel disease. The use of transgenic bacteria expressing IL-10 was studied in a phase I trial in patients with Crohn disease, but did not show therapeutic benefit.[90] IL-10 was shown to suppress gliadin-induced T-cell activation ex vivo in cultured celiac intestinal biopsies.[91] However, similar results were not seen in a pilot study in which recombinant IL-10 was administered subcutaneously with subsequent intestinal biopsies in patients with RCD.[92]

Anti-CD3

The CD3 protein complex is a coreceptor of the T-cell receptor. Anti-CD3 monoclonal antibodies are used to treat transplant rejection, and they are currently in clinical evaluation for type I diabetes and ulcerative colitis.[93–95] Anti-CD3 therapy for celiac disease has the theoretical potential to eliminate inflammatory T-cells while inducing regulatory T cells. However, its side-effect profile may limit repeat application.

Anti-CD20

Anti-CD20 therapy has been used successfully to treat B-cell malignancies, rheumatoid arthritis, and multiple sclerosis.[96] In celiac disease, B cells may play a pathogenic role as potent antigen-presenting cells for immunogenic gluten peptides, thereby fueling the Th1 inflammatory T-cell response. However, anti-CD20 does not eliminate the generation of immunoglobulin A–producing plasmablasts.[97] Therefore, the true therapeutic role of anti-CD20 therapy remains unclear. Several anti-CD20 monoclonal antibodies, including Rituximab, Tositumomab, and ibritumomab have been approved for clinical use but none have been systematically evaluated in celiac disease.[9]

Cladribine

Treatment of RCD II has relied mainly on conventional immunosuppressants, such as azathioprine and corticosteroids, and no standard therapeutic regimen exists.[98] A modified treatment strategy has included cladribine. Cladribine (2-CdA) is a synthetic purine nucleoside that is cytotoxic to both proliferating and nonproliferating lymphoid cells.[99] It is metabolized to its pharmacologically active metabolite, cladribine triphosphate, which induces lymphoid cell DNA/RNA synthesis and apoptosis. Cladribine, which is typically used to treat hematologic malignancies and selected autoimmune disorders, including multiple sclerosis, was studied in an open-label, prospective cohort study of 32 patients with RCD II.[100] Outcome measures included rate of survival, occurrence of EATL, clinical course, and histologic and immunologic response rates. Patients were followed for a median of 31 months. Eighteen of 32 patients responded favorably, with statistically significantly increased survival compared with unresponsive patients. No control group was included in the study. Sixteen patients with RCD II progressed to EATL despite therapy, and all died.

Bone Marrow Transplantation

The classic CHOP protocol (doxorubicin, cyclophosphamide, vincristine, prednisone) has been largely ineffective for the treatment of EATL, and survival remains poor. Autologous hematopoietic stem cell transplantation (auto-SCT) has been used to treat patients with RCD II and induce remission in patients with EATL.[101] In a single-center study, 18 patients with RCD II unresponsive to cladribine were preconditioned with high-dose chemotherapy followed by auto-SCT. Thirteen patients were transplanted successfully with a 4-year survival rate of 66%. One patient developed EATL after 4 years of follow-up. Auto-SCT after conditioning with high-dose chemotherapy in patients with RCD II unresponsive to cladribine may hold promise as a therapeutic option. Unfortunately, relapses are common because of the presence of residual cells in the transplanted autologous bone marrow.[102,103] Therefore, allogeneic stem cell transplantation could hold more promise but also may introduce more risk. Currently no studies are evaluating allogeneic bone marrow transplantation for the treatment of RCD II or EATL.

Mesenchymal Stem Cell Therapy

Mesenchymal stem cells can be produced in large quantities ex vivo from human donors. They have low immunogenic potential because they lack HLA class I or II molecules and also lack costimulatory molecules. Mesenchymal stem cell transplantation offers a safe and promising therapeutic option for patients unresponsive to auto-SCT.[104] This cell population homes preferentially to sites of organ damage, where they suppress the proliferation of lymphocytes. Mesenchymal stem cell transplantation has been investigated in various inflammatory gastrointestinal diseases, including therapy-resistant inflammatory bowel disease and fibrotic liver disease. This form of therapy has potential applications for the management and treatment of patients with RCD and EATL. Currently no clinical trials are investigating mesenchymal stem cell therapy in celiac disease.

SUMMARY

This article outlines recent advances in nondietary therapies for celiac disease. A greater understanding of the pathogenesis of celiac disease has led to improvements in the development of preclinical models for testing. Ongoing and future clinical trials will help determine the validity of these models. The GFD remains the only currently available therapy for celiac disease. Novel strategies provide promise of alternative, adjunctive treatment options but also raise important questions regarding safety, efficacy, and monitoring of long-term treatment effects. The development of surrogate markers for celiac disease activity should be a concomitant priority along with ongoing drug development.

REFERENCES

1. Di Sabatino A, Corazza GR. Coeliac disease. Lancet 2009;373:1480–93.
2. Maki M, Mustalahti K, Kokkonen J, et al. Prevalence of celiac disease among children in Finland. N Engl J Med 2003;348:2517–24.
3. Fasano A, Berti I, Gerarduzzi T, et al. Prevalence of celiac disease in at-risk and not-at-risk groups in the United States: a large multicenter study. Arch Intern Med 2003;163:286–92.
4. Schuppan D, Junker Y, Barisani D. Celiac disease: from pathogenesis to novel therapies. Gastroenterology 2009;137:1912–33.

5. Schuppan D. Current concepts of celiac disease pathogenesis. Gastroenterology 2000;119:234–42.
6. Sollid LM. Coeliac disease: dissecting a complex inflammatory disorder. Nat Rev Immunol 2002;2:647–55.
7. Maiuri L, Ciacci C, Ricciardelli I, et al. Unexpected role of surface transglutaminase type II in celiac disease. Gastroenterology 2005;129:1400–13.
8. Gianfrani C, Auricchio S, Troncone R. Adaptive and innate immune responses in celiac disease. Immunol Lett 2005;99:141–5.
9. Sollid LM, Khosla C. Novel therapies for coeliac disease. J Intern Med 2011;269: 604–13.
10. Dubois PC, Trynka G, Franke L, et al. Multiple common variants for celiac disease influencing immune gene expression. Nat Genet 2010;42:295–302.
11. van Heel DA, Franke L, Hunt KA, et al. A genome-wide association study for celiac disease identifies risk variants in the region harboring IL2 and IL21. Nat Genet 2007;39:827–9.
12. Petronzelli F, Bonamico M, Ferrante P, et al. Genetic contribution of the HLA region to the familial clustering of coeliac disease. Ann Hum Genet 1997;61:307–17.
13. Elli L, Bergamini CM, Bardella MT, et al. Transglutaminases in inflammation and fibrosis of the gastrointestinal tract and the liver. Dig Liver Dis 2009;41:541–50.
14. Dieterich W, Ehnis T, Bauer M, et al. Identification of tissue transglutaminase as the autoantigen of celiac disease. Nat Med 1997;3:797–801.
15. Aeschlimann D, Thomazy V. Protein crosslinking in assembly and remodelling of extracellular matrices: the role of transglutaminases. Connect Tissue Res 2000; 41:1–27.
16. Shan L, Molberg O, Parrot I, et al. Structural basis for gluten intolerance in celiac sprue. Science 2002;297:2275–9.
17. Fasano A, Not T, Wang W, et al. Zonulin, a newly discovered modulator of intestinal permeability, and its expression in coeliac disease. Lancet 2000;355:1518–9.
18. Clemente MG, De Virgiliis S, Kang JS, et al. Early effects of gliadin on enterocyte intracellular signaling involved in intestinal barrier function. Gut 2003;52:218–23.
19. Schumann M, Richter JF, Wedell I, et al. Mechanisms of epithelial translocation of the alpha(2)-gliadin-33mer in coeliac sprue. Gut 2008;57:747–54.
20. Man AL, Prieto-Garcia ME, Nicoletti C. Improving M cell mediated transport across mucosal barriers: do certain bacteria hold the keys? Immunology 2004;113:15–22.
21. Rashtak S, Murray JA. Review article: coeliac disease, new approaches to therapy. Aliment Pharmacol Ther 2012;35:768–81.
22. Akobeng AK, Thomas AG. Systematic review: tolerable amount of gluten for people with coeliac disease. Aliment Pharmacol Ther 2008;27:1044–52.
23. Lanzini A, Lanzarotto F, Villanacci V, et al. Complete recovery of intestinal mucosa occurs very rarely in adult coeliac patients despite adherence to gluten-free diet. Aliment Pharmacol Ther 2009;29:1299–308.
24. Aziz I, Evans KE, Papageorgiou V, et al. Are patients with coeliac disease seeking alternative therapies to a gluten-free diet? J Gastrointestin Liver Dis 2011;20:27–31.
25. Troncone R, Ivarsson A, Szajewska H, et al. Review article: future research on coeliac disease - a position report from the European multistakeholder platform on coeliac disease (CDEUSSA). Aliment Pharmacol Ther 2008;27:1030–43.
26. Auricchio S, De Ritis G, De Vincenzi M, et al. Effects of gliadin-derived peptides from bread and durum wheats on small intestine cultures from rat fetus and coeliac children. Pediatr Res 1982;16:1004–10.

27. Frisoni M, Corazza GR, Lafiandra D, et al. Wheat deficient in gliadins: promising tool for treatment of coeliac disease. Gut 1995;36:375–8.

28. Zandonadi RP, Botelho RB, Araujo WM. Psyllium as a substitute for gluten in bread. J Am Diet Assoc 2009;109:1781–4.

29. van Herpen TW, Goryunova SV, van der Schoot J, et al. Alpha-gliadin genes from the A, B, and D genomes of wheat contain different sets of celiac disease epitopes. BMC Genomics 2006;7:1.

30. Di Cagno R, De Angelis M, Lavermicocca P, et al. Proteolysis by sourdough lactic acid bacteria: effects on wheat flour protein fractions and gliadin peptides involved in human cereal intolerance. Appl Environ Microbiol 2002;68:623–33.

31. Di Cagno R, De Angelis M, Auricchio S, et al. Sourdough bread made from wheat and nontoxic flours and started with selected lactobacilli is tolerated in celiac sprue patients. Appl Environ Microbiol 2004;70:1088–96.

32. Rizzello CG, De Angelis M, Di Cagno R, et al. Highly efficient gluten degradation by lactobacilli and fungal proteases during food processing: new perspectives for celiac disease. Appl Environ Microbiol 2007;73:4499–507.

33. Yokoyama K, Nio N, Kikuchi Y. Properties and applications of microbial transglutaminase. Appl Microbiol Biotechnol 2004;64:447–54.

34. Stepniak D, Spaenij-Dekking L, Mitea C, et al. Highly efficient gluten degradation with a newly identified prolyl endoprotease: implications for celiac disease. Am J Physiol Gastrointest Liver Physiol 2006;291:G621–9.

35. Pyle GG, Paaso B, Anderson BE, et al. Effect of pretreatment of food gluten with prolyl endopeptidase on gluten-induced malabsorption in celiac sprue. Clin Gastroenterol Hepatol 2005;3:687–94.

36. Marti T, Molberg O, Li Q, et al. Prolyl endopeptidase-mediated destruction of T cell epitopes in whole gluten: chemical and immunological characterization. J Pharmacol Exp Ther 2005;312:19–26.

37. Pyle GG, Paaso B, Anderson BE, et al. Low-dose gluten challenge in celiac sprue: malabsorptive and antibody responses. Clin Gastroenterol Hepatol 2005;3:679–86.

38. Mitea C, Havenaar R, Drijfhout JW, et al. Efficient degradation of gluten by a prolyl endoprotease in a gastrointestinal model: implications for coeliac disease. Gut 2008;57:25–32.

39. Gass J, Vora H, Bethune MT, et al. Effect of barley endoprotease EP-B2 on gluten digestion in the intact rat. J Pharmacol Exp Ther 2006;318:1178–86.

40. Gass J, Bethune MT, Siegel M, et al. Combination enzyme therapy for gastric digestion of dietary gluten in patients with celiac sprue. Gastroenterology 2007;133:472–80.

41. Ehren J, Moron B, Martin E, et al. A food-grade enzyme preparation with modest gluten detoxification properties. PLoS One 2009;4:e6313.

42. Siegel M, Garber ME, Spencer AG, et al. Safety, tolerability, and activity of ALV003: results from two phase 1 single, escalating-dose clinical trials. Dig Dis Sci 2012;57:440–50.

43. Tye-Din JA, Anderson RP, Ffrench RA, et al. The effects of ALV003 pre-digestion of gluten on immune response and symptoms in celiac disease in vivo. Clin Immunol 2010;134:289–95.

44. Liang L, Pinier M, Leroux JC, et al. Interaction of alpha-gliadin with polyanions: design considerations for sequestrants used in supportive treatment of celiac disease. Biopolymers 2010;93:418–28.

45. Pinier M, Verdu EF, Nasser-Eddine M, et al. Polymeric binders suppress gliadin-induced toxicity in the intestinal epithelium. Gastroenterology 2009;136:288–98.

46. Warny M, Fatimi A, Bostwick EF, et al. Bovine immunoglobulin concentrate-clostridium difficile retains C difficile toxin neutralising activity after passage through the human stomach and small intestine. Gut 1999;44:212–7.

47. Elliott DE, Summers RW, Weinstock JV. Helminths as governors of immune-mediated inflammation. Int J Parasitol 2007;37:457–64.

48. Summers RW, Elliott DE, Urban JF Jr, et al. Trichuris suis therapy for active ulcerative colitis: a randomized controlled trial. Gastroenterology 2005;128:825–32.

49. Daveson AJ, Jones DM, McSorley H, et al. Effect of hookworm infection on wheat challenge in celiac disease - a randomized double-blinded placebo controlled trial. PLoS One 2011;6(3):e17366.

50. McSorley HJ, Gaze S, Daveson J, et al. Suppression of inflammatory immune responses in celiac disease by experimental hookworm infection. PLoS One 2011;6(9):e24092.

51. Maurano F, Siciliano RA, De Giulio B, et al. Intranasal administration of one alpha gliadin can downregulate the immune response to whole gliadin in mice. Scand J Immunol 2001;53:290–5.

52. Marietta EV, David CS, Murray JA. Important lessons derived from animal models of celiac disease. Int Rev Immunol 2011;30:197–206.

53. Senger S, Luongo D, Maurano F, et al. Intranasal administration of a recombinant alpha-gliadin down-regulates the immune response to wheat gliadin in DQ8 transgenic mice. Immunol Lett 2003;88:127–34.

54. Huibregtse IL, Marietta EV, Rashtak S, et al. Induction of antigen-specific tolerance by oral administration of lactococcus lactis delivered immunodominant DQ8-restricted gliadin peptide in sensitized nonobese diabetic Abo Dq8 transgenic mice. J Immunol 2009;183:2390–6.

55. van Elburg RM, Uil JJ, Mulder CJ, et al. Intestinal permeability in patients with coeliac disease and relatives of patients with coeliac disease. Gut 1993;34: 354–7.

56. Sapone A, de Magistris L, Pietzak M, et al. Zonulin upregulation is associated with increased gut permeability in subjects with type 1 diabetes and their relatives. Diabetes 2006;55:1443–9.

57. Drago S, El Asmar R, Di Pierro M, et al. Gliadin, zonulin and gut permeability: Effects on celiac and non-celiac intestinal mucosa and intestinal cell lines. Scand J Gastroenterol 2006;41:408–19.

58. Duerksen DR, Wilhelm-Boyles C, Veitch R, et al. A comparison of antibody testing, permeability testing, and zonulin levels with small-bowel biopsy in celiac disease patients on a gluten-free diet. Dig Dis Sci 2010;55:1026–31.

59. Tripathi A, Lammers KM, Goldblum S, et al. Identification of human zonulin, a physiological modulator of tight junctions, as prehaptoglobin-2. Proc Natl Acad Sci U S A 2009;106:16799–804.

60. Paterson BM, Lammers KM, Arrieta MC, et al. The safety, tolerance, pharmacokinetic and pharmacodynamic effects of single doses of AT-1001 in coeliac disease subjects: a proof of concept study. Aliment Pharmacol Ther 2007;26: 757–66.

61. Kelly CP, Green PH, Murray JA, et al. Intestinal permeability of larazotide acetate in celiac disease: results of a phase IIB, 6-week gluten-challenge clinical trial [abstract]. Gastroenterology 2009;136(Suppl 1):M2048.

62. Beaurepaire C, Smyth D, McKay DM. Interferon-gamma regulation of intestinal epithelial permeability. J Interferon Cytokine Res 2009;29:133–44.

63. Chaturvedi LS, Marsh HM, Basson MD. Role of RhoA and its effectors ROCK and mDia1 in the modulation of deformation-induced FAK, ERK, p38, and

MLC motogenic signals in human Caco-2 intestinal epithelial cells. Am J Physiol Cell Physiol 2011;301:C1224–38.

64. McKerracher L, Higuchi H. Targeting Rho to stimulate repair after spinal cord injury. J Neurotrauma 2006;23:309–17.

65. LoGrasso PV, Feng Y. Rho kinase (ROCK) inhibitors and their application to inflammatory disorders. Curr Top Med Chem 2009;9:704–23.

66. Zhao J, de Vera J, Narushima S, et al. R-spondin1, a novel intestinotrophic mitogen, ameliorates experimental colitis in mice. Gastroenterology 2007;132: 1331–43.

67. Esposito C, Caputo I, Troncone R. New therapeutic strategies for coeliac disease: tissue transglutaminase as a target. Curr Med Chem 2007;14:2572–80.

68. Molberg O, McAdam S, Lundin KE, et al. T cells from celiac disease lesions recognize gliadin epitopes deamidated in situ by endogenous tissue transglutaminase. Eur J Immunol 2001;31:1317–23.

69. Choi K, Siegel M, Piper JL, et al. Chemistry and biology of dihydroisoxazole derivatives: selective inhibitors of human transglutaminase 2. Chem Biol 2005; 12:469–75.

70. Silano M, Di Benedetto R, Maialetti F, et al. A 10-residue peptide from durum wheat promotes a shift from a Th1-type response toward a Th2-type response in celiac disease. Am J Clin Nutr 2008;87:415–23.

71. Silano M, Leonardi F, Trecca A, et al. Prevention by a decapeptide from durum wheat of in vitro gliadin peptide-induced apoptosis in small-bowel mucosa from coeliac patients. Scand J Gastroenterol 2007;42:786–7.

72. Silano M, Di Benedetto R, Trecca A, et al. A decapeptide from durum wheat prevents celiac peripheral blood lymphocytes from activation by gliadin peptides. Pediatr Res 2007;61:67–71.

73. Biagi F, Ellis HJ, Parnell ND, et al. A non-toxic analogue of a coeliac-activating gliadin peptide: a basis for immunomodulation? Aliment Pharmacol Ther 1999; 13:945–50.

74. Xia J, Bergseng E, Fleckenstein B, et al. Cyclic and dimeric gluten peptide analogues inhibiting DQ2-mediated antigen presentation in celiac disease. Bioorg Med Chem 2007;15:6565–73.

75. Kapoerchan VV, Wiesner M, Hillaert U, et al. Design, synthesis and evaluation of high-affinity binders for the celiac disease associated HLA-DQ2 molecule. Mol Immunol 2010;47:1091–7.

76. Berlin C, Berg EL, Briskin MJ, et al. Alpha 4 beta 7 integrin mediates lymphocyte binding to the mucosal vascular addressin MAdCAM-1. Cell 1993;74:185–95.

77. Rivera-Nieves J, Ho J, Bamias G, et al. Antibody blockade of CCL25/CCR9 ameliorates early but not late chronic murine ileitis. Gastroenterology 2006; 131:1518–29.

78. Walters MJ, Wang Y, Lai N, et al. Characterization of CCX282-B, an orally bioavailable antagonist of the CCR9 chemokine receptor, for treatment of inflammatory bowel disease. J Pharmacol Exp Ther 2010;335:61–9.

79. Ghosh S, Goldin E, Gordon FH, et al. Natalizumab for active Crohn's disease. N Engl J Med 2003;348:24–32.

80. Parikh A, Leach T, Wyant T, et al. Vedolizumab for the treatment of active ulcerative colitis: a randomized controlled phase 2 dose-ranging study. Inflamm Bowel Dis 2011;18(8):1470–9.

81. Villablanca EJ, Cassani B, von Andrian UH, et al. Blocking lymphocyte localization to the gastrointestinal mucosa as a therapeutic strategy for inflammatory bowel diseases. Gastroenterology 2011;140:1776–84.

82. Booth V, Keizer DW, Kamphuis MB, et al. The CXCR3 binding chemokine IP-10/CXCL10: structure and receptor interactions. Biochemistry 2002;41:10418–25.
83. Di Sabatino A, Rovedatti L, Vetrano S, et al. Involvement of CD40-CD40 ligand in uncomplicated and refractory celiac disease. Am J Gastroenterol 2011;106: 519–27.
84. Ciccocioppo R, Di Sabatino A, Bauer M, et al. Matrix metalloproteinase pattern in celiac duodenal mucosa. Lab Invest 2005;85:397–407.
85. Pender SL, Tickle SP, Docherty AJ, et al. A major role for matrix metalloproteinases in T cell injury in the gut. J Immunol 1997;158:1582–90.
86. Reinisch W, de Villiers W, Bene L, et al. Fontolizumab in moderate to severe Crohn's disease: a phase 2, randomized, double-blind, placebo-controlled, multiple-dose study. Inflamm Bowel Dis 2010;16:233–42.
87. Gillett HR, Arnott ID, McIntyre M, et al. Successful infliximab treatment for steroid-refractory celiac disease: a case report. Gastroenterology 2002;122: 800–5.
88. Costantino G, della Torre A, Lo Presti MA, et al. Treatment of life-threatening type I refractory coeliac disease with long-term infliximab. Dig Liver Dis 2008;40: 74–7.
89. Yokoyama S, Watanabe N, Sato N, et al. Antibody-mediated blockade of IL-15 reverses the autoimmune intestinal damage in transgenic mice that overexpress IL-15 in enterocytes. Proc Natl Acad Sci U S A 2009;106:15849–54.
90. Braat H, Rottiers P, Hommes DW, et al. A phase I trial with transgenic bacteria expressing interleukin-10 in Crohn's disease. Clin Gastroenterol Hepatol 2006;4: 754–9.
91. Salvati VM, Mazzarella G, Gianfrani C, et al. Recombinant human interleukin 10 suppresses gliadin dependent T cell activation in ex vivo cultured coeliac intestinal mucosa. Gut 2005;54:46–53.
92. Mulder CJ, Wahab PJ, Meijer JW, et al. A pilot study of recombinant human interleukin-10 in adults with refractory coeliac disease. Eur J Gastroenterol Hepatol 2001;13:1183–8.
93. Herold KC, Gitelman S, Greenbaum C, et al. Treatment of patients with new onset Type 1 diabetes with a single course of anti-CD3 mAb Teplizumab preserves insulin production for up to 5 years. Clin Immunol 2009;132:166–73.
94. Wiczling P, Rosenzweig M, Vaickus L, et al. Pharmacokinetics and pharmacodynamics of a chimeric/humanized anti-CD3 monoclonal antibody, otelixizumab (TRX4), in subjects with psoriasis and with type 1 diabetes mellitus. J Clin Pharmacol 2010;50:494–506.
95. Hale G, Rebello P, Al Bakir I, et al. Pharmacokinetics and antibody responses to the CD3 antibody otelixizumab used in the treatment of type 1 diabetes. J Clin Pharmacol 2010;50:1238–48.
96. Edwards JC, Szczepanski L, Szechinski J, et al. Efficacy of B-cell-targeted therapy with rituximab in patients with rheumatoid arthritis. N Engl J Med 2004;350:2572–81.
97. Mei HE, Frolich D, Giesecke C, et al. Steady-state generation of mucosal IgA+ plasmablasts is not abrogated by B-cell depletion therapy with rituximab. Blood 2010;116:5181–90.
98. Abdallah H, Leffler D, Dennis M, et al. Refractory celiac disease. Curr Gastroenterol Rep 2007;9:401–5.
99. Al-Toma A, Goerres MS, Meijer JW, et al. Cladribine therapy in refractory celiac disease with aberrant T cells. Clin Gastroenterol Hepatol 2006;4:1322–7 [quiz: 1300].

100. Tack GJ, Verbeek WH, Al-Toma A, et al. Evaluation of Cladribine treatment in refractory celiac disease type II. World J Gastroenterol 2011;17:506–13.
101. Tack GJ, Wondergem MJ, Al-Toma A, et al. Auto-SCT in refractory celiac disease type II patients unresponsive to cladribine therapy. Bone Marrow Transplant 2011;46:840–6.
102. Al-Toma A, Verbeek WH, Visser OJ, et al. Disappointing outcome of autologous stem cell transplantation for enteropathy-associated T-cell lymphoma. Dig Liver Dis 2007;39:634–41.
103. Al-toma A, Visser OJ, van Roessel HM, et al. Autologous hematopoietic stem cell transplantation in refractory celiac disease with aberrant T cells. Blood 2007;109:2243–9.
104. Garcia-Castro J, Trigueros C, Madrenas J, et al. Mesenchymal stem cells and their use as cell replacement therapy and disease modelling tool. J Cell Mol Med 2008;12:2552–65.

Index

Note: Page numbers of article titles are in **boldface** type

Gastrointest Endoscopy Clin N Am 22 (2012) 833–844
http://dx.doi.org/10.1016/S1052-5157(12)00117-1
1052-5157/12/$ – see front matter © 2012 Elsevier Inc. All rights reserved.

giendo.theclinics.com

United States Postal Service

Statement of Ownership, Management, and Circulation
(All Periodicals Publications Except Requestor Publications)

1. Publication Title	2. Publication Number	3. Filing Date
Gastrointestinal Endoscopy Clinics of North America	0 1 2 - 6 0 3	9/14/12

4. Issue Frequency	5. Number of Issues Published Annually	6. Annual Subscription Price
Jan, Apr, Jul, Oct	4	$319.00

7. Complete Mailing Address of Known Office of Publication (Not printer) (Street, city, county, state, and ZIP+4®)

Elsevier Inc.
360 Park Avenue South
New York, NY 10010-1710

Contact Person
Stephen R. Bushing
Telephone (Include area code)
215-239-3688

8. Complete Mailing Address of Headquarters or General Business Office of Publisher (Not printer)

Elsevier Inc., 360 Park Avenue South, New York, NY 10010-1710

9. Full Names and Complete Mailing Addresses of Publisher, Editor, and Managing Editor (Do not leave blank)

Publisher (Name and complete mailing address)

Kim Murphy, Elsevier, Inc., 1600 John F. Kennedy Blvd. Suite 1800, Philadelphia, PA 19103-2899

Editor (Name and complete mailing address)

Kerry Holland, Elsevier, Inc., 1600 John F. Kennedy Blvd. Suite 1800, Philadelphia, PA 19103-2899

Managing Editor (Name and complete mailing address)

Sarah Barth, Elsevier, Inc., 1600 John F. Kennedy Blvd. Suite 1800, Philadelphia, PA 19103-2899

10. Owner (Do not leave blank. If the publication is owned by a corporation, give the name and address of the corporation immediately followed by the names and addresses of all stockholders owning or holding 1 percent or more of the total amount of stock. If not owned by a corporation, give the names and addresses of the individual owners. If owned by a partnership or other unincorporated firm, give its name and address as well as those of each individual owner. If the publication is published by a nonprofit organization, give its name and address.)

Full Name	Complete Mailing Address
Wholly owned subsidiary of	1600 John F. Kennedy Blvd., Ste. 1800
Reed/Elsevier, US holdings	Philadelphia, PA 19103-2899

11. Known Bondholders, Mortgagees, and Other Security Holders Owning or Holding 1 Percent or More of Total Amount of Bonds, Mortgages, or Other Securities. If none, check box ☐ None

Full Name	Complete Mailing Address
N/A	

12. Tax Status (For completion by nonprofit organizations authorized to mail at nonprofit rates) (Check one)
The purpose, function, and nonprofit status of this organization and the exempt status for federal income tax purposes:
☐ Has Not Changed During Preceding 12 Months
☐ Has Changed During Preceding 12 Months (Publisher must submit explanation of change with this statement)

PS Form 3526, September 2007 (Page 1 of 3 (Instructions Page 3)) PSN 7530-01-000-9931 PRIVACY NOTICE: See our Privacy policy in www.usps.com

13. Publication Title		14. Issue Date for Circulation Data Below
Gastrointestinal Endoscopy Clinics of North America		July 2012

15. Extent and Nature of Circulation			Average No. Copies Each Issue During Preceding 12 Months	No. Copies of Single Issue Published Nearest to Filing Date
a. Total Number of Copies (Net press run)			614	558
b. Paid Circulation (By Mail and Outside the Mail)	(1)	Mailed Outside-County Paid Subscriptions Stated on PS Form 3541. (Include paid distribution above nominal rate, advertiser's proof copies, and exchange copies)	261	239
	(2)	Mailed In-County Paid Subscriptions Stated on PS Form 3541 (Include paid distribution above nominal rate, advertiser's proof copies, and exchange copies)		
	(3)	Paid Distribution Outside the Mails Including Sales Through Dealers and Carriers, Street Vendors, Counter Sales, and Other Paid Distribution Outside USPS®	98	106
	(4)	Paid Distribution by Other Classes Mailed Through the USPS (e.g. First-Class Mail®)		
c. Total Paid Distribution (Sum of 15b (1), (2), (3), and (4))			359	345
d. Free or Nominal Rate Distribution (By Mail and Outside the Mail)	(1)	Free or Nominal Rate Outside-County Copies Included on PS Form 3541	80	71
	(2)	Free or Nominal Rate In-County Copies Included on PS Form 3541		
	(3)	Free or Nominal Rate Copies Mailed at Other Classes Through the USPS (e.g. First-Class Mail)		
	(4)	Free or Nominal Rate Distribution Outside the Mail (Carriers or other means)		
e. Total Free or Nominal Rate Distribution (Sum of 15d (1), (2), (3) and (4))			80	71
f. Total Distribution (Sum of 15c and 15e)			439	416
g. Copies not Distributed (See instructions to publishers #4 (page 63))			175	142
h. Total (Sum of 15f and g)			614	558
i. Percent Paid (15c divided by 15f times 100)			81.78%	82.93%

16. Publication of Statement of Ownership

☐ If the publication is a general publication, publication of this statement is required. Will be printed in the October 2012 issue of this publication.

Publication not required.

17. Signature and Title of Editor, Publisher, Business Manager, or Owner

Stephen R. Bushing

Stephen R. Bushing – Inventory Distribution Coordinator

Date: September 14, 2012

I certify that all information furnished on this form is true and complete. I understand that anyone who furnishes false or misleading information on this form or who omits material or information requested on the form may be subject to criminal sanctions (including fines and imprisonment) and/or civil sanctions (including civil penalties).

PS Form 3526, September 2007 (Page 2 of 3)

Moving?

Make sure your subscription moves with you!

To notify us of your new address, find your **Clinics Account Number** (located on your mailing label above your name), and contact customer service at:

Email: journalscustomerservice-usa@elsevier.com

800-654-2452 (subscribers in the U.S. & Canada)
314-447-8871 (subscribers outside of the U.S. & Canada)

Fax number: 314-447-8029

Elsevier Health Sciences Division
Subscription Customer Service
3251 Riverport Lane
Maryland Heights, MO 63043

*To ensure uninterrupted delivery of your subscription, please notify us at least 4 weeks in advance of move.